THE ULTIMATE
BACK BOOK

Understand, Manage, and
Conquer Your Back Pain

JUDYLAINE FINE

Stoddart

TORONTO • BUFFALO

Published in 1997 by
Stoddart Publishing Co. Limited

Distributed in Canada by
General Distribution Services Inc.
30 Lesmill Road
Toronto, Canada M3B 2T6
Tel. (416) 445-3333
Fax (416) 445-5967
e-mail Customer.Service@ccmailgw.genpub.com

Distributed in the United States by
General Distribution Services Inc.
85 River Rock Drive, Suite 202
Buffalo, New York 14207
Toll free 1-800-805-1083
Fax (416) 445-5967
e-mail gdsinc@genpub.com

01 00 99 98   2 3 4 5

Cataloging in Publication Data

Fine, Judylaine
The ultimate back book: understand, manage, and conquer your back pain

Includes index
ISBN 0-7737-5863-1

1. Backache – Popular works.   2. Backache – Treatment.
I. Title.

RD768.F55 1997   617.5'64   97-930273-0

The information in this book is not intended to replace the services of a physician. While most
back pain is of a chronic nature, any pain can be the result of a disease that should be diagnosed
and treated only by a physician. Regardless of which type of health-care professional you choose
to help you cope with your back problem, the author and publisher strongly recommend that
you consult a medical doctor about your back pain, if only to rule out the possibility of disease
as opposed to chronic degenerative processes. Any application of the treatments set forth in this
book is at the reader's discretion and sole risk.

For information about the Back Association of Canada and its educational materials, contact the
Back Association of Canada, 83 Cottingham Street, Toronto, Ontario, M4V 1B9.

Medical illustrations by Dorothy Irwin, used by permission; "Jan and Joan" illustration, page
227, used by permission of RJL Systems, Michigan; cartoons by Peter Honor, used by permission;
other illustrations copyright Whitehall-Robins, or by Tannice Goddard, used by permission.

Cover design: Bill Douglas @ The Bang
Text design: Tannice Goddard

Printed and bound in Canada

To Whitehall-Robins,
in recognition of its commitment to
back pain education

Contents

Prelude

I hate people who write two books on the same subject. But I get *seriously* annoyed when that subject is back pain — and that's precisely what I told the editor who urged me to write a sequel to *Your Guide to Coping with Back Pain* several years after it was published in 1985.

My opinion was that most "second volume" back pain books were little more than rehashes of the original version. (In some cases, authors devised unusual structures to disguise the similarities, but that never fooled me.) I also felt that most of these books were slapped together for money rather than love, and that sat poorly with me as well. My view is that far too many people exploit back pain for financial gain without authors entering the fray.

Now I am doing exactly what I complained about.

I have a line of defense, however. A dozen years have passed since *Your Guide to Coping with Back Pain* was published, and since then the diagnosis and treatment of back pain have undergone momentous changes. This, by the way, is unusual in medical science, a field where advances are generally made in increments.

Because of this about-face, I decided to write a second book.

I should warn you right off the bat that, when it comes to back trouble,

I am opinionated. One of my opinions is that I am entitled to my point of view. Back pain has been a part of my personal and professional life for seventeen years. Furthermore — and I hate to admit this — I've come to realize that I'm in the back business for the duration — both as a back pain sufferer and as an educator and advocate.

Despite the wry tone of voice in my writing, helping back pain sufferers live happy lives is a vocation I'm honored to be married to. My only regret is that such a devastating ailment is so seriously underfunded in terms of research and education. My friends say that's why this cause has become mine.

But I don't want you to get the impression that I'm totally selfless. My own back started to kill me in 1981 and, as is my wont, I got angry because there were facts I needed to know. To learn those facts, I founded the Back Association of Canada (BAC). Of course, a number of North American organizations try to educate back pain sufferers, but to this day BAC is the only registered charitable organization whose goal is to provide information from an unbiased point of view — in as much as it is possible for human beings to be utterly unopinionated! Nevertheless, I feel very proud.

The day the BAC was incorporated was the day I became its voluntary executive vice president. (A number of the volunteers I work with refer to me as its chief bottle-washer, but let me assure you that's not true!) Executive vice president is the title I hold and the title I intend to hold until I accomplish my goal. Thank God my seventeen-year "job" has never been boring — a fairly amazing statement for a journalist to make.

The diversity of my plate holds my interest. I research and write a quarterly newsletter called *Back to Back*, as well as brochures and other educational material. This affords me the opportunity to schmooze with the most interesting back pain specialists on Earth, as well as to devour stacks of fascinating articles from scientific journals. (My only complaint is that so few researchers are able to write in plain English.)

I sit on the advisory board of the Vermont Back Research Center of the University of Vermont — the only federally funded back pain research program in the whole of the United States of America. (I am the only

Canadian on this board, but that has never stopped me from being the most vociferous member!) I also write a monthly column on back pain for the *Toronto Star*.

Plus, I often get angry, which increases the circulation of my blood, which, in turn, reduces muscle spasm in the lumbar region of my spine — the region that causes me grief.

When I mouth off my theme rarely varies. I believe that as back pain sufferers we *must* come to understand the nuances of our multifaceted ailment. (Health-care professionals, I might add, could use some education as well.)

I also believe that those of us who suffer from back pain ought to be regarded as stakeholders when it comes to setting policy about diagnosis and treatment. I intend to convey this idea to the powers that be if it kills me — and it probably will.

But I do not mean to sound negative. Many individual health-care professionals have evolved to the point of treating back pain sufferers with respect. It's the institutions that are still living in the Dark Ages. The most obvious example are Canada's provincial Workers' Compensation Boards (WCBs). It is my opinion that, for the most part, they are a pain in the ass. (For a prime example of why this is so, see Chapter 12.)

In the meantime, I beg you to consider these grim statistics:

- The most common reason why people visit their family physicians (almost a third of visits) is the common cold — a virus that doctors can usually diagnose but not cure. The *second* most common reason is back pain, which, in the majority of cases, doctors can't even diagnose, let alone cure!
- It has been estimated that, in Canada, 9.5 million work days are lost annually because of back pain.
- The Ontario WCB currently has an unfunded liability of $9.5 billion, about 40 percent of which is related to back pain. Yet over the past four years, the board has spent a total of only $10,000 per year on printed educational materials for back pain sufferers, all of which is created and produced in a small bedroom of a small house in

downtown Toronto: the office of BAC. This particularly irks me each time the Ontario WCB issues a press release that stresses the importance of education.

- In Canada, a CT-scan diagnostic test (which almost every back pain sufferer believes he or she is entitled to at the very least) costs approximately $350. A magnetic resonance imaging (MRI) test (which people prefer if they are given the choice) costs about $1,200. In the vast majority of cases, neither of these tests reveal anything more than what was found during the clinical exam! (See Chapter 4.)

Clearly, the cost of back pain to our society is enormous.

Over the past seventeen years I have come to another immutable conclusion: as a back pain sufferer, *you* must take on some of the responsibility for reducing these costs. In order to do so, you need knowledge.

Providing it is the *raison d'être* of this book.

Judy Laine

Introduction

In a perfect world, you would be reading this book to prevent back pain from becoming a part of your life. In *this* world, it's more likely that you're reading it because your back already hurts. Unfortunately, it's human nature to be uninterested in back pain until the nether regions of your anatomy begin to cause you grief.

Luckily, when it comes to back trouble, painful is not synonymous with serious. Your back may hurt like hell, but it is likely that the problem is relatively minor. Furthermore, it's probable that you can become pain-free, or almost pain-free — and if it's the latter, you can certainly find ways to cope.

To do this you need to get a handle on how human backs ought to work, as well as why they so often don't work. Plus you need to calm down. In my opinion, the calming down is the hardest part. It took me years — and if this book can shorten the journey for you I will consider it a success.

GROUPS OF BACK PAIN SUFFERERS

Every back problem is unique. Nevertheless, I've come to think of back pain sufferers as members of one of two groups: "first-timers" and "old-timers."

To my way of thinking, the first time you experience an acute bout of back pain is the scariest. For some people — and this is what happened to me — episode number one strikes without warning. You've never had a backache in your life, then suddenly you are a "first-timer" in agony.

Other people say that their backs niggled at them for years but not seriously enough to grab their attention. If you're in this group, your back may have ached after a game of tennis or an afternoon of gardening, but it always settled down after a couple of days. People in this group tend to promise themselves to be more diligent about warming up before playing sports, for example, but they never get around to it. Nor do they take the trouble to consult a health-care professional. Then when they get leveled by an acute attack of shocking intensity, they are keen to listen up.

Among the "old-timers" are people who have long suffered from chronic mild discomfort. Several times each year, however, they must face an acute flare-up. If you are in this group, you may have done a bit of reading and/or tried an exercise program. But now you're ready to take your back seriously because it has taught you the meaning of the word "respect."

Another group of old timers have also been experiencing acute bouts of dreadful back pain several times a year, but in between they are totally pain-free. If you fall into this category, you likely have a little bit of knowledge and now you are keen to learn a lot more, and to take some action. But this time you mean it!

Still others have been experiencing back pain all or most of the time, but not so severely that it has cramped their style. At least it never used to. If you fall into this category, you probably have learned some coping skills along the way, but lately they don't seem to do the trick. The time between acute flare-ups may be getting shorter or the chronic pain between acute bouts may be getting more severe. Or both. In any case, it's clear that your back is not going to put up with you unless you put in an effort.

Or perhaps you are a chronic back pain sufferer who manages to keep your pain under control in the sense that it doesn't wreck your life. You work, you participate in activities with your family and friends, but coping is downright draining. The writing is on the wall: learn better coping skills or you're going to be in enormous trouble. (People in this group usually experience occasional acute flare-ups as well.)

Then there are chronic back pain sufferers whose back pain rules their lives. If you are in this group, you have probably stopped doing some or most of the activities you used to enjoy. Most likely you are depressed and you have good reason to be. It's a tough position to be in, but I've been there myself and I'm prepared to assure you that, while you may never become pain-free, you *can* turn your life around.

WHEN AND WHERE TO GET HELP

Although it is very rare, a back problem can constitute a medical emergency that warrants a trip to the nearest hospital, pronto. An example is back pain that produces either bowel or bladder incontinence. If you are in doubt, my opinion is that you should call your family physician and describe your signs and symptoms to him or her.

If you can't move one single inch, don't! But, as I explain in Chapter 12, bed rest is no longer prescribed for more than a few days and even during those first few days, it's important to do some gentle stretching. It's also better to crawl to the bathroom than to use a bedpan. (See Chapter 17 for tips on how to get out of bed without exacerbating your pain.)

After a couple of days, you should begin to return to your regular activities — gradually. Then, once you are more or less back to normal, you should be thinking about preventing a recurrence. That's pretty straightforward. The hard part is how.

The answer depends upon whom you ask. Most health-care professionals have particular biases — see Chapter 3 for more on this issue. My own current answer is a product of personal evolution. Two decades ago, which is when I started to ponder the wily mysteries of back pain, I was convinced that there was indeed One Answer. (In Chapter 5 you can read about my search for a guru to bestow it upon me!)

About ten years ago, it started to dawn on me that there was neither one guru nor one answer. I can't claim responsibility for this step forward; at the time, lots of people were concluding the same thing — that different methods worked for different people. Ultimately, most back pain sufferers and health-care professionals came to accept this philosophy.

About five years ago, I changed my tune again, but no one gave me the time of day. Nevertheless, I persevered because I believed that what I was trying to promulgate was eminently sensible: Yes, different treatment methods work for different people, but in addition, *all back pain sufferers require a variety of "treatments"* in order to cope. In other words, the answer is a mix, and my mix is different from yours. A person's mix may include:

- *exercise*, meaning specific (remedial) back exercises. Examples you may have already heard of are: the pelvic tilt, extension stretches, and sit-ups. Some work for everyone; others are helpful for some conditions but detrimental to others.
- *aerobic exercise*, which is quite different from the remedial exercises just mentioned. Aerobic exercise serves a different purpose vis à vis the healing process, and again, which type of aerobic exercise works best depends upon what's wrong with your back. However, aerobic exercise of some kind is crucial if you want to have a fit back, and a fit back is less susceptible to injury than a back that's out of condition. Oddly enough, it has only been during the past few years that exercise specialists have acquired a strong enough voice to spread this fact.
- *ergonomic knowledge*, for example, an understanding of good posture and what kind of chairs promote it. Understanding *dynamic* posture is essential as well. This means that it's important to learn how to use your body without throwing it around. A variety of techniques address this issue: good old-fashioned western posture tips; yoga; the Alexander technique; the Feldenkrais method — all of these pursue the same thing, incredible as it sounds!
- *pain management*, which includes stress management. This may involve the use of medication for acute back pain as well as some of the dozens of techniques that can help you cope with stress. Some will feel right for you; others won't.
- *passive techniques* for coping with pain and muscle spasm. (Exercise is an active technique.) There's something special when a human

being works with you to relieve your pain. This is generally referred to as "the power of touch." Passive techniques include massage, acupuncture, and manipulation. (I'm going out on a limb by including manipulation in this list; personally I believe it can accomplish far more, but you'll have to read Chapters 15 and 16.)

ABOUT THIS BOOK

The human spine is a marvellous and amazing structure. It blows me away. However, understanding how it's built and how it functions and malfunctions takes effort. If you are going to control your own back problem, the only route is to put your nose to the grindstone and learn what's happening inside your back. Part I of this book, *BACKground*, will help you do this. You may find it easier to read a few other chapters before tackling Chapters 1 and 2; I don't mind a bit as long as you eventually buckle down!

Part II, *Diagnosis*, deals with the next obvious topic. Chapter 3 explains the complexities of diagnosing back pain, with an emphasis on the five commonly recognized categories. Chapter 4 discusses high-tech diagnostic testing — the "miracle" of the 1980s that has ultimately failed to produce all the answers.

Part III, *Pain*, looks at this fascinating subject from several points of view: the physiological phenomenon of pain (Chapter 5); the contribution of stress (Chapter 6); chronic pain (Chapter 7); and medication for pain (Chapter 8, which is accompanied by a back medication chart).

The rest of the book was a little harder to organize. Part IV is called *Helping Yourself: Posture, Fitness, and Exercise.* In Chapters 9 and 10, I discuss posture (sitting and moving, respectively). Chapter 11 deals with ergonomics — the science of designing your environment to fit your needs rather than the other way around.

Chapters 12 and 13 deal with physical activity — in the first I explain why it's so important, and why, as the title says, bed rest is for the birds. This chapter also introduces the philosophy of early active treatment. The second gives practical advice about fitness and exercise.

Part V, *The Health-Care Pros and Their Wares*, begins with a chapter on dealing with health-care professionals generally (Chapter 14). Then I talk about the major disciplines: physiotherapy (Chapter 15), chiropractic (Chapter 16), surgery (Chapter 17), and massage (Chapter 18).

In my last book, alternative disciplines, such as the Alexander technique, got entire chapters, while in this book, I've given them far less space. The reason is that, these days, I hear a lot less about such techniques because we are in the midst of a research revolution whose buzzword is "evidence-based." Everyone is hot to prove, in a scientific way, what works, and unfortunately there is a dearth of funds (not to mention a lack of keen interest) in alternative therapy research. Personally, I sense that, where alternative therapies for back pain are concerned, we are at a watershed. In a sense, the pages of the last chapter for this section are still blank.

Part VI, *Back in the Future*, is devoted to a few topics that I believe are going to have a major impact on our society in the coming years. Chapter 19 deals with rehabilitation in the workplace; Chapter 20 discusses neck problems, which are on the rise as motor vehicle accidents increase exponentially. Chapter 21 deals with osteoporosis, which as our population ages, threatens to reach unheard-of proportions.

Finally, I've included a bibliography of sorts — not an exhaustive list of every work I've used while writing this book, but an attempt to point you in the right direction if you would like more information. And, of course, there is a comprehensive index at the end of the book.

Throughout the book, you will occasionally come across commentary that is more political and social than medical. You may find this information fascinating; or you may ask why you should care. If you are in the latter group, I leave you with this thought: As a back pain sufferer, you are part of a large phenomenon in motion — something like a cog in a wheel. We all know that institutions vie for power and that their decisions are not always made with your best interests at heart. The same sometimes holds true for health-care professionals. And both groups can forget that, as sufferers of back pain, we too are stakeholders and warrant a voice. I pray that this book inspires you to take up that challenge and run with it. Okay, walk with it. And to keep the faith.

1

BACKGROUND

1

Back to Anatomy

I have what can best be described as a love/hate relationship with my back. I hate my back because it has forced me to give up tennis (among other things) and because it has caused me more pain than any other part of my anatomy. On the other hand, now that my back problem is more or less under control, I must also admit that I love this mysterious and complex structure. It has taught me a lot about life.

For example, my spine has forced me to learn to balance work time with leisure time; to manage stress; and to cope with my fear of both pain and disability. I have come to realize that I am capable of putting up with a lot more discomfort than I thought.

I have also come to respect my back for all it manages to do despite what it puts up with from the likes of me! The truth is that my inactive, sedentary lifestyle has wreaked havoc on my spine on a daily basis for decades — and I bet that your lifestyle has wreaked havoc on yours. It's amazing that our backs didn't pack up on us a whole lot sooner.

Years ago, before I understood this, I used to tell people that I had one bone to pick with Mother Nature. Being the genius that she is, why couldn't she have given us *two* backs instead of one? If spinal columns came in pairs like arms and legs, we could let one spine do the work while the sore one had a chance to rest up. Although I still find this idea intriguing from an intellectual stand-point, I now see that the human spine is such a feat of engi-neering that Mother Nature deserves two gold medals for pro-viding each of us with

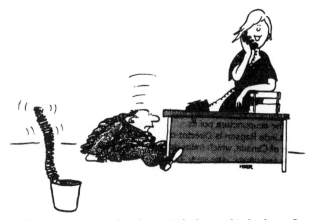

"He can't come to the phone. He's thrown his back out."

just one! I mean, think about it. When it is functioning the way it is sup-posed to work, your spinal column is so flexible that you can bend it forward to form two-thirds of a circle. At the same time, this stack of bones is able to support your head (12 to 16 pounds) and your torso (90 to 120 pounds). Your lower spine has a lifting capacity of up to 300 pounds per square inch. And, as if all that weren't enough, your spine operates your body's entire communication system.

THE COMPONENTS OF A SPINE

The first step in understanding your back pain is understanding your back. Take a look at Figure 1.1, a side view of the human spine. As the drawing shows, normal spines have three gentle curves. The two forward curves — one at the top and the other near the base of the spine — are called **lordotic curves,** or **lordosis.** The other curve, called a **kyphotic curve,** or **kyphosis,** arches the opposite way.

These curves develop shortly after you are born. When they are in bal-ance, they help absorb shock while you stand at rest or move about. If these curves are either excessive or inadequate, however, the muscles, ligaments, and tendons of your back and abdomen have to work a lot harder in order to keep you from toppling over.

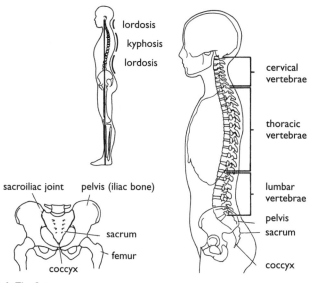

Figure 1.1 The Spine

All together, your spinal column is made up of twenty-four mobile bones, called **vertebrae**, which are stacked one on top of the other. To prevent bone from grinding upon bone, each pair of vertebrae is separated by a kind of cushion, or pouch, called a **disc**.

The top seven vertebrae, which form the lordotic curve in the neck, are called the **cervical** vertebrae. The next twelve, which form the kyphosis, are the **thoracic** vertebrae; each is attached to a pair of ribs. The lowest five vertebrae, which form the lower lordotic curve, are called the **lumbar** vertebrae. It is in this lumbar area that the vast majority of back problems occur.

To make talking about vertebrae easier, back experts have developed a system of labeling them. The cervical vertebrae are labeled C1 to C7. The thoracic vertebrae are labeled T1 to T12. The five lumbar vertebrae are labeled L1 to L5.

Below the lowest vertebra is the **sacrum**. It is attached by strong ligaments, several on either side, to the two large bones of the pelvis, which are called the **ilia**. Hence the name for these two joints: **sacroiliac**, or **SI**, **joints**. When you are born, your sacrum is made up of five separate vertebrae. During your first few years of life they fuse together into one arrowhead-shaped bone. Even when they have fused, however, it is easy to see where each section of the sacrum begins and ends, so these bones too have labels: S1 to S5.

At the very base of the spine, below the sacrum, is the **coccyx** — the word is pronounced "cock-six." This is all that human beings have left of what was once a tail. The coccyx consists of four (occasionally three) small vertebrae. By the time you reach the age of twenty, these vertebrae usually fuse together as well.

Some health-care professionals describe the spine as having thirty-two or thirty-three vertebrae. To reach that total, they add the five bones of the sacrum and the three, or four, bones of the coccyx to the twenty-four mobile vertebrae. Others prefer to call the total number of vertebrae twenty-six; they count the mobile vertebrae as twenty-four, and add one for the sacrum and one for the coccyx.

THE MOBILE VERTEBRAE

Although they differ in size, the twenty-four mobile vertebrae are all fairly similar in design. (Exceptions are the top two vertebrae, which are some-what different in shape; these are described in detail in Chapter 19.)

Figure 1.2 gives you a pretty good idea of what all the mobile segments look like and how they function.

Each vertebra is made up of two parts. The **anterior** section is the part closest to the front of your body; the **posterior** section is the back part.

The anterior section of each vertebra is shaped like a drum. The bottom **endplate** of one drum is solidly attached to the top of the disc below it. The top endplate of the drum below is attached to the bottom of the same disc. You could compare two vertebrae to the two slices of bread in a sand-wich and say that the disc between them is the filling. Nutrients move into the discs and waste products move out via the endplates; more on this in the section on discs, below.

The function of this drum-shaped section of each vertebra is to bear weight. As I have already mentioned, the largest ones, in your lumbar

POSTERIOR

lamina

superior articular process

spinal canal

ANTERIOR

transverse process

spinous process

end plate

spinous proces

intervertebral
foramen

intervertebral disc

facet joint

vertebral body

transverse process

inferior articular process

facet of inferior process

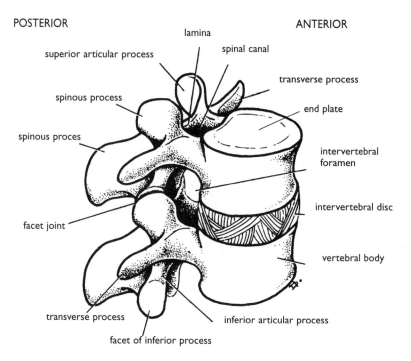

Figure 1.2 Normal Vertebrae, Lateral (Side) Oblique View

spine, can support up to 300 pounds per square inch — surely an accomplishment that deserves a round of applause.

The posterior section of a vertebra is more complex (see Figure 1.3). It consists of a tube-shaped piece of bone which, when lined up with all the other vertebrae, forms the **spinal canal**. The back section of the spinal canal is called the **lamina**.

FACET JOINTS AND PROCESSES

Seven projections, called **processes**, emerge from the lamina of each vertebra. The two at the top are called the **superior articular processes** and the two at the bottom are the **inferior articular processes**. At the end of each of the four articular processes is a **facet**, which, like the facet of a diamond, is smooth.

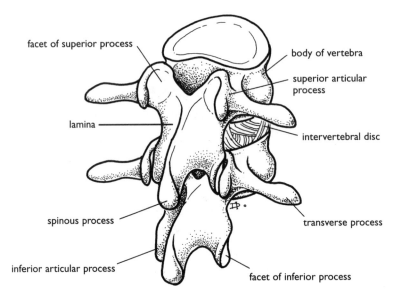

Figure 1.3 Normal Vertebrae, Posterior (Rear) Oblique View

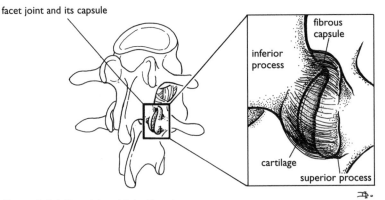

Figure 1.4 A Facet Joint with Its Capsule

The two superior articular processes of each vertebra join with the two inferior articular processes of the vertebra above. The resulting structure is called a **facet joint** (see Figure 1.4). Each facet is capped with smooth cartilage to help it move almost frictionlessly against its partner, and each facet joint is encased in a strong, fibrous **joint capsule** that prevents the facets from coming apart. The joint capsules, however, are roomy enough for the facets to move.

Of the three other processes on each mobile vertebra, the two that stick out sideways, like wings, are the **transverse processes** and the other one, which is called the **spinous process**, points back, with a downward slant. These spinous processes are what you can feel when you run your fingers up and down someone's back.

THE DISCS

The twenty-four mobile vertebrae are separated by twenty-three discs. If you were to pile all the discs together they'd measure approximately six inches, with the discs of the lumbar spine being slightly thicker — *plumper* might be a better word — than the ones at the top. Each disc creates a space, called the **intervertebral foramen**, between two vertebrae. (See Figure 1.2. I'll have more to say about this space later on.) Discs also act as shock absorbers.

Discs are identified by the vertebrae above and below them. For example, the disc between the first and second lumbar vertebrae is called L1-L2, or just L1-2. The disc between the lowest lumbar vertebra and the sacrum is called L5-S1; this label cannot be shortened.

Each disc is made up of two sections, shown in Figure 1.5. The outer section is called the **annulus fibrosus**, and is composed of tough, criss-crossed, fibrous layers — much like the layers of a radial-belted tire. When I say tough, I mean *tough*. If you fell off a roof or were hit by a bus, the trauma would more likely result in a fractured vertebra than a damaged disc.

As you move toward the center of each disc, the layers gradually become less fibrous. Finally, they turn into the **nucleus pulposos** — a compartment filled with a pulpy mass that looks like jelly when you are an infant and crabmeat by the time you reach adulthood. Because this mass is mostly water, it is very elastic; whenever you bend in any direction, it changes its shape and then returns to its original form.

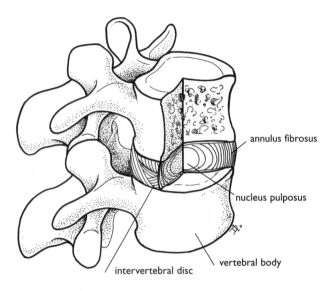

Figure 1.5 An Intervertebral Disc

When you are born, the water content of each nucleus is something like 90 percent. As you age, this percentage gradually decreases; at age seventy, the water content of your discs' nuclei is more like 70 percent.

Discs absorb and lose water on a daily basis. The way this happens makes me think of a sponge soaking up water and then being wrung out. During the day, while gravity is exerting its force on your body, water leaves the discs' centers and they lose a bit of height. While you are sleeping, water containing nutrients soaks into the discs from the blood. This is why the average person is slightly taller in the morning than at night. After eighty-four days in the zero gravity of Skylab, astronaut William Pogue had "grown" almost four inches. When he came down to earth, however, he went back to his normal size.

THE LIGAMENTS OF THE SPINE

Ligaments are tough bands of connective tissue that bind one bone to another (see Figure 1.6). They support the spine and also help prevent you

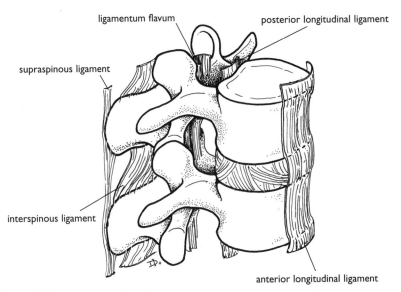

Figure 1.6 The Ligaments of the Spine

from making excessive movements that may be damaging, such as moving a facet joint beyond its normal range. The **ligamentum flavum** (sometimes called the **yellow ligament** because of its color), the **interspinous ligament**, and the **supraspinous ligament** provide support for your facet joints. The two **longitudinal ligaments** provide support for your discs and vertebrae.

The *anterior* longitudinal ligament runs the length of the spinal column. It is attached to the front section of the vertebral bodies and discs. The *posterior* longitudinal ligament also runs the length of the spinal column, but it is attached to the back of the vertebral bodies and discs. No back expert will disagree that both these ligaments are essential for spinal stability; however, the extent and nature of the role they play in back pain is the subject of some debate.

THE MUSCLES OF THE SPINE

Muscles, as you probably know, are highly elastic tissues that expand and contract to allow your body to move. Spinal muscles come in three basic sizes: short, medium, and long.

The shortest muscles, which are also the farthest from the surface, enable you to make delicate movements. They also support your spine. Some of these little muscles are attached to the processes; as they lengthen and shorten, the processes are pulled and released like levers. This allows your body to bend and twist within the limitations set by the ligaments.

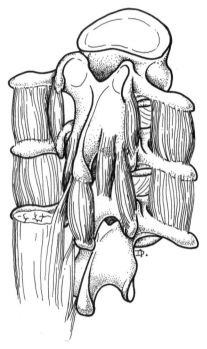

Other short muscles are attached to the facet joints (see Figure 1.7). When these lengthen and shorten, the facet joints are pulled and released. But in this case, the plane of each facet joint determines its ability to move forward, backward, sideways, or to rotate. Those at the top of the spine, for example, are more horizontally oriented than those of the lumbar region and, because of this, they are better suited for rotational movements. That's why your neck has a greater rotational range than your lower spine.

Above the short muscles are many layers of medium-length muscles. They stretch from one

Figure 1.7 Some Short Muscles of the Back

vertebra to another vertebra several inches away.

Covering these medium-length muscles is the group of long muscles. These run the entire length of your spine and are called the **erector spinae** (see Figure 1.8). When this group of muscles is contracted, your spine arches backward. When the long muscles on only one side are tightened, the spine bends sideways. The erector spinae muscles also brace your spine from the rear and prevent you from falling forward. Some people find it helpful to visualize a flagpole with its guy wires holding it erect.

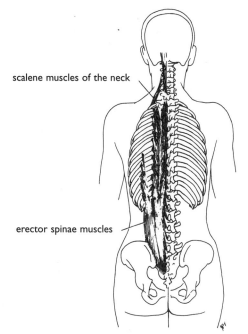

scalene muscles of the neck

erector spinae muscles

Figure 1.8 The Erector Spinae Muscles

THE MUSCLES OF THE ABDOMEN

If you look at Figure 1.9, you'll see that very few muscles are attached to the front of the vertebrae to help your spine bend forward. (The **psoas** muscle is an exception, but its main function is to move your legs rather than your spine.) This means that the job of bending forward falls to the abdominal muscles. There are several layers of these running in different directions.

The innermost layers, the **obliquus internis** and the **obliquus externis**, are not visible in Figure 1.9. They run diagonally from the hip bones to the ribs. The middle layer, the **transversus abdominis**, crosses the innermost layer. The outermost layer, the **rectus abdominis**, runs vertically. When you contract all of them, your spine bends forward.

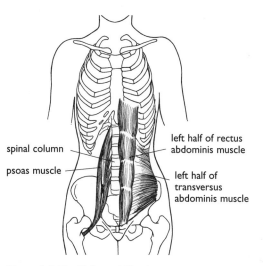

spinal column

psoas muscle

left half of rectus abdominis muscle

left half of transversus abdominis muscle

Figure 1.9 The Abdominal Muscles

Your abdominal muscles have other responsibilities as well. For example, when you contract only those on one side, your spine is pulled sideways. Most importantly, however, they provide the other side of the guy wire system, which means that they keep you from toppling backward. When the erector spinae and the abdominal muscles are more or less equal in strength, they work in tandem and your body finds maintaining an erect posture relatively easy. When your abdominal muscles are considerably weaker than your back muscles — and this is true of the vast majority of people who lead sedentary lives, including me — the spine is more vulnerable to wear and tear, and to injury.

THE SPINAL CORD AND NERVES

The most complex part of your back is your **spinal cord**, which, together with your brain, forms your central nervous system. The cord itself runs from the base of your brain down through the spinal canal, which as I've mentioned is formed by the tubelike structure toward the rear of each vertebra. Several layers of fibrous tissues cover and protect the spinal cord within the canal. The innermost layer is called the **pia mater**. The outermost layer is the thick, fibrous **dura mater**. In between is the **arachnoid**. (See Figure 1.10.)

Before birth, in the early stages of an embryo's development, the spinal cord extends from the brain all the way to the sacrum. The vertebrae, however, grow faster than the spinal cord, and by the time you are born your spinal cord only spans the area from your brain to your third lumbar vertebra. This uneven growth continues during your developing years; by the time you are twelve, the end of your spinal cord, called the **conus medullaris**, is located at L1 (see Figure 1.11).

The spinal cord branches off into thousands of **nerves**, which run to and from every organ and inch of tissue from the top of your head to the tips of your toes. They deliver messages to and from the organs and tissues of the body. These develop from sixty-two main branches (thirty-one on each side of the cord) called **nerve roots**. Each nerve root emerges from your spinal column through an intervertebral foramen, which as you may recall is the space between two vertebrae. Just past the point where it emerges,

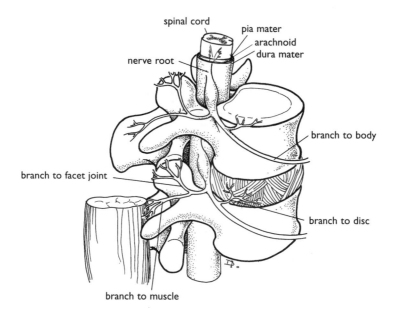

spinal cord

pia mater
arachnoid
dura mater

nerve root

branch to body

branch to facet joint

branch to disc

branch to muscle

Figure 1.10 The Spinal Cord, Nerve Roots, and Nerve Branches

each nerve root splits into several smaller branches; these are your **nerves**. One of these nerve branches delivers messages to and from the nearest facet joint, another to the disc nearby, and another to the closest muscle. But another, much longer branch winds away from the spine and branches, rebranches, and combines with other nerves. Some of these nerves supply power to your muscles. Others supply sensation — both normal touch and pain — to your skin. Still others supply information to your organs. This network is bewildering in its complexity, like the telephone system of a huge city; Figure 1.11 shows a much simplified representation.

The branches of the nerve roots in the cervical region send and receive messages to and from the upper regions of the body, and the branches of the lumbar nerve roots send and receive messages to and from the lower regions of the body. For example, branches of the nerve roots that exit from between C3 and C4 wind all the way to the arms, passing between the muscles that move the shoulders.

The nerve roots that emerge from between L4 and L5, as well as the four pairs of nerve roots below, merge together at hip level, beneath the

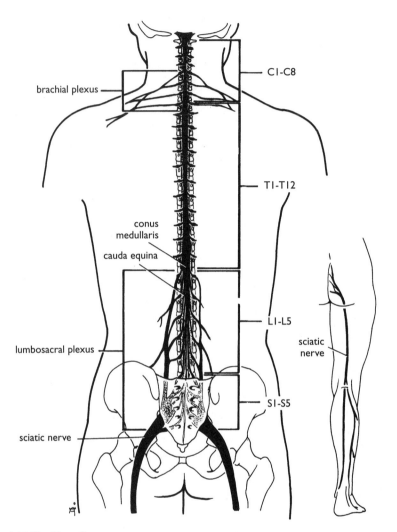

brachial plexus

C1-C8

conus medullaris

cauda equina

T1-T12

L1-L5

lumbosacral plexus

sciatic nerve

S1-S5

sciatic nerve

Figure 1.11 The Nerve Roots

gluteus maximus muscle. This combination forms the thickest nerve of the body: the **sciatic nerve**.

The sciatic nerve runs down the back of each thigh and divides into two just above the knee. One of these branches runs down the front of the shin into the big toe; the other branch divides again, running down the back of the leg to the heel and winding again toward the front of the leg to the smaller toes, and so on. Each one has many, many tiny offshoots.

Because the spinal cord ends at L1, the nerves that eventually exit from between the lower lumbar and sacral vertebrae must run down the length of the spinal canal for longer and longer distances. These strands of nerves running through the spinal canal are called the **cauda equina**, which means "horse's tail" in Latin.

Many nerve endings are sensitive to pain, but some are not. It is only recently that researchers have begun to study the various tissues of the body in general and the spinal column in particular to see which ones contain pain receptors. For example, there are pain receptors in the nerve endings that branch to the facet joints, to the dura mater, to the blood vessels that supply the muscles of the back, and to the ligaments of the spine. There are, however, no pain receptors in the nerves that supply the nuclei of the discs. Likewise, there are none in those that supply the annuli, except at the point where each annulus is attached to the posterior longitudinal ligament. And, amazing as it may sound, there are no pain receptors in muscles. As well, there are more pain receptors in some structures than in others. The significance of pain receptors is explained in more detail in Chapter 5, but it's a good idea to keep it in mind when you are reading Chapter 2, which explains how everything works — and what can go wrong!

2

Function and Malfunction: What Goes Wrong?

When you consider the complexity of your back and all the things you ask it to do for you on any given day, it's no wonder there's a wide range of things that can go wrong with it. The $64,000 question, of course, is always: what is causing your particular pain?

More often than not, the answer is actually: not much. This is one of the least endearing aspects of back ailments — a minor problem can hurt like hell.

Most often the lumbar, or lowest, area of the spine (L2 to S1 — I'll assume from now on that you've read Chapter 1 and are familiar with basic back anatomy terms and labels) suffers because it bears the most weight. Problems with the cervical spine (the neck) are treated separately in Chapter 19, because they tend to be quite different from low back problems.

THE FIVE MOST COMMON CATEGORIES OF BACK PAIN

These days, the most common causes of low back pain are generally divided into five main categories:

1. strains and sprains of the muscles, ligaments, and tendons, which,

according to many health-care professionals, account for between 80 and 90 percent of all back pain;

2. disc problems, including bulging discs and herniated discs;
3. facet joint problems, often referred to as facet joint syndrome;
4. osteoarthritis, a natural process during which growths of bone form on the vertebrae; and
5. spinal stenosis, which occurs in many different forms but generally has to do with irritation due to a narrowing of spinal structures.

In this chapter I'll discuss each of these categories in detail, then describe many of the other common causes of back pain. But first, I think it will be helpful to explain how back pain relates to age and aging.

Although there are lots of exceptions, the categories outlined above tend to follow general age-related trends. For instance, most people with disc problems are between the ages of about 25 and 45. (Some health-care professionals would lower the top end to 40.) Most people with severe osteoarthritis and/or spinal stenosis are over the age of 40 or 45. Facet joint problems tend to occur over a broader age range, but I think it's fair to say that the majority of them occur when people are between 25 and 50. And, although strains and sprains can and do occur at any age, most elderly people don't tend to strain their backs for the simple reason that they tend to live less active lives. As well, their spines are more stable and less flexible.

THE NATURAL AGING PROCESS OF THE SPINE

By the time you reach your mid-twenties, the bones of your spinal column will have attained their mature size. When this occurs, your spine immediately begins to degenerate — an unfortunate term used by many health-care professionals to describe a perfectly normal process. If you think about it for a moment, the word *degenerate* is not particularly ominous; it simply means the opposite of *generate*, which means "grow." Cells in your body are constantly wearing out and being replaced, but during the growth years, bone and other tissue is created faster than it is destroyed with the net result of generation. After maturity, however, slightly less bone and other tissue is produced than destroyed. The net result is, technically, **degeneration**.

In this sense, the spine is no different from any other organ of your body. The trouble is, if you don't understand its literal meaning, the word conjures up images of vertebrae crumbling to dust, or discs disintegrating into nothingness. I don't think I'm exaggerating when I say that mistaken notions of the "degenerating spine" have left thousands of people in fear for their long-term well-being and, in some cases, their very lives.

It is also true, however, that degeneration can cause severe back pain in spite of the fact that the actual physical problem is usually minor and certainly no more life-threatening than the common cold. (Cases where the spinal cord itself is damaged are an extremely rare exception.) What this boils down to is that more than 90 percent of us back pain sufferers have a problem that is manageable.

In many respects, what is happening here can be compared to the natural process your skin begins to go through at about the same time. In the case of your spine, however, this process is ultimately helpful in the majority of cases. If you're like most people, you'll find that by the time you've reached the sixth or seventh decade of life, the degenerative changes in your spine have rendered it less flexible, more stable, and *less* susceptible to both injury and pain. The majority of back pain sufferers are in their late twenties, their thirties and forties, or their early fifties. **Epidemiologists** (researchers who study health problems in large groups of subjects) say back pain tends to get better with age rather than worse.

But let's take a closer look at the aging skin analogy. When you hit your mid-twenties, your skin begins to dry out and sag. Tiny lines — minuscule cracks, actually — appear around your eyes. Your skin's tautness, which is another characteristic of youth, also begins to diminish. Meanwhile, in your spine, the water content of each disc's nucleus begins to decrease. The fibers of the annulus also begin to wear out; like the plies of a slightly worn radial-belted tire, they sometimes fray and may develop tiny tears, which usually start near the center and work their way toward the outer edge.

When an annulus tears, it tends to do so near its posterior (back) section rather than toward the front; generally, the back section is weaker — only Mother Nature knows why! The fibers at the front may weaken rather than tear, and this weakness can also contribute to back pain.

At the same time, your body's ability to lubricate its facet joints diminishes as the body becomes gradually less efficient at taking in nutrients and expelling waste products. As a result, your facet joints may begin to suffer from general wear and tear.

Meanwhile, your spinal ligaments begin to lose some of their strength; a good way of putting it is to say that they become *lax*. This may create a sort of chicken-and-egg problem, since lax ligaments can also contribute to the wear and tear of facet joints for the simple reason that these joints rely on ligaments for support. (Facet joints themselves were not designed to bear weight.)

Try to visualize the beginning of this vicious cycle: your ligaments begin to sag, often due to chronic strain caused by poor posture; the facet joints become less stable (and more poorly aligned); in turn, this causes the ligaments to be strained further. Most professionals believe that once a spinal ligament has lost its tautness, this process cannot be reversed completely, even if you correct your posture — which most of us never do. In fact, our modern, sedentary lifestyle promotes the kind of posture that speeds this process up.

The story continues. Once your ligaments have lost some of their ability to support your spine, your muscles must bear an increased load. Therefore, as you age, it is more important than ever to have strong muscles that can help compensate for weak ligaments. Unfortunately, most people's muscles tend to get weaker rather than stronger — again because of our lifestyle and the natural consequences of aging. Weak muscles are common among people who get little or no exercise — and are thus more likely to have strained ligaments to begin with. To add insult to injury, until recently millions of back pain sufferers were put to bed, which caused their muscles to become weaker still (see Chapter 12).

Weak muscles also have a greater tendency to go into spasm. The extra burden they must bear due to the degenerative changes of the discs, ligaments, and joints is simply too much for them. From your body's point of view, muscle spasm makes a lot of sense; it is Mother Nature's way of protecting a strained area by limiting movement. On the down side, Mother Nature is not always so clever at knowing when to let go. In a lot of cases, this sort of spasm becomes chronic, continuing to some degree long after the original injury has healed. And as most of us know only too well, muscle spasm can be terribly painful.

There is an up side, however. Unlike your ligaments, your muscles have great adaptive powers. By correcting your posture and exercising, you can regain your previous muscle strength and endurance and even increase these abilities. The effort is well worth it, since it greatly decreases your chances of recurrent muscle strain.

AS WE CONTINUE TO AGE . . .

Changes such as the ones just described cause other changes. For example, where a disc is attached to the vertebra above and below it, bone projections called **osteophytes** begin to form, causing irritation to adjoining structures. Bone growths may also appear around your facet joints. Over the years, these changes diminish the flexibility of your spine, but leave your vertebra and joints less susceptible to the problems caused by degeneration, less lubrication, and general wear and tear. This increased stability is why back pain eventually tends to decrease.

In the same category as the regrettable term "degenerate" for the natural aging process of your spine's discs and joints is the term **osteoarthritis**. This word is used — more or less interchangeably with **arthritic changes** or simply **arthritis** — by physicians and other health-care professionals to describe the development of osteophytes.

Let's break these words down. The syllable *arth* is a derivative of the Greek word *arthron*, which simply means "joint." *Itis* means "an inflammation of" and *osteo* means "bone." Hence *osteoarthritis* is an inflammation of a bony joint.

Arthritic changes are normal and very common. And yet, the mere mention of the word "arthritis" often frightens people, conjuring up images of totally unrelated ailments such as rheumatoid arthritis. Because of this, thousands of back pain sufferers who are told that osteoarthritis is at the root of their problem react as if they are being handed a death sentence rather than a description of a very natural occurrence.

While natural processes will cause almost everyone to experience some back pain in their lives, it is also true that many people could avoid, or at least diminish, much of their pain if they understood more about these processes and how to mitigate their effects. Of course, if, like cavemen, we had a life expectancy of less than three decades, back problems would pose less of a problem for human beings. But personally, I'm willing to take the trade-off!

Now that you have a general understanding of the aging process underlying most back problems, let's examine the five most common categories more closely. Remember, however, that more than one category may be involved in one person's problem, because the functioning of the discs, facet joints, muscles, and ligaments, as well as the formation of osteophytes, are interdependent. In fact, the complexity of this interdependence is one of the factors that makes the diagnosis of back pain so difficult.

CATEGORY 1: STRAINS AND SPRAINS OF THE MUSCLES, LIGAMENTS, AND TENDONS

The easiest way to make sense of this category is to first take a look at how your ligaments function. The main job of your spinal ligaments is to support your spine. Unlike muscles, which are designed to lengthen and shorten, ligaments are only slightly elastic. They can stretch, on average, about a quarter of their length. If you try to stretch them more they will tear, generally only partially. A partially torn ligament is called a **sprain**.

But sprained ligaments are not usually the thorn in the back pain sufferer's side. Ligaments will only stretch beyond their 25 percent limit under *extreme* stress, and ligaments of the spine are rarely torn. If you take a bad fall while skiing, you may tear some of the ligaments of your knee.

If you stumble on an unexpected bump, you may sprain an ankle. But if you fall on your back, it's unlikely that you will tear your spinal ligaments.

Chronic ligament **strain** is far more common in your spine. This usually results from years of misuse rather than a sudden trauma. If, year after year, you sit all day in a chair that provides your back with little or no support, a number of your spinal ligaments will be strained. (See Chapter 9.)

Have another look back at Figure 1.6. It's easy to see that bending forward strains the back sections of the lumbar discs, and we hear about this all the time. But this posture also puts stress on the posterior longitudinal ligament, the supraspinous ligament, the ligamentum flavum, and the interspinous ligament. If these ligaments are stressed for years on end, they lose some of their ability to support your spine.

Chronically strained ligaments can also cause pain. For one thing, like muscles and nerves, ligaments have pain receptors (see Chapter 5). Under chronic strain, the firing rate of these receptors may increase. This means that they send a lot of messages to your brain informing it that there is trouble down below.

Strained ligaments can also lead to other painful problems. For example, while the four ligaments mentioned above stretch during prolonged sitting, the anterior longitudinal ligament shortens. As well, while the capsules at the back of the facet joints stretch, their front sections shorten. **Adaptive shortening** is the term professionals use to describe the tightening up that happens to chronically contracted tissue. A **misaligned facet joint**, i.e., with its capsule stretched at the back and shortened at the front, cannot function properly.

Another posture that tends to strain the ligaments of the spine is standing for long periods of time, especially if you tend to hyperextend, or arch, your lower back — a posture that exaggerates the lordotic curve of the lumbar spine. Chronic hyperextension leads to a different type of adaptive shortening, in which the anterior longitudinal ligament stretches while the others shorten. The front part of the facet joint capsule also becomes stretched, while the back part shortens. But the alignment of these joints is still affected and, usually, the result is pain.

(It's almost impossible, by the way, to avoid hyperextension if you wear high heels.)

As I have already mentioned, when ligaments under chronic strain become lax, they lose some of their ability to support your spine. Eventually, without the assistance of the appropriate ligaments, the other parts of the back will be forced to take over the ligaments' job. This includes the facet joints, the discs, and, of course, the muscles.

Strained Muscles

Your muscles, unlike your ligaments, are extremely elastic. They lengthen and shorten all the time, which is how your body moves. (If you're interested, I've included an explanation of the mechanics of *how* muscles contract at the end of this subsection. Personally, I find the process fascinating, but if you don't enjoy mechanical descriptions, skip it!)

Muscles, therefore, tend to overstretch rather than tear. A strained muscle can cause severe pain.

How frequently strained muscles are the cause of back pain has been debated for decades. The issue is difficult to resolve. For one thing, muscles (like ligaments and discs) are composed of soft tissue, which does not show up on plain X-rays, making it difficult to prove a diagnosis of muscle strain. When deep muscles (as opposed to those nearer your skin) are in question there is even less evidence available, since clinicians can neither see them nor feel them — at least not directly.

There is another confusing aspect to the controversy. As I've already mentioned, some of the small, deep muscles may go into spasm, immobilizing an area where a facet joint or a disc is causing a problem. But is most of the actual pain caused by the muscle spasm? Or is it coming from the joint or the disc? Another question: Is it appropriate to say that the *source* of the pain — the bottom-line cause — is the muscle spasm, the joint, or the disc? And if some muscle spasm remains after the joint or disc has healed, what do you call that? As well, do muscles sometimes go into spasm when there is nothing wrong with a facet joint or a disc? Can stress — either emotional or physical overexertion — cause muscle spasm when there is no evidence of significant degeneration?

Considering how many young athletes experience back pain, the answer is probably yes.

Finally, how significant is what some health-care professionals call **hypersensitivity** of muscles? In other words, if a muscle that has been in spasm for a long time relaxes partially, can a small amount of strain send it back into spasm?

Different experts will give you different answers to all these questions. However, most of the health-care professionals I've asked believe that, when muscles are involved in back pain, they are the secondary rather than the primary cause. What they mean is that, in almost all cases, the root cause is the degeneration of ligaments, discs, or facet joints; the muscles go into spasm as a protective response, incidentally causing more pain to the owner of the spine. It is also my experience that physiotherapists and massage therapists, for example, usually believe that the contribution of muscle spasm to back pain is far more significant than do health-care professionals from other disciplines. This makes sense when you remember that these peoples' training concentrates more on soft tissue. Orthopedic surgeons, on the other hand, tend to focus on bones and on specific anomalies: herniated discs, severely worn joints, etc. For a further discussion of the points of view from which different groups of experts operate, see Chapter 3.

Whether their discipline is physiotherapy or surgery, however, most health-care professionals agree that muscle strain tends to subside on its own after a few days or weeks, assuming the injury has a chance to heal. Nevertheless, although it may not generally be long-lived, or a sign that something is terribly amiss, muscle spasm can cause extremely severe pain. Recent studies have shown that the complex system of blood vessels that run throughout the muscles of the spine are dense with pain receptors.

At times, when my back is especially painful, I remember a simple experiment that never fails to bring tears to my eyes as well as make me smile. A physiotherapist showed it to me years ago and it helped put my frazzled psyche to rest. I urge you to try it.

Hold a copy of a formidable book in your hand — a concise version of *Webster's Dictionary* will do nicely — and then extend your arm in front of you so that it is parallel to the ground. Now count to sixty, extremely slowly.

By the time a minute has passed, the pain caused by the strain and fatigue of the muscles in your hand and arm should convince you that, as I mentioned at the opening of the chapter, severe pain doesn't necessarily mean that something serious is wrong physically. Usually the pain will subside when the stress is removed. In the case of this experiment, simply put down the book. There — don't you feel better already?

Reducing the stress on your back is not quite so simple, alas. I have come to learn that it takes a number of things in most cases, and some of them don't work all of the time. But you *can* reduce strain with such actions as changes in posture, back exercises combined with aerobic exercise, understanding stress and learning ways of coping with it, and understanding the nature of pain, which allows you to deal with your fear. When necessary, and for a time-limited period, you can also rely on passive modalities such as acupuncture (discussed in Chapter 5), manipulation (Chapter 16), or massage (Chapter 18).

Anatomy of a Muscle Contraction

Many researchers believe that increased muscle tension plays an important role in back pain. Exactly what happens, however, is not totally understood.

There are theories. For example, some scientists talk about the nerve "pathways" that carry messages such as pain from the site of an injury to the brain. They believe that, sometimes, the brain "remembers" this pathway long after the injury has healed. Even years later, a minor irritation will reactivate the old pathway, causing the previously injured muscles to contract. This is even more likely to happen if, as sometimes happens, the injury has not in fact healed 100 percent.

Many health-care professionals believe that emotional stress can be just as "irritating" as physical stress caused by a fall. When you fall, the pain signal probably begins at the site of the injury. When emotional stress is the culprit, however, the pain message may be triggered by the brain and actually begin there.

Explaining what happens in the muscle is easier than trying to explain the complex workings of the brain. Every time you move, you contract certain muscles. This is what is known as a **voluntary contraction**. That is, the contraction is under your control. There are also **involuntary contractions**. This, of course, is what is happening when muscles go into spasm after an injury. In order to prevent further movement (which Mother Nature realizes could increase the damage), the muscles in the area tighten up — like a natural splint.

Pain produces an electrical signal. This signal travels along the nerve and up the spinal cord to the brain. Then a signal goes back down the nerve to the muscles in the area and "tells" them what to do. (This process is explained in more detail in Chapter 5.)

If the signal is strong enough, it enters the muscle fibers connected to the nerve. This causes calcium, which is stored in the muscles, to be released.

To understand what happens next, you have to be able to picture a relaxed muscle as it looks to the naked eye, as well as under a microscope. Look at Figure 2.1. Muscles run from one tendon to another tendon. They are made up of many fibres that together make up thousands of small compartments called **sarcomeres**. Forget the word; I can't even pronounce it! What's important is how these compartments are constructed and what happens inside them. Sarcomeres are divided from one another by **Z lines**. Think of these as the vertical posts in a fence: they provide both strength and support.

Running the other way — between Z lines — are thinner filaments called **myosin** and **actin**. (You can compare these to the fence's horizontal boards.) As you can see in the diagram, these filaments come in many different lengths.

Other filaments — they look like little lollipops! — run from the myosin to the actin, creating a kind of ratchet system. When a muscle is relaxed, however, the link is incomplete. This is because

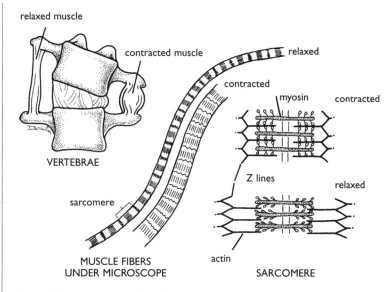

Figure 2.1 Anatomy of a Muscle Contraction

a chemical called an **inhibitor** prevents the connection from being made.

The release of calcium allows these connections to be completed. The myosin bonds chemically with the actin. Next, energy that has been stored in the muscle is released. A kind of twisting motion takes place, causing the actin and myosin to slide over one another and the Z lines to move closer together: a contraction.

All that happens each and every time a muscle contracts — pretty darn amazing, if you ask me.

CATEGORY 2: DISC PROBLEMS

Disc Degeneration

As I've already mentioned, around the time you reach the third decade of your life, the daily process whereby discs absorb water containing nutrients and expel water containing waste products gradually begins to fail. Slightly less water goes in than goes out, with the net result that the percentage of water in your discs begins to decline. At the same time, the annulus of each disc tends to weaken.

As it dries out, each disc loses a bit of thickness, or height — on average, about an eighth of an inch over the years, although the lumbar discs (which are larger and bear more weight) tend to lose a bit more height than the ones higher up. An eighth of an inch may seem like a meager amount, but when you multiply it by twenty-three discs you'll understand why, at the age of eighty, people tend to be about three inches shorter than they were at seventeen.

Losing a couple of inches in height is normal and inconsequential, except perhaps from vanity's point of view. It's no different from your hair turning gray. Other consequences of those twenty-three shock absorbers ending up looking more like raisins than grapes can, however, cause back trouble. Loss of disc height may, for example, stimulate the growth of osteophytes, and these bone growths sometimes come into contact with pain-sensitive tissue. When the annulus is weak as well, the alignment of the facet joints may be affected.

But the good news is that the drying out process of the discs' nuclei probably eliminates more back problems than it causes, at least in the long run. Try to imagine these two aging processes going on simultaneously: the disc's nucleus is drying out and its annulus, or outer shell, is beginning to weaken and, perhaps, fray. It makes sense that, as its water content diminishes, the nucleus will exert less force against the fibers of its annulus, which translates into less stress.

Here's an analogy that might help: Picture a balloon. The more air you pump into it, the more important it is that the rubber be firm in all places so that it can withstand the pressure of the air. But if you leave that blown up balloon for a few days, some of the air will leak out. The pressure will diminish and the rubber will not give way as easily, even if one spot happens to have a weakness.

The Herniated Disc

In the best of circumstances, the nuclei and the annuli of your discs will age in harmony. One disc's annulus will lose some of its strength and, as

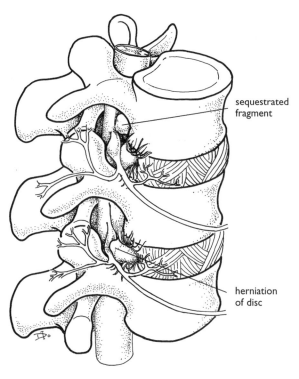

sequestrated
fragment

herniation
of disc

Figure 2.2 A Herniated Disc and a Sequestrated Disc

if it knows to compensate, its nucleus will lose a percentage of its water content, therefore exerting less stress.

Sometimes, however — though it's really not all that common — nature's balancing act fails completely, resulting in a herniated disc. (Bulging discs, which are described next, are far more common.) Almost all cases of disc herniation involve a lumbar disc.

In a **herniation**, the annulus weakens *before* its nucleus has had a chance to dry out. Then, one day — sometimes after doing nothing more strenuous than bending over, or coughing — the annulus ruptures, like a tire blowing. The nucleus (or part of it) oozes out, as in the lower disc in Figure 2.2.

It is interesting to note that, except where they attach to the posterior spinal ligament, there are no pain receptors in the discs themselves. Therefore, a herniated disc can be completely painless if the bit that oozes out does not happen to come into contact with a nerve root. When it does meet up with a nerve root, however, the pain of a true disc herniation can be excruciating. (In almost all cases, it will cause more leg pain — called **sciatic pain** — than back pain.) If the nerve's ability to function is actually disrupted by the bit of disc pressing against it, muscle atrophy will occur. Sometimes there is numbness rather than pain.

Herniated discs are often referred to as **slipped discs**. By now it should be clear to you that this term is a total misnomer, however, since nothing whatsoever slips.

Sometimes a disc will herniate because its annulus is **congenitally weak**. This means that the patient was born with the weakness; some studies suggest that a disc's propensity to herniate may be related to genetics. In other instances, the cause is a mystery. Some studies suggest that a life of hard labor increases your risk of a disc herniation, while other studies suggest that a sedentary existence places you in an even higher risk category.

Whatever the causes, true disc herniations are not all that common. Many orthopedic surgeons have told me that far fewer than 10 percent of the back pain patients referred to them for consultation are actually suffering from a herniated disc that is pressing against a nerve. To me this suggests that perhaps 1 or 2 percent of the back pain sufferers who go to see their family physicians have a herniated disc. And yet, if you're like most back pain sufferers, there are times that you've probably been certain that you fall into that category. Ask ten uneducated back pain sufferers to explain the source of their pain and I guarantee that at least eight will inform you that they have a disc pinching a nerve. Many of these people also have the erroneous idea that their back has "gone out." Now that you know some back anatomy, however, you'll realize that a human disc can't move into and out of place like a computer disk in your A-drive!

A frayed annulus can repair itself; the process, although slow, is the same as with any kind of injury: over the course of time scar tissue forms. One of the problems with scar tissue is that it is neither as strong, nor as flexible, as ordinary tissue, although doing gentle stretching exercises during the healing process can certainly help. (Why this is so is explained in Chapter 12.)

However, in a few cases, the bit of nucleus that has oozed through the annulus actually breaks away completely from the rest of the disc and becomes lodged against a nerve root in the spinal canal, a short distance away. In this situation, the herniated portion of the nucleus will remain in the spinal canal even after the annulus heals. This type of herniation is called a **sequestrated disc** (see the upper disc in Figure 2.2); the word simply means "isolated," from the same root as "sequester" — what we do to a jury while it ponders its verdict. Totally sequestrated discs are fairly rare, however. More frequently, the bit of nucleus that has herniated through the annulus remains attached, even just by a hair, to the rest of the nucleus.

In one respect, if you happen to be one of the small percentage of people who do have a true disc herniation, you're lucky. You are one of the few back pain sufferers whose back pain is due to a specific, localized problem. In many instances, with time and rest combined with conservative treatment, a herniated disc will heal. When this doesn't happen, its location can be pinpointed by a CT scan or magnetic resonance imaging (MRI) and the disc can be surgically removed. Because surgical and diagnostic techniques have improved so much over the years, the success rate is high; this invasive procedure usually eliminates the problem and, with it, all or most of the pain — at least that portion of the pain that comes from the pinched nerve.

Sometimes, however, surgery fails. In at least some cases, the technical skill of the surgeon is to blame. But in other cases the finger must be pointed toward **adhesions** that were not spotted (and therefore not removed) at surgery. The theory goes like this: When the injury occurs — that is, when the herniation actually takes place — there is a lot of swelling at the site. Due to poor circulation, or muscle tension, this fluid may not dissipate over a period of months as it should. When this happens, it dries out and becomes a sticky, viscous mass that "adheres" to pain-sensitive tissue such as a nerve. It is only recently that we have learned how gentle stretching exercises done during the healing process help to dissipate this fluid. (See Chapter 12.)

In still other cases, health-care professionals feel that some of the pain remains because of scarring; while the surgery fixes one problem, it actually creates another. This usually has more to do with how a person's tissue heals than the skill of the surgeon.

The final reason for failure is the most complex. It relates to stress, depression, and other kinds of emotional problems that so often go hand in hand with chronic back pain, especially when it has gone on for many years. In fact, many surgeons are reluctant to operate on back pain patients whose problems have been going on for more than two years. (For more on long-term pain, see Chapter 7.)

If you do have a herniated disc, it is likely that it is one of the two lowest discs of your lumbar spine — either the L4-L5 disc or the L5-S1 disc. As I've already mentioned, the rear portion of a disc's annulus tends to be weaker than the front portion. Therefore, when a disc herniates, it tends to do so at the back, near the intervertebral foramen. This is bad luck for two reasons. First of all, the rear portion of the annulus is the only part of the disc that contains pain receptors. Second of all, this is where the nerve roots exit from the spinal canal.

If you take another look back at Figure 1.11, you'll recall that branches of the nerves exiting from between L4-L5 and L5-S1 join together in the hip area with other nerve branches to form the sciatic nerve — one on each side. These nerves run down the leg all the way to the foot, which is why the pain or numbness that accompanies a disc herniation is so often felt in the buttock and leg rather than in the back. Depending upon the extent of the pressure against the nerve, the pain or numbness may extend down the leg to the knee or even as far as the heel or big toe.

In many cases, however, patients with a herniated disc experience some pain in the back as well. Some health-care professionals believe that, because nerve branches are so interconnected, the brain may get confused about the source of the pain (see the discussion of referred pain in Chapter 5). Others believe that the back pain emanates from the ligaments and/or muscles in the damaged area.

Some herniated disc patients, however, experience no back pain at all; they arrive at their doctor's office complaining of burning pain shooting down one leg, and are shocked when they are told that the source of the pain is in the lumbar spine.

The Bulging Disc
In the majority of cases, the nucleus of a disc doesn't actually herniate. Rather, the annulus weakens before its nucleus has had a chance to dry

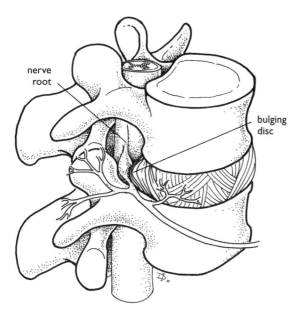

Figure 2.3 A Bulging Disc

out, and the pressure of the nucleus against the annulus causes it to **bulge**. (See Figure 2.3.) Such a bulge may be minor or severe, but as long as the annulus remains intact, the technical term "herniate" should not be used.

Even a bulging disc can come into contact with a ligament or a nerve root. Most often, however, a disc that is bulging doesn't exactly *pinch* a nerve root sufficiently to interfere with its functioning; a better way of describing the situation is to say that it *irritates* the pain-sensitive tissue.

Nevertheless, an irritated nerve root can certainly cause pain, numbness, or a tingling sensation in your back, buttock, or leg, and such symptoms can be quite severe. In most cases the sensation does not extend all the way to the foot; if it does, the feeling below the knee is difficult to pinpoint. When a ligament is irritated, the pain receptors in it will fire more frequently. In turn, this can also cause painful, protective muscle spasm.

If your back problem is caused by a weak annulus that has a propensity to bulge, you will most likely suffer from the type of annoying backache and/or leg pain that comes and goes. Many people also experience acute flare-ups several times a year. And because, as I have already mentioned, the back of the annulus tends to be the weakest part, prolonged **flexion**, or forward bending, will usually be the cause of a flare-up. For instance, every fall, I plant a few hundred bulbs, and for a few days afterward, I cope with back pain.

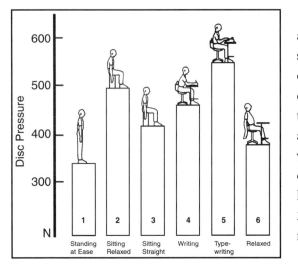

Dr. Alf Nachemson, a Swedish orthopedic surgeon who is famous for his work on discs, designed a study to demonstrate the amount of strain that various postures place on the discs of the lumbar spine. Figure 2.4 shows some of the results.

Most people are surprised to learn that sitting puts more strain on the lumbar discs than standing. Sitting hunched over a desk, or standing bent over a table, a shovel, or a vacuum cleaner strains your lumbar discs even more, often causing a weak annulus to bulge.

In many cases, a minor bulge will subside after a couple of days, along with the pain. Other times, however, a bulging disc can take months to subside completely. In some cases, the pain drags on for much longer than seems logical. Studies have shown that even a badly herniated disc will generally heal within nine months. When the pain continues after this amount of time, some health-care professionals blame adhesions. Their feeling is that while the bulge itself may have subsided, the adhesions caused by the injury have not dissipated. Some doctors believe that adhesions can take up to several years to dissipate completely, and that sometimes they never totally subside. Again, I can't overemphasize the importance of gentle stretching exercises during the healing process.

It can be very difficult to diagnose a bulging disc with total certainty, and even tougher to pinpoint it as the source of your pain. (For more detail, see Chapters 3 and 4.)

At this point, I would like to add two more comments about discs. The first is that everyone of us who has experienced severe back pain has wished on occasion that a disc problem could be diagnosed and cured surgically. It's the magic bullet solution, requiring no effort on our part! It would, however, be unethical to prescribe an invasive procedure whenever there is *some* evidence of a bulging disc. Before you can be considered a candidate for disc surgery, there must be conclusive evidence of a true herniation or a very large bulge that has not responded to conservative treatment. The diagnosis must also be corroborated by both clinical and radiological findings.

The second comment is that, in most cases, a bulging disc will stabilize over the years rather than herniate. As the nucleus dries out and loses a bit of height, osteophytes will develop, limiting mobility; as well, there will be less pressure for the annulus to bear. The trick is to find the conservative treatment that works for you while your discs are going through this process.

CATEGORY 3: FACET JOINT PROBLEMS

How Facet Joints Become Worn

As I've just explained, once a disc's nucleus begins to dry out, less pressure is exerted on its annulus. That's the up side of the equation. The down side is that, at least for a time, there may be *more* strain on the facet joints.

Look back at Figure 1.2, which shows a lumbar disc of a twenty-year-old. Because its nucleus is still plump, the disc has not lost any height. As we age, the disc loses a bit of height and the vertebrae above and below settle closer together. The result is that the facet joints at the back of the vertebra move closer together as well. Try to picture what's happening in your mind's eye.

Other degenerative changes can cause facet joints to settle closer together. As discussed earlier, ligaments that have stretched from years of poor posture can no longer support the facet joints as they were intended to. Without this support, these joints must bear additional weight, and since they were never intended to be weight-bearing joints, this additional strain can cause the same sort of settling effect. A third cause of facet joint strain has to do with the front portion of the annulus stretching. If your back tends to hurt after **extension** (backward arching), it may be an indication of a facet joint problem. High heels, for example, cause overextension, and women who stand around in them for hours at a time often suffer because of it.

And the results of this kind of settling? To put it very simply, if the two parts of a joint move closer, their alignment will change. This may cause them to rub against each other when they move. If this goes on for long enough, the smooth cartilage lining such joints will suffer from wear and tear, often causing pain.

The thought of having a couple of your facet joints rub together every time you move is as frightening to think about as the degeneration of a disc, or as osteophytes growing on a vertebra — until you stop for moment and think calmly about what actually occurs.

For one thing, we're talking about a process that can take decades to develop; facet joints don't settle and start rubbing together overnight. For another thing, just as they form on a vertebra, stabilizing osteophytes frequently form around worn facet joints, ultimately limiting their mobility.

Fortunately, worn facet joints grinding together like two gears that don't mesh are even less common than herniated discs. Again, the more common situation is not grinding but irritation. As two facet joints begin to settle, they stop functioning as well as they once did. Just as a disc bulges slightly because its annulus is weak, worn facet joints lose a bit of their youthful ability to operate frictionlessly. In most cases, nothing more than this goes wrong — a very minor physical problem.

However, there are pain receptors in facet joints. While bending forward will aggravate a disc that has a tendency to bulge, the opposite motion — arching your back into extension — can aggravate worn facet joints. When you extend your back, you bring the facet joints closer together. If they're already a bit worn, it makes sense that this posture will accentuate the problem. On the other hand, reducing your spine's lower lordotic curve (for example, by doing the pelvic tilt described in Chapter 13, exercise 3) will ease this kind of pain.

Just as a bulging disc can cause leg pain as well as back pain, most health-care professionals believe that worn facet joints can cause leg pain as well. In fact, several studies during which a saline solution has been injected into a facet joint have confirmed that sensations from facet joints can actually refer pain all the way to the foot! Usually, however, the pain is less severe and far less specific than the neurological pain caused by a disc pressing against a nerve. Patients generally describe leg pain that originates from a facet joint as "vague." Sometimes they can't even pinpoint exactly where the pain is. On the other hand, the leg pain caused by a herniated disc often shoots down the leg and patients frequently describe it as electric, or burning.

To understand more about how facet joint pain can radiate into the leg, take a look back at Figure 1.10. While one branch of the nerve runs down the leg, another branch moves off toward the facet joint, a third supplies the muscles nearby, and yet another serves the outer layers of the adjacent disc.

As an example, let's imagine a woman with a slightly worn pair of lumbar facet joints who wears high heels to a cocktail party where she ends up standing around for several hours. This posture, of course, will accentuate her lumbar lordotic curve.

By the end of the party, this lady's anterior longitudinal ligament will be feeling the strain, and this may cause some pain. But more likely, the source of her pain will be her worn facet joints. Because her back is arched, these joints will be taxed even more than usual. Basically, this irritation produces signals, which travel to the spinal cord via the nerve branch that serves the facet joints. At the spinal cord, this information is processed and then relayed to the brain where it is registered as pain. (For more detail, see Chapter 5.)

But while your body's communication system is brilliant in many respects, like most systems it tends to exhibit the odd flaw. One flaw is that it sometimes gets confused about the precise source of a signal. On occasion, your nervous system may think that signals which are emanating from one source are coming from another. In other words, it has become confused about which nerve branch is sending the information. When this happens, we say that the pain is being **referred**.

Imagine that you are in a train station looking down the tunnel as a train is pulling in. Trains arrive at this station from many places; you can't always determine the origin of this particular train. Your brain sometimes has the same problem.

Sometimes a situation like this can become even more complex. At the same time as the signal is getting its wires crossed, an impulse, which travels via the nerve branch that serves the muscles in the area, will alert those muscles that there is trouble afoot. They respond by going into spasm in an attempt to limit movement and thus ease the irritation. However, when these muscles go into spasm, others frequently tighten up to compensate, and the painful area becomes even more widespread.

Your brain often finds this kind of response extremely confusing. Sometimes it can't answer the question: "Where did the problem begin?" All it knows is that a branch of a branch of another branch of a nerve has delivered a message that spells *pain*. It realizes that the pain is coming from the left side of the body rather than the right, and from below the waist rather than above. But much more than this may be difficult to compute. By the time you arrive at the doctor's office with pain that originates from a worn facet joint, which is referring pain to your leg and causing muscle spasm as well, it's frequently very difficult to pinpoint the source of the pain.

Another type of facet joint problem can also cause pain. Sometimes, if you twist very suddenly or move beyond your normal range, the capsule surrounding these joints gets nipped by the joint itself. Try to visualize the capsule as a balloon that has lost some air after sitting around for a couple of days. It will be loose and a bit saggy, which in the case of facet joints is beneficial, since this roominess allows the joints to move. But because it is loose, the capsule sometimes gets nipped between the two ends of bone, in the same way that the inside of your cheek sometimes gets nipped between your teeth. This can bruise the capsule. Inflammation may follow, which leads to protective muscle spasm in the area. This is what is often happening when you twist suddenly, then feel a twinge of pain.

A third type of facet joint problem, which is probably more common, is very poorly understood. It has to do with the synovial fluid contained within the capsules of facet joints. Prior to a storm, barometric pressure frequently drops suddenly, causing the synovial fluid to expand. You would think that discovering exactly how this mechanism works, and why it so frequently causes back pain, would be a topic that researchers would be lining up to address. But over the past seventeen years, despite inquiries and searches through databases across the world, I have yet to come across a single documented research study that deals with this well-known phenomenon as it relates to back pain. (The small amount of information that does exist has to do with migraines.)

Irritation, muscle spasm, and pain caused by overstraining worn facet joints or bruising facet joint capsules usually subside soon after the source of the irritation is removed. Most health-care professionals agree that when facet joints cause pain, the acute stage does not generally last as long as an acute bout caused by a bulging disc. More common is low-grade chronic pain. If the woman at the party goes home, gets a good night's rest, wears sensible shoes, and avoids arching her back for several days, chances are that the pain will return to its normal dull roar. Likewise, if you twist badly while playing a sport, the pain will likely be gone after two or three days. As well, once the storm breaks, the increased back pain caused by a sudden drop in barometric pressure almost always subsides.

The trick is to incorporate the needs of your slightly worn joints, or discs, into your lifestyle so that you can avoid beginning a new bout of pain almost as soon as you have gotten over the last one. While you are learning to do this, Mother Nature will also be at work to diminish your vulnerability to back pain. It will be busy stabilizing your spine, a process that will ultimately limit your susceptibility to the pain caused by degenerative changes such as these.

Category 4: Osteoarthritis

As we saw earlier in the chapter under the discussion of the aging process, this scary term simply refers to the development of osteophytes, or bony growths, on vertebrae.

A number of years ago, the spines of 195 Swedish men and women were X-rayed. Some of these people suffered from back pain; others did not. Several interesting things showed up on the films.

Of those who were in their forties, 72 percent had evidence of osteophytes growing on the rims of the vertebral bodies, near the facet joints, or in both areas. Of those who were in their sixties, 97 percent had evidence of osteophytes. And yet, curiously enough, there was very little correlation between the degree of degeneration and the incidence of back pain.

Osteophytes, which are also called **bone spurs** (because of their shape), or **lipping**, are ultimately an aid to back pain rather than the cause of it. Once their shape has become established and they have actually accomplished their purpose of stabilizing the discs, or joints, on which they are growing, osteophytes limit mobility, which usually causes the pain to subside. There may be stiffness, particularly in people over the age of sixty-five. But as far as actual pain is concerned, most health-care professionals believe that osteophytes are the villain in relatively few cases.

When osteophytes do cause trouble, they can lead to a form of spinal stenosis, discussed below.

CATEGORY 5: SPINAL STENOSIS

Spinal stenosis is another term that many people find scary, when in fact its meaning is rather benign. *Steno* is from the Greek word *stenos*, which means "narrow." And *osis* means "a condition of" or "a process." Basically, this highfalutin term means nothing more than "a condition where there is narrowing." There are many different types of spinal stenosis; I will discuss the most common two types only here.

Central Spinal Stenosis
The first type, **central spinal stenosis**, has to do with the spinal canal itself, through which the spinal cord runs. If you are suffering from this condition, it means that your canal is narrower than normal in a particular area (see Figure 2.5). Sometimes, central spinal stenosis is congenital.

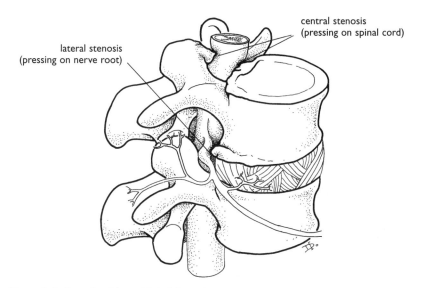

Figure 2.5 Central and Lateral Spinal Stenosis

There are different opinions about whether or not a congenitally narrow canal actually causes back pain or simply *predisposes* a person to it. I think the best idea is to think of a narrowish spinal canal as, if you will, less forgiving than one that is normal in size.

The results of a study that was done by two British physicians seem to confirm this. While studying the spines of pain-free patients as well as those who suffer from back pain, these physicians discovered that about 10 percent of the population have lumbar spinal canals that are less than half an inch wide. At the opposite extreme, about ten per cent of the population have lumbar spinal canals that are nearly three-quarters of an inch wide. The most interesting aspect of the study, however, was that a large proportion of people who suffered from back pain fell into the small group of people with very narrow canals. Out of 154 patients who suffered from sciatic pain, 56 percent had spinal canals less than half an inch wide!

Central spinal stenosis can be so mild that it remains undetected. At other times it can cause severe back pain. When severe central spinal stenosis is suspected, a CT scan or an MRI is in order.

Lateral Spinal Stenosis

What's involved with **lateral spinal stenosis** is a narrowing of an inter-vertebral foramen, the space at the back of a vertebra out of which the nerve roots exit (see Figure 2.5). Many things can cause lateral spinal stenosis: an injury, severe settling of the facet joints due to a disc that has lost an abnormally large amount of height, spondylolisthesis (discussed later), or an abnormal variation in the shape of a vertebra.

Osteophytes, however, are the most common cause. When they form around the edges of a vertebra, they may sometimes encroach into the spinal canal. These bony growths may then irritate a nerve root as it makes its exit through the foramen, which is now narrower than normal.

When the encroachment is minimal, the back pain caused by lateral spinal stenosis is usually minor — perhaps the occasional ache after strenuous activity. In the rare instances when it is severe (that is, when a nerve root is actually being pinched by bone), it can be corrected by surgery (see Chapter 17) to remove the excess bone.

OTHER SPECIFIC CAUSES OF BACK PAIN

Arachnoiditis

As I explained in Chapter 1 (see Figure 1.10), three layers of tissue protect the nerves that run through the spinal canal. The middle layer, which is a fine, cobweb-like membrane, is called the arachnoid. For various reasons, the outermost layer, called the dura, can become damaged. Thick scar tissue is produced, which impinges into the arachnoid layer as well, and the nerves within the spinal canal become compressed. This condition is called **arachnoiditis**. Sometimes only a small number of nerves are affected. Other times, the damage is extensive.

Patients who suffer from arachnoiditis develop severe pain in both the back and the legs, and sometimes, if the arachnoiditis is extensive, right up into their necks and arms. Many patients complain of a burning or "pins and needles" sensation in their legs. Some patients also experience a loss of motor control, and if the nerves to the bladder or bowel are affected —

which is rare — they may become partially or completely incontinent. Other patients develop a **syrinx**, a tubular cavity that fills up with spinal cord fluid and, in turn, further decompresses the nerves. Obviously, this is one of the most serious and devastating back conditions.

Until about twenty years ago, doctors thought that arachnoiditis was caused by infections of the spine. Most likely this is true in some instances; for example, some people who suffer from an infection called meningitis, if it is not caught early enough, develop arachnoiditis. Starting in the 1970s, however, a number of people who had undergone a diagnostic test called a myelogram (see Chapter 4) went on to develop arachnoiditis, and doctors now believe that a reaction to the oil-based dye that was used for this test back in those days actually caused the problem. (Today, myelograms are performed far less frequently, and when they are done, a water-based dye — which has not caused any problems as far as we know — is used.) It is also thought that there are people suffering from arachnoiditis who have never been properly diagnosed.

A small number of arachnoiditis patients have undergone surgery to remove the scar tissue. Unfortunately, a significant number of them end up with even worse problems when, a number of months later, scar tissue reforms.

This is obviously not a pretty picture. The only bright side is that research is being conducted and, perhaps, the future will bring with it the chance of a cure.

Cancers of the Spine

Primary cancers of the spine, which are cancers that develop in a vertebra, the bone marrow, or the muscles of the spine, are extremely rare. When they do occur, however, the main symptom is usually pain that does not respond to conservative treatment or rest. If a patient complains of unrelenting back pain that is worse throughout the night, a physician may suspect a cancerous growth, or **tumor**. Because the cells in a cancerous tumor (also called **malignant**; harmless tumors are known as **benign**) divide more quickly than normal cells, they can be detected by means of a bone scan. However, this test is not always conclusive, so other tests —

usually blood tests, and X-rays, and sometimes a biopsy — will also be done. Surgery (if the tumor is accessible), radiation therapy, and chemotherapy are all used in the treatment of primary cancer of the spine.

Although **secondary cancers of the spine** are also rare, it is more common for a cancer that has developed in another organ of the body to spread, or **metastasize**, to the spine than to originate in the spine. Breast cancer, for example, sometimes spreads to the bones of the spine, as do cancer of the prostate and the lung. The diagnosis and treatment of secondary cancer of the spine is similar to that for primary cancer of the spine.

Fibromyalgia

A syndrome also known as **FM**, **fibromyalgia**, is a condition of unknown cause. It affects women far more often than men. Patients complain that they ache all over, although upon examination, specific areas of tenderness, called **tender points**, can be found in particular locations. (Tender points are different from trigger points, which are related to myofascial pain, discussed later in this section.) FM is also characterized by fatigue, morning stiffness, sleep disturbances, depression, and headaches. Most people complain of backache as well.

Until recently, many researchers considered this ailment to be largely psychogenic (of the mind) rather than a specific physical problem. Controversy over whether an ailment is physical or mental often arises when its diagnosis is based on the exclusion of other disorders that cause some of the same symptoms. In other words, you suffer from FM when every other possibility has been ruled out.

Today, there is a more precise definition of FM. According to the American College of Rheumatology, there are two basic criteria. One is widespread pain, which is still a pretty vague symptom. But the other is that the patient must experience pain in at least eleven of eighteen specific tender points when these points are palpated by the examiner.

Some researchers believe that the pain of FM is related to deconditioned muscles. Others are more specific, saying that the muscles of FM sufferers are prone to **microtrauma**, which means that even slight exertion can cause microscopic tears. Still other researchers suggest that the brains of fibromyalgia sufferers produce low levels of neurotransmitters such as serotonin, and that this affects the way their brains process pain signals. And finally, there is a group of researchers who believe that FM sufferers do not get enough deep sleep and that their symptoms tend to subside when their sleep patterns improve.

FM is generally treated with controlled, gentle exercise. Aqua aerobics and walking (see Chapter 13) have been found to be particularly useful. Sometimes antidepressants are prescribed, both for depression and to help patients sleep.

Lumbago

Of all the stupid terms that have been coined and used to describe back ailments, this takes the cake. It's even less meaningful than spondylosis! Basically, **lumbago** means "pain in the lumbar region," and you already knew you had pain in the lower back before you consulted a health-care professional!

Myofascial Pain

This type of myofascial pain used to be discussed along with fibromyalgia but more recently these two conditions have been described and treated as separate syndromes. Patients suffering from **myofascial pain** syndrome have what are called **trigger points** (not to be confused with the tender points discussed under FM, above). Trigger points are tiny, taut nodules located in muscle tissue that, when probed by the examiner, cause referred pain to another part of the body rather than just within the muscle itself. Quite often the pain can be very sharp. An example: A trigger point in the neck may refer pain to the head, causing a headache.

As with FM, the cause of myofascial pain is unknown. Also like FM, it is controversial. One study concluded that trigger points don't exist because different examiners couldn't find the same points in the same patients. However, a more recent study, in which the examiners were first trained to recognize trigger points, yielded better results.

Treatment for myofascial pain includes an exercise program that concentrates more on stretching than strengthening exercises. Aerobic exercise is important to improve overall fitness and to improve sleep patterns. Most patients do better if they exercise for short periods throughout the day rather than exercising for one long session. Massage is also very helpful if it is done by someone who understands the syndrome.

Osteoporosis

Another important cause of back pain, especially in older women, is osteoporosis, in which bones get brittle and frail. This ailment is important enough in our aging society that I've given it its own chapter — see Chapter 21.

Pregnancy as a Cause of Back Pain

The increase in the hormone progesterone that occurs during pregnancy causes several changes to take place. The broad ligaments that support the uterus and hold it in place relax so that the uterus can expand. As well, the connective tissue linking the right and left sections of the abdominal muscles soften so that the abdomen can expand. As the abdomen expands, the body's center of gravity changes and many women develop an excessively lordotic or hyperextended posture, which frequently causes muscle spasms in the lower back. In addition, many women experience pain from the strained sacroiliac ligaments (part of the pelvic girdle) where the uterus is located.

Rotational movements in particular put excessive strain on the sacroiliac joint ligaments. Much of this pain can be avoided or at least reduced if rotational movements are avoided as much as possible. Here are a few tips:

- When you get out of bed, first roll to one side and use your arms to push your body into a sitting position; then sit for a moment before standing.
- When doing household chores, it's more important than ever to move your feet to face your task rather than twisting your upper body.
- Try to carry two light bags of groceries, one on either side, rather than one heavy bag.
- Avoid bending over with your legs straight and pay particular

attention to lifting techniques, especially if you have a young child. (For more on back-friendly movement, see Chapters 10 and 13.)

Rheumatoid Arthritis

Unlike osteoarthritis, which is a local problem, **rheumatoid arthritis** is a body-wide illness. It attacks the joints — specifically, the synovial membranes. The hands, wrists, elbows, knees, ankles, feet, hips, and/or sometimes the facet joints of the spine may become severely inflamed, swollen, and painfully stiff. Unlike osteoarthritis, rheumatoid arthritis will usually destroy a joint as it progresses, as well as the tissue nearby.

Rheumatoid arthritis can be crippling. For reasons that are not known, it strikes three times as many women as men. In fact, the cause of the disease is largely unknown, although recent research points to a genetic disorder that may be triggered by a virus but only when a person is particularly susceptible because of a deficiency in his or her immune system. Stress may also play a role in the onset, or exacerbation, of the disease or its symptoms.

Rheumatoid arthritis can begin at any age; even young children are sometimes stricken. The disease can also be difficult to diagnose, but usually a physician will be alerted by an antibody called the **rheumatoid factor** that is present in the blood. In some patients, however, the rheumatoid factor is not present and the diagnosis is "confirmed" only when all other diseases that produce similar symptoms have been ruled out.

At present there is no cure, only treatments that can reduce, or slow down, the onset of symptoms. Once damage has been done to a joint, it is largely irreversible. However, for reasons that are not understood, a patient with rheumatoid arthritis will sometimes go into remission for years at a time.

Until a cure is found, the treatment will continue to focus on controlling the disease. Specialists, called **rheumatologists**, supervise the treatment, which consists of drug therapy to relieve the pain and inflammation, exercise to prevent the affected joints from stiffening further, and resting splints to prevent or reduce deformities. Aspirin, gold salts, cortisone, and other anti-inflammatory drugs are all used, the choice depending upon the individual's tolerance and reactions. In severe cases of rheumatoid arthritis, a destroyed joint can be replaced surgically.

Sacroiliac Joint Problems

In the 1920s, before it had been linked to disc problems, back pain was frequently attributed to sprains and strains of the ligaments of the sacroiliac (SI) joints — which, you may recall, attach the sacrum to the hipbone, one on each side (see Figure 1.1). Then, during the 1930s, disc trouble was "discovered" by two American surgeons and sacroiliac strain went out of fashion. Fashions, however, almost always return if you wait long enough, and over the past few years, strains of the ligaments of the SI joints have been receiving more press.

The main symptom of SI joint strain is pain, which is often very localized. (In some cases, the tender area is no larger than the size of a quarter.) The patient usually feels pain when sitting; walking generally relieves it.

A host of ligaments attach the ilium to the sacrum on each side. No one disputes this fact. The bone of contention is that some health-care professionals believe that, other than during pregnancy because of hormonal changes, the SI joints scarcely move at all; in their opinion, only a severe trauma such as a car accident could exert enough force on these ligaments to cause them to become strained. Therefore, they do not believe that the contribution of SI joints to back pain is significant.

Others — notably chiropractors — disagree, insisting that SI joint strain is a significant cause of low back pain for many people, with athletes in particular (high jumpers who land on one leg make a good example) at higher risk than people who do not engage in stressful activities.

Chiropractors diagnose SI joint strain by doing a motion palpation test, which, if positive, will usually reproduce the pain. If they do discover strain, they will manipulate these joints, and they find this works for many patients. It also works quite quickly — often after just one or two treatments. If there is no change after several treatments, it is likely that some other problem is at the root of the pain.

A number of physicians (they call themselves orthopedic physicians) also manipulate the SI joints and sometimes use a technique called

sclerosing as well. Sclerosing involves the injection of a thickening agent — a mixture of phenol and glucose — into these stretched ligaments. The result is a sterile inflammation, which causes the stretched ligaments to thicken and shorten.

Scoliosis

The medical term **scoliosis** signifies a spine that curves sideways. About 12 percent of the population suffers from scoliosis but it is often so minimal that it remains undiagnosed. There are four types of scoliosis:

- **Congenital scoliosis** is present at birth. Usually, the spinal vertebrae and ribs are poorly formed.
- **Neuromuscular scoliosis** is an umbrella term for a wide variety of conditions; however, there is always some damage to nerves and muscles, usually caused by such diseases as polio or cerebral palsy.
- **Traumatic scoliosis** is caused by an injury to a previously normal spine. A spinal fracture, unrelated surgery, radiation treatment, or injury to muscles and tissues at the side of the spine can all cause traumatic scoliosis.
- **Idiopathic scoliosis** accounts for 70 to 80 percent of all cases of scoliosis. Despite extensive research, the precise cause is unknown. Recent studies point to genetic factors, but further investigation needs to be done to confirm this theory. In children with idiopathic scoliosis, the spine is normal at birth and starts to curve just before or during the adolescent growth spurt. This type of scoliosis affects both boys and girls, but almost all of the severe cases occur in girls.

Scoliosis conditions of all types are categorized according to the severity of the curve. A curve of 30 degrees or less is considered mild and may remain undetected until the person is examined for unrelated backache later in life. For mild scoliosis which does not appear to be progressing, serial observation will usually suffice. There is no active treatment; the doctor simply examines the patient at regular intervals to ensure that the condition is not getting worse.

Curves of between 30 to 60 degrees or so are considered moderate. In this category there is a noticeable deformity and, in most cases, pain eventually develops. Children whose curves are moderate are usually treated with a brace and exercise — known as conservative observation. Sometimes, a technique called electro-spinal stimulation is used as well.

Curves of more than about 60 degrees are considered severe and can cause heart failure, severe arthritis, or early death from heart and/or lung problems caused by constriction of the chest cavity. For extremely severe curves, surgery is an option, but these days, very few people are treated this way. During surgery, the curve is reduced and the spine is stabilized. To make the back straighter, metal rods are implanted on either side of the spine; then the spine is fused in the areas of the scoliosis.

If you think that your back pain may be caused by mild scoliosis there are some exercises that you can do. Swimming, for instance, will increase your flexibility and strengthen your trunk muscles without stressing your body. Many people also find that yoga exercises are very helpful. You should first be checked out by a family physician, however, in case something more than exercise is required.*

Spina Bifida

Like spondylolysis, **spina bifida** is a condition that rarely causes back pain and often remains undetected. It is at least as old as the mummies of Egypt, in whose vertebral remains "holes" have been found.

The condition sounds much worse than it is. Basically, in the process of developing, the bony ring that forms the back of each vertebra fails to close completely; a tiny gap is left at the rear. Generally this gap is filled with scar tissue (see Figure 2.6) and is so minimal — less than a sixteenth of an inch — that it is totally insignificant. Only on very rare occasions is the gap wide enough to be a serious birth defect.

Spondylitis

Itis means "inflammation" and *spondyl* means "spine." **Spondylitis** refers

---

* For more information on scoliosis, contact the Alberta Scoliosis Association at (403) 782-5205.

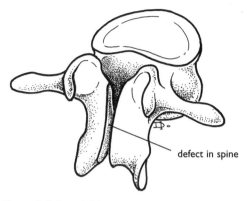

Figure 2.6 Spina Bifida

to the inflammation usually caused by an infection or a reaction to a chemical.

Bacteria can sometimes be the cause of such a spinal infection. When bacteria invade the spine, the term *osteomyelitis* is generally used. This condition can be caused by an infection elsewhere in the body spreading to the spine, or it can result from surgery when an incision becomes infected after the operation. Treatment generally consists of antibiotics and rest. In rare circumstances, spondylitis can take several years to subside completely.

In other rare cases, the cause is a chemical that irritates the spine. For example, when a diagnostic test such as a myelogram (see Chapter 4) is conducted, a chemical is injected in the spine and there is a small chance the patient will develop an infection. These types of infections are also treated with antibiotics and rest. (See also the section on arachnoiditis, above.)

Ankylosing spondylitis, or Marie-Strumpell Disease, is a rare condition that affects men twice as often as women and usually begins when people are in their late twenties. *Ankylosing* means "stiffening."

The symptoms of ankylosing spondylitis include severe inflammation of the spinal joints, which stiffen and become extremely painful. The hip and knee joints are also frequently affected. Eventually some, or all, of the vertebrae fuse together (see Figure 2.7).

Typically, this disease begins at the base of the spine and affects the sacroiliac joints first. The lumbar vertebrae are affected next. Over a period of years the disease progresses up the spinal column and, when more than a few of the vertebrae become fused, the afflicted patient will actually become hunched over until he or she can barely see ahead. At this point, the fused joints resemble a bamboo rod, so the disease is sometimes referred to as **bamboo spine**. The cause is unknown, although recent

(defect in spine)

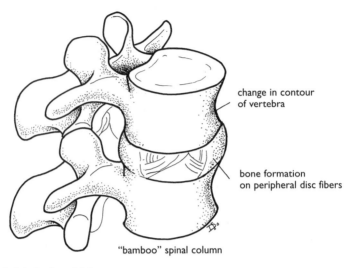

change in contour
of vertebra

bone formation
on peripheral disc fibers

"bamboo" spinal column

Figure 2.7 Ankylosing Spondylitis

research points to genetic factors. It is also unknown why patients who suffer from this disease sometimes go into remission spontaneously.

Analgesics (painkillers) and anti-inflammatory drugs, as well as exercise and attention to posture, are used to treat this disease. Only in extremely severe cases will surgery be performed. If the disease is not severe, a person with ankylosing spondylitis can live a nearly normal existence in terms of function.

Spondylolysis and Spondylolisthesis

Spondyl, you will remember, comes from the Greek word for "vertebra." *Olisis* comes from the Greek word for "loosen." Put them together and you have a condition called **spondylolysis**, in which a defective vertebra becomes loose or wobbly because it has cracked (see Figure 2.8).

Spondylolysis occurs across the back of a vertebra. Usually, the crack or fracture is hairline — so minor that it remains undetected unless an X-ray is taken for another reason. Spondylolysis is surprisingly common; in North America, it is estimated that one in twenty people have a mild spondylolysis. In some populations, notably the Eskimo population of northern Alaska, nearly 30 percent of the people have spondylolysis.

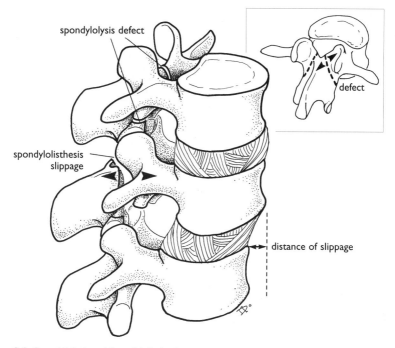

spondylolysis defect

defect

spondylolisthesis slippage

distance of slippage

Figure 2.8 Spondylolysis and Spondylolisthesis

Although the cause of spondylolysis is unknown, some researchers speculate that it is related to a hereditary weakness combined with prolonged stress. The crack often occurs in early childhood and fails to heal.

Generally speaking, mild spondylolysis causes neither back pain nor mechanical problems.

In rare instances the hairline crack will widen; this wider crack is called a **spondylolisthesis**, which can cause back trouble. This condition sounds unpronounceable, but once again, if you break it down it will make sense. *Spondyl* means "vertebra" or "spine" and *olisthesis* is from the Greek word meaning "slip." Ironically, the misnomer "slipped disc" is used more frequently to describe a herniated disc than for this condition, where actual slippage does take place.

For a person to develop spondylolisthesis, spondylolysis (see above) must first exist. If the spondylolysis crack widens sufficiently, the front portion of the vertebra, which is detached from the rear, can gradually slip forward in relation to the vertebra below. (See Figure 2.8.)

In its very mild form, spondylolisthesis may remain undetected. More severe cases usually respond to conservative treatment, which consists of rest during a flare-up and some form of exercise to strengthen the area when the acute pain subsides. A flare-up may be caused by physical overexertion. In extremely severe cases, surgery may be performed to fuse the slipping area (see Chapter 17).

Spondylosis

Once again, take the word apart. *Spondyl* means "spine" and *osis* means a "condition of." This gets you to the meaning of the term **spondylosis** — which is no meaning at all! Unfortunately, it is sometimes used by health-care professionals who forget that to most lay people medical jargon can produce fear and anxiety. If you hear it, ask the person who has used it what he or she means and keep asking until you are told it means nothing.

11

DIAGNOSIS

3

Pinning Down That Pain

Most back pain sufferers start out with the idea that their problem can be, and therefore should be, *precisely* diagnosed. I certainly did, and because of my conviction, I ran from health-care professional to health-care professional, certain that *somewhere* (at the top of Mount Kilimanjaro, if need be!) existed a human being who could pin my pain down. Like millions of other back pain sufferers, I wasted a huge amount of time and energy (not to mention health-care dollars) trying to locate him or her.

To begin with, my conviction was not true. It was not true when my back problem began in 1975, before the advent of high-tech diagnostic tests such as the CT scan, and it is still not true today. Like the vast majority of back pain sufferers, I have had to learn to be content with my problem being merely categorized. (The main categories are described in Chapter 2.) Unless you are one of the under 10 percent of back pain sufferers who are candidates for surgery, in all probability you will have to be satisfied with a category, too. Furthermore, you are unlikely to require a high-tech test, since the best method of discovering what category you fit into is the good old, tried and true, clinical exam (discussed later in this chapter).

This is not bad news, however. In order to control your back problem, you only *need* to be fitted into a category in order to determine appropriate treatment. Nevertheless, a ton of money is spent every year by back pain sufferers in hot pursuit of what I've come to call the "Holy Diagnostic Grail." Canadians are less culpable than Americans, who spend literally billions of dollars annually on unnecessary diagnostic tests. (In many cases, their doctors order these tests because they are trying to cover themselves in the event of a lawsuit.) But we all overspend, that's for sure.

FIRST, A BIT OF BLACK HUMOR

A couple of years ago, I was trying to find a way of explaining all this to Morris Dobson, a member of the Back Association of Canada (BAC). (His name has been changed slightly to protect the guilty.) I tried logic. But this guy was convinced that one of his discs had herniated, and he would have found a way to fly to the *moon* if he thought the man in the moon could discover which disc it was. Here on Earth, he'd managed to get himself three CT scans as well as a magnetic resonance imaging (MRI) test, none of which indicated any evidence of disc trouble.

I showed him studies. Some explained why high-tech tests are not the be-all and end-all for back pain sufferers. (Two of them concluded that herniated discs often show up on the CT scans of people who've never suffered from back pain in their lives!) None of this, however, impressed Morris Dobson one bit.

Next I tried a history lesson, explaining how opinions about what, other than strains and sprains, causes most back pain have changed over the years. This too failed to impress him. His attitude was that, if clinical examinations were the gold standard, then his family physician should have been able to determine from his symptoms exactly what was going on. I threw my hands up in frustration.

That night (due, I'm sure, to a guilty conscience), I woke up at 3 a.m. with a terrible backache and, while I was meandering around in an attempt to work it out, I hit upon a way to make clear even to a numbskull like him the uselessness of clinging to diagnostic exactitude.

I remembered a take-off of a game show performed by the *Firesign Theatre* on the radio decades ago. (I warn you: if you have no stomach for black humor, stop reading this chapter right now!) *Beat the Reaper* was based on *Beat the Clock*. You remember *Beat the Clock*: two contestants tried to perform a certain task as the clock ticks away — Tick! Tock! Tick! Tock! — and, if they got the chore done before the time ran out, they won a prize. But *Beat the Reaper* added a sick twist to this theme. In the skit, just before the clock started ticking, the contestant was injected with a lethal dose of some horrendous disease. If, using the symptoms as clues, the contestant guessed the name of the ailment before the clock ran out, the host injected the antidote. If the clock ran out . . . well!

It went something like this:

Tick! Tock! Tick! Tock!

"I feel cold. No, dizzy! No, wait, there's no feeling in my legs!"

Tick! Tock! Tick! Tock!

"I've got . . . pains in my chest. No, not my chest!"

Tick! Tock! Tick! Tock!

"A burning sensation. Numbness . . . "

And so on, until the buzzer sounded and the game show host (in a purring voice) announced to the prostrate body of the dead contestant, "I'm sorry, Sir! You had the plague."

Well, this story did penetrate the thick skull of my intransigent BAC member. He soon let his obsession with diagnosis go and started to spend his time and energy on learning ways to control his back problem. Finally, I had found a way of making it clear to him how difficult back pain is to diagnose . . . and I hope that, by now, I've made it clear to you as well!

SYMPTOMS VS. SIGNS

Symptoms, as the unfortunate *Beat the Reaper* contestant discovered, are often impossible to pin down. They can be different from one moment to the next; even different from one patient to another. Of course, this is maddening, since symptoms are our main ally when we are trying to describe our back problem to a health-care professional who just might be able to make it go away.

It will probably turn your head around even farther if I tell you that, when they are trying to make a diagnosis, health-care professionals are not even all that interested in symptoms. Well, they're *interested* (or at least they should be). But what they are really looking for — and what they must rely on — are not symptoms but signs.

A **sign** is something unusual, or abnormal, that someone who is examining you can observe and measure. Signs are both *objective* and *quantitative*. Examples are: a scoliosis (sideways curvature of the spine); the loss of muscle power in a foot; evidence of reduced mobility when you try to bend forward.

Symptoms, on the other hand, are not visible. They are what you — the patient — report, and are thus both subjective and qualitative. The most common symptom is pain. But when you describe how your back pain depresses you, or makes you anxious, you are not providing your health-care professional with useful information. For one thing, different people react very differently to the same amount of pain. (There is more on this subject in Chapter 5.) Recent studies have also shown that, when it comes to back ailments, pain varies from patient to patient more than for any other medical condition. In other words, you and your neighbor could have the same injury and you might have a lot of pain whereas your neighbor may simply complain of discomfort.

To make matters even more complicated, even signs can be misleading. Broadly speaking, there are two types of signs: specific and nonspecific. Specific signs are generally less ambiguous than nonspecific signs, but even they aren't always worth their weight in gold. For example, the loss of muscle power — a specific sign — indicates that a certain nerve that ought to be carrying messages to a certain muscle isn't working properly. (A common test is to see if a patient can raise the big toe of one foot upward against the downward pressure applied by the doctor.) In the majority of cases, the L5 nerve will be at fault. But precisely what is *causing* this specific sign is often extremely difficult to determine. It could be a disc; it could be bone.

To make matters worse, most of the signs that back problems exhibit are nonspecific: reduced mobility in one or more directions; stiffness in the lower spine. Quite often, the physician cannot figure out the cause of a nonspecific sign.

Imagine a patient shows up at the doctor's office with a nonspecific sign, say reduced mobility when she tries to bend sideways. The problem could be caused by an irritated joint in her spine, which might or might not have been caused by a bit of disc degeneration, something that might or might not have been caused by ligaments that have stretched because of chronic lousy posture . . . any of which may or may not be causing muscle spasm, which may or may not be the actual cause of the back pain.

The patient asks "What's wrong?" and expects a forty-second explanation as to why she feels like a pretzel. You can see why the physician is at a loss for words.

You can also see by now, I hope, that your best bet is to find out which category, or categories, your back problem falls into. Unfortunately, until very recently this down-to-earth concept has received short shrift. Many health-care professionals do try to explain the complexities of diagnosing back pain to sufferers who don't want to hear that they don't have cut-and-dried answers to all of our questions. In some cases, however, health-care professionals are to blame for our hang-ups about diagnosis. When they can find no precise signs, they somehow manage to give you the impression that your back problem is not real, or is at least being exaggerated. It comes across in a tone of voice, or the manner in which you are hustled out the door. In other cases, health-care professionals use vague labels because they find it uncomfortable to admit that they don't know what's wrong. Or sometimes they simply begrudge their patients the time it takes to explain that medical science isn't always in the know.

The Professional's Point of View

To make the whole diagnostic can of worms even more confusing, all health-care professions have particular ways of looking at human backs, and these biases color the approach that their members take to diagnosis and to treatment. Professionals begin to acquire these points of view the moment they begin their training. These viewpoints can be so basic, and so deep-rooted, that it's sometimes appropriate to think of them as philosophies. I've also come to realize that some health-care professionals — particularly those who practise "alternative" types of therapies — aren't even aware that they promote a particular point of view.

Therefore, it is up to you, the patient, to put what any health-care professional has to say into context, which is no easy task. It's particularly difficult if you are new to the world of back pain and poorly versed in its language — which also, by the way, differs from one discipline to another!

Let me illustrate what I mean about points of view by giving you a couple of examples. Then I'll try to explain what I mean about the use of language.

Take surgeons. If you go to see an orthopedic surgeon or neurosurgeon, you'll get far more out of the consultation by bearing in mind that you are consulting a professional who is looking for a specific abnormality that can be corrected by surgery. When you stop to think about it, this should not be so surprising. Apart from diagnosing back problems, operating on backs is what back surgeons do. Nevertheless, millions of back pain sufferers hobble into the offices of surgeons expecting to learn about muscle strain or poor posture . . . and hobble out half an hour later, disappointed.

It's the rare surgeon who feels comfortable telling patients that his or her strong suit is not the conservative (i.e., noninvasive) management of back pain. Nor are most of them very good at explaining that, if conservative treatment is what you need, you're better off consulting someone else. This is a pity, since, when a surgeon can get it together to explain these things, most patients feel as if a huge burden has been lifted from their shoulders: "Yes, there is something wrong with your back, Mr. Jones. No, it does not require surgery. Yes, there is a therapist out there who can help you. But I'm a surgeon and my role in life is to perform surgery. So that therapist ain't me!"

Another example: Because of *their* training, physiotherapists tend to gravitate toward soft tissue injuries when they diagnose and/or treat back pain. They feel comfortable talking about strained ligaments and worn joints, which can be treated conservatively. They do not, in the majority of cases, take a look at a back pain patient, then send him or her off to a surgeon — at least not until a trial of conservative care has proven to be unsuccessful. Since surgery is inappropriate for more than 90 percent of back pain patients, this particular attitude works almost all of the time. Nevertheless, it is a way of thinking based on some preconceptions, and if you consult a physiotherapist, you should bear it in mind.

Practitioners of holistic types of therapies (for example, the Alexander technique and the Feldenkrais method) use very general labels when the subject of "diagnosis" comes up. This is because they tend to treat everyone in more or less the same way. This is fine when it works . . . but it doesn't always work, and it drives me up the wall when such people urge back patients to persist, that they are "not trying hard enough," or "not giving their technique enough time."

Years ago, before I knew what I was talking about, I personally endured such an experience. At the time, I was going through my first acute bout of back pain, which was radiating into my leg. What I needed was encouragement and a bit of rest combined with a regime of *gentle* stretching exercises, increased gradually. Instead, a practitioner who shall remain nameless insisted that the *only* way I'd ever get better was if I immediately and totally immersed myself in a "treatment" that required me, just for openers, to change my posture dramatically. This was simply too much for my back, never mind my ennervated psyche, at the time.

As the days wore on, I got worse and he got tougher. This was not a case of "working through the pain," which I wholeheartedly advocate when appropriate. This was a case of a professional acting like a guru; his demand for devotion was so total that it prevented him from considering me as an individual with particular needs. Today I'd have enough confidence to resist; back then I didn't, and I suffered for it.

Now, back to my point about language. In many instances, I think language is at the root of professional biases. The fact that different professionals use different words to describe the same thing does not help us patients make sense of what's going on. Nor does it help professionals from different disciplines try to communicate with each other.

Posture makes a great example. Years ago, I was interviewing various professionals about the diagnosis of back pain, particularly the contribution of poor posture. The first person I spoke to was a physiotherapist. She talked about the fact that so many people's knowledge of "biomechanics" — how, for instance, to stand without straining the lower back — was lacking. Next I talked to a massage therapist who added that slouching, which *is* poor body mechanics, is so frequently connected to one's self-image — the need to hide feelings such as anger or sadness. In her view, you can't correct one without correcting the other. The Alexander technique teacher I interviewed used the term "disorganized" to describe lousy posture; he also pointed out that slouching actually requires an enormous amount of unnecessary muscle strain. The next day, a yoga teacher talked about poor posture in terms of "lost unity"; in our modern sedentary society, she explained, people have become almost totally unaware of how they use their bodies. A Feldenkrais practitioner related posture to "efficiency," using first-class levers as an example (the founder of this discipline was a physicist). A psychologist talked about "pain behavior." A psychiatrist talked about the effects back pain caused by poor posture can have on one's self-esteem, sounding a lot like the massage therapist. A chiropractor talked about lousy posture in terms of "poorly aligned" spines.

Anyone looking at my notes would have thought every one of those interviews was on a different topic! That same evening my family physician, a man I adore and respect, bowled me over when he said simply that people's backs would hurt less if they sat up straight. Well!

To sum up this point and add some humanity to this theme, I thought it would be interesting to include some comments on diagnosis from several professionals from different disciplines. Michael Schwartz is a neurosurgeon; George Wortzman, a radiologist; Ahmed Sakoor, a family practitioner; Linda Woodhouse, a physiotherapist; and Christine Sutherland, a massage therapist. In my mind they are all stars in their particular fields and I have enormous respect for each of them.

A Neurosurgeon's Perspective
MICHAEL SCHWARTZ

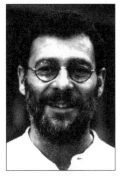

Dr. Michael Schwartz,
Sunnybrook Medical
Centre, Toronto

A lot of back pain patients don't really understand why they are referred to a surgeon, or even what a surgeon is looking for in terms of diagnosis. In general, when it comes to back pain, the job of a surgeon is to relieve nerve compression. In plain English, this means that when we discover a neurological problem, we perform an operation to decompress — remove the pressure that's preventing the nerve from functioning properly. Lay people often call this a "pinched" nerve.

However, less than a third of the back pain patients who are referred to me actually have a compressed nerve — and that's after all of them have first been screened by a family physician. Usually, after examining someone for half an hour, it is clear to me if he or she doesn't have one.

Often, it's difficult to tell these patients that there is nothing I can offer because they don't need surgery. When I try to explain this, many people look very disappointed. They are in a lot of pain and I suppose they are hoping that, because I'm a specialist, I will somehow know about a magic drug, a brilliant physiotherapist, or a special exercise. Often people don't think through the fact that surgeons only have surgery to offer. I also think that a lot of people believe that, in 1997 — the era of high tech — there must be an instant way to relieve their problem. This is simply not true.

I almost always examine people when they come into my office, even if they have brought an X-ray with them. I think people like, as well as need, to be examined clinically. They like to know that I've checked all their reflexes and found them to be present, or that I've discovered one that is absent and is therefore a clue to the problem.

Generally, I can tell a lot from the clinical exam, and yet just about everyone feels that they should also have an MRI or, at the very least, a CT scan. Even people with simple muscle spasm with no clinical evidence of nerve involvement want a high-tech test. Many of them are not happy until they get one, even though it's completely unnecessary.

If I had to choose just one thing to get across to back pain patients about diagnostic imaging it would be this: surgeons do not make the decision to operate on the basis of an X-ray or other high-tech finding. We decide on clinical grounds and we use X-ray, CT scan, and MRI findings to *confirm* the signs and symptoms we discover when we examine you. I look for concordance between what I find during my clinical examination and what I see on the X-ray. But I must stress that the clinical picture is what I base my final decision on. A diagnostic test, like a CT scan, confirms my decision and provides me with what you might call a "surgical road map" or guide.

A Physiotherapist's Perspective
LINDA WOODHOUSE

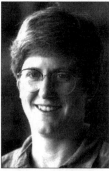

Linda Woodhouse,
Orthopaedic and
Arthritic Hospital,
Toronto

Physiotherapists are less concerned than surgeons with the precise reason for a patient's back pain. Once it's been established that you are not one of the rare back pain sufferers who will require surgery, then physios more or less leave the specific diagnosis arena behind.

We are far more interested in function. In other words, what is your ability in terms of being able to stand, sit, and walk? What is your range of motion in various directions? Can you care for yourself in the sense of managing day-to-day activities? Can you go to work? The trouble is that many nonsurgical back pain patients are under the impression that getting an exact diagnosis is what matters most. In a lot of cases this is simply not true, because the therapeutic program for a person with a bulging disc at L5-S1 is exactly the same as it is for a person with a disc problem a couple of levels up.

Sometimes we get patients who are clearly not going to need surgery but who for one reason or another are waiting for a CT scan or an MRI. (At times, this happens because the patient is so anxious, so desperate for the family physician to DO SOMETHING that he or she orders a high-tech test just to calm the patient down.) But sometimes this presents a problem. The patient comes in for therapy, the CT scan isn't going to happen for a month, but no matter what you say, you can't convince the person to begin therapy while waiting for the scan. These people are too scared to do anything until all the results are in — and by that time their general level of fitness has declined as well. Now they've got two problems to deal with!

What back pain patients need to understand is that there are people out there in terrible pain whose X-rays show only the most minor degenerative changes. At the same time, there are people who jog five miles a day and never feel a twinge, although when you look at their X-rays you can't figure out how they've managed to get out of bed! For this reason, how a person responds to treatment is far more important for the majority of back pain patients than all the high-tech tests in the world.

A Family Physician's Perspective
AHMED SAKOOR

A lot of back pain patients have this notion that they need to know exactly what is wrong as well as the exact number of days it will take them to get better. But the truth is that, in the vast

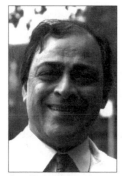

Dr. Ahmed Sakoor,
Raxlen Clinic, Toronto

majority of cases, the most you're going to get is a general idea of what's wrong. And no matter how many fancy X-rays you order, you're not going to learn a whole lot more.

As a family physician — and usually the first health-care professional to see the patient — my first job is to rule out anything that might constitute a medical emergency, or a serious neurological problem. Then I try to explain why it's likely that you haven't done anything very serious, even though your back hurts like hell. I try to reassure people that what's happening is normal in the sense that this kind of excruciating pain is what people often feel when they injure their backs. I think reassurance is one of the most important aspects of treatment for a back pain patient.

Next I explain that what I'm looking for is a pain pattern, which will tell me what general category the problem falls into. Basically, there are five categories, although there is often some overlap. (These categories are described in Chapter 2.) The funny thing is that nerve compression — which is least common by far — is the category almost everyone is positive they fall into! In plain language, everyone seems to think that they must have a pinched nerve because nothing less serious could possibly hurt so much.

Plus, these days, people want you to DO SOMETHING! They say to me, "Doc, how do you know what's going on when you haven't even taken an X-ray?"

Well, first of all, a plain X-ray isn't, in all probability, going to give any additional clues at all. People have to realize that you can look at the X-rays of a hundred people who have no back pain at all and a hundred people who have terrible back pain and you won't be able to tell which set of X-rays belongs to which group!

So, generally, I wait a month. Then, if we're not getting anywhere, I might try a plain X-ray even if I suspect that I won't learn anything that I don't already know. I might order a CT scan, but only if I suspect that there is some nerve root involvement. In this case, I'll also make a referral to a specialist.

But you still get people who say: "Why can't I have an MRI? I read in the newspaper that this Blue Jay got an MRI and I want one too. . . ." All I can do is try to explain that these high-tech diagnostic tests are really only useful for the handful of back pain patients who are likely to require surgery. And if you're not a candidate for the operating room, the therapy you need — education, exercise, and instruction about good posture — will depend upon the category you fit into and that's about it.

A Radiologist's Perspective
GEORGE WORTZMAN

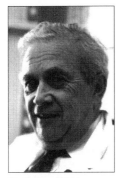

Dr. George Wortzman, Mount Sinai Hospital, Toronto

As a radiologist, I've seen an amazing evolution in terms of diagnostic tests for back pain. We can certainly do some amazing and wonderful things, when they should be done. But if we did an MRI on every back pain patient, first of all we'd need thousands of MRI machines, and second of all, in the vast majority of cases, we wouldn't learn anything we didn't already know. What most back pain patients need is a good clinical diagnosis, a good therapeutic program, and time. What they want, however, is a picture — an X-ray or a high-tech scan — which, for some reason, they seem to have more faith in.

Just because you see something on a high-tech X-ray does not mean that it is the cause of your back problem. Huge numbers of people with no back pain at all have spinal abnormalities that show up on CT scans and MRIs.

In the late 1950s I, myself, had a terrible back problem. I was a radiology resident at the time. I went to see an orthopedic surgeon who took an X-ray. From it, he concluded that I had a spondylolisthesis — a type of crack — and said that I needed spinal fusion right away. Instead, I took some 292s, went to bed for a few days and got better. I later learned that 5 percent (one out of twenty!) of North American males have this condition.

To my way of thinking, this underscores the point: X-rays should provide a road map for surgery. They should not be what the decision to operate is based upon.

In a way, a radiologist is the doctor's doctor. But sometimes we only get a short note about the patient along with a request for a certain test. There are times when I wish there were more opportunities for consultations with the doctors who order these tests. I've had requests that don't even tell me what the referring doctor thinks he or she is looking for! On the other hand, if the referral comes from a doctor working in this hospital, we can discuss what we've found, or what we are trying to find. That kind of communication can certainly be of enormous help to the patient whose diagnosis is problematic or complex.

A Massage Therapist's Perspective
CHRISTINE SUTHERLAND

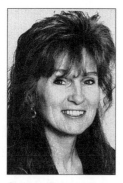

Christine Sutherland,
Registered Therapist,
Nelson, B.C.

When someone with back pain is hung up on getting a diagnosis, I tell them the bad news right away: they're asking the wrong person! Massage therapists are not tied to diagnosis in the same way as, for example, orthopedic surgeons. It's not that we're not interested. It's just that finding a label — this worn facet joint, or that bulging disc — isn't so important because it doesn't make an enormous difference to the way we work.

Bear in mind that massage therapists work on groups of muscles. We try to reduce muscle spasm, which goes hand in hand with most back problems. But muscle spasm is not limited to one specific spot in the same way as, for example, a fractured bone. Muscles are connected to one another — and so, while I might position you a little differently on the table depending on your problem, I begin in more or less the same way for everyone.

I don't think there's anything so new about this way of looking at diagnosis. In the "olden days" people also lifted things poorly and sustained impact injuries. They might have been pitching a bale of hay (rather than lifting a block of concrete) or they might have been struck by a falling tree (rather than a car). The point is, the people who tried to help them didn't know exactly what the problem was and, for the majority of back pain patients, that's still true today. What "healers" concentrated on back then — and what modern health-care professionals still base their choice of treatment on — is function: what you can and cannot do.

But that's not to say that, when I put my hands on your back for the first time, it feels like everyone else's back. Quite the contrary. You may, for instance, have a hot spot caused by inflammation. (This has to do with increased cell division in a place where your body is attempting to repair damaged tissue.) Of course this is a very subtle thing. It can be difficult to translate into words.

There are, however, some basics. To begin with I do investigative strokes. One is called **effleurage**. Now, there's a massage therapist's diagnostic word for those of you who feel you need one! To put it as simply as possible, an effleurage is one general stroke up the back. I do it with flat hands, palms down. From this kind of touch, I can tell if you have a cement back, an iron back, a back that's like the Rocky Mountains, or a back that's functioning better on one side than the other. As well, as I just mentioned, I will pick up warm areas, if there are any.

I also do another investigative stroke with my fingertips, which is a bit like playing the piano. I use my fingertips to play the affected areas with a kind of "poke-and-press" technique; a pianist might call it "staccato." What I'm doing is traveling the keyboard of skin and developing a tactile database, which I use to make a therapeutic plan.

Then I start hunting for what I call "hitching posts." Hitching posts are connected to other hitching posts, which eventually can lead me to the center of the pain. But I don't look for hitching posts with the objective of coming up with a diagnostic label. I do it because, quite often, you have to "unlock" a line of hitching posts before you can start to work on the center of the pain — even if you have sensed right from the beginning where that center is.

So, with pain, muscle spasm, reduced mobility, and of course, feedback from you, the patient, as my clues, I unravel some of the mystery of the story and make a map which will lead to recovery via massage. Is diagnosis involved in this process? It's an interesting question. The answer, of course, depends on your definition of the word!

My final word (in this chapter) on the subject of professional bias is that back pain sufferers are too often expected to fit into the world view of the professionals we consult, rather than the other way around. But that's the way it is. Don't go to an acupuncturist expecting an ergonomic assessment of your work station. Don't consult a practitioner of the Feldenkrais method with the hope that he or she will watch you move, then conclude that you have a bulging disc. Don't go to a chiropractor if manipulation does not appeal to you; chiropractors perform manipulation almost all of the time because it's part of their belief system.

With all that said, I do think that health-care professionals are, on average, more open-minded than they used to be, and I hope things will continue to improve. It will happen a lot faster if, as "customers," we become better educated and more demanding.

THE M.D.'S CLINICAL DIAGNOSIS

Now that I have you thoroughly convinced of the difficulty of diagnosing back pain, I'd like to be a little more optimistic and look at what *can* be done. For most of us, the first stop once we decide we need help with back pain is the family physician. He or she will perform a clinical examination, the main purpose of which is to rule out the possibility that something serious is wrong, including anything that may constitute a medical emergency. In fact, for far more than 90 percent of cases, nothing serious is wrong.

If, in addition to back pain, you have pain that radiates into your buttock or leg, your physician will perform a **neurological examination** (nerve-related tests), or send you to a specialist for this purpose. In more than 90 percent of cases, this exam will also produce a big fat zero, which means you are not a good candidate for surgery. However, a *good* clinical diagnostician who communicates well should also be able to send you home with a pretty good idea of at least what category your problem falls into. In some cases, I believe that a thorough clinical exam is done mostly to calm us down. In any case, the clinical exam will mean more if you understand what your physician is looking for and how complicated it can get. So here goes.

Taking the History

To begin with, your physician will want to hear an account of your back pain as well as a description of your symptoms: when the pain began; what it feels like; where it hurts; which activities or postures make it better as well as which make it worse; whether you recently injured your back or the pain developed for no particular reason; whether the onset was gradual or sudden; whether or not you've experienced any signs — such as loss of bowel or bladder control — that might suggest a medical emergency; and whether resting relieves your pain, at least to some degree. As I have mentioned, medical doctors (and surgeons in particular) tend to look for specific neurological signs: a muscle group that has lost a substantial degree of power, or has atrophied; an area that has lost its sense of touch because messages are not being ferried to it due to nerve compression. These are the types of back problems that, if they are corroborated by a high-tech test, can often be corrected by surgery.

Most of the time, however, severe specific signs will not be found. As Dr. Michael Schwartz has explained to me, some medical doctors will then say, "I can find nothing wrong with your back!" What they really mean, and should say, is that they can find nothing wrong *that makes you a good candidate for surgery*. The lack of serious neurological signs does not mean that you have nothing wrong with your back, or that you are making too much out of nothing.

But most of us at least start out thinking that we have a serious neurological problem, so let's look at a couple of examples of what often shows up when in fact a patient *is* suffering from nerve damage.

Let's say that you are in your mid-thirties and you come into your doctor's office explaining that this is the first time you've ever had back pain in your life. You can't remember doing anything that could have caused your back to hurt — that is, you have not had a trauma such as a fall, and you didn't wrench your back during a squash game. You just woke up one morning last week with severe back pain and, a couple of days later, the pain started to radiate down your leg into your heel. Now your heel is numb.

From a description like this, your doctor would get a pretty good idea that you have a herniated, or severely bulging, disc. He or she would also bet that the S1 nerve root is involved because the numbness is in your heel; if, for instance, the L5 nerve was being pinched, the pain would most probably be radiating into your toe. This information will alert your doctor to be on the look-out for other signs that will point to the same thing.

An osteophyte, or bone growth, can also be the cause of a pinched nerve, but most back pain patients with severe osteoarthritic changes are over the age of thirty-five or forty, while most patients with a disc problem are under the age of forty. In addition, the onset of pain caused by bone is not usually as sudden as the onset of pain from a herniated disc. Still, you can see that the information you provide your doctor is not always enough to make a diagnosis as clear-cut as you'd like it to be.

This can be frustrating for everyone, especially if you're pressing for precision.

Here's another example. Let's say your back has been bothering you off and on for years but a recent game of golf caused the pain to radiate into your leg and increase to a level that's unbearable. In this case, your doctor would likely be inclined to suspect a flare-up of a chronic facet joint problem. However, this situation can also be ambiguous. You *can* get leg pain from a facet joint problem, although in most cases, the pain that's referred to the leg from a worn facet joint is different than the pain caused by a pinched nerve. Neurological pain is often described as "electric" or "burning," although some people experience tingling or numbness instead. Worn facet joints don't cause "burning" pain or "electric" pain. A further clue is that many patients with a facet joint problem find it difficult to pinpoint the exact location of their referred pain, which in most cases will not extend below the buttocks, and almost never past the knee.

Now, if it's a disc that's pinching the nerve, your pain will likely increase with flexion (bending forward), for example, coughing or vacuuming. On the other hand, if you have a worn facet joint, your pain will probably increase when you extend (or arch) your spine.

Most of the time, back and/or leg pain will subside, at least to some extent, when you are lying down. If, however, a few days of rest accomplishes nothing, and your pain in fact gets worse at night, your doctor *might* begin to think about the possibility of a tumor. In such a situation, a bone-scan X-ray, which can locate tumors, would be ordered. (See Chapter 4.) However, I personally have gone through periods where my back pain has prevented me from sleeping, and I believe this is true for many people. In my case, there was never a question of a tumor. The point is that severe muscle spasm, especially when it is exacerbated by anxiety and stress, can certainly keep you up at night.

The Physical Exam

After listening to your history, your doctor will begin the clinical exam. Different physicians may vary the order in which they conduct this exam, but the following description is more or less standard.

To begin with, you will be asked to stand so that your doctor can inspect your entire back. What he or she is looking for are red spots, muscle spasm, or deformities such as scoliosis, abnormal kyphosis, or abnormal lordosis, any of which may, or may not, be contributing to your pain.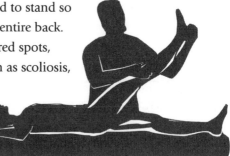

Next, the doctor will flex your neck forward, which puts stress on your spinal cord. If you do have a herniated disc, flexing your neck may cause pain to shoot down your leg. Next, with your neck still flexed, you will be asked to cough, which puts even more strain on your spinal nerves. If coughing provokes leg pain, your doctor will look out for further evidence of a herniated disc. If not, it's more likely that a facet joint problem, or perhaps spinal stenosis, is the cause.

Pressing the carotid arteries in your neck puts pressure on the jugular veins behind them. This changes the pressure within the spinal fluid, and that is what many physicians do next. This too may also produce leg pain. If it does, your doctor will have found another sign to substantiate the suspicion of a herniated disc. The thing to keep in mind is that, for every problem, there are at least several tests; your doctor is looking for correlation — the *same* indication from different tests.

The next part of the procedure involves putting your spine through its range of motions. The first is bending forward, although this test can be ambiguous since even people with totally fused spines (ankylosing spondylitis) can almost touch their toes by rotating their hip joints. The trick is to watch your spine carefully to see if each level moves. As I've already mentioned, flexion is also a test for a herniated disc. If, when you bend forward a little bit, and then stand upright again, severe pain shoots down your leg and your back goes into spasm, then you've got another checkmark for a herniated disc.

The next movement is extension, or bending backward. If you are suffering from spinal stenosis, extension will likely increase your pain. This happens because the space in the spinal canal out of which the nerves exit (the intervertebral foramen) becomes narrower when you're in extension. You might also feel numbness or tingling in your legs or toes. Once your doctor suspects that spinal stenosis may be your problem, he or she will want to know if walking a couple of blocks exacerbates your symptoms. What makes the diagnosis of spinal stenosis so difficult, however, is that pain from a worn facet joint, or from osteophytes on a facet joint, will also increase with extension. It may be necessary to verify the clinical picture of spinal stenosis with a CT scan or an MRI. (A severely degenerated facet joint with osteoarthritic changes can usually be confirmed by a plain X-ray, although a CT scan is sometimes preferable.)

The third range of motion test is for lateral or side bending. When you bend to one side, your hand should be able to reach slightly beyond the level of your knee without causing pain. Once again, if lateral bending causes pain to shoot down your leg, your doctor will likely think of a disc problem. (This test, however, is less conclusive than some of the others.)

The last range of motion test is rotation. With your feet on the floor, you should be able to turn a full 90 degrees to both the right and the left. If your range is restricted, a facet joint problem is quite likely the cause. On the other hand, if rotation causes the kind of electric nerve pain described above, then it's more likely that you're looking at a disc problem. Both worn facet joints and spinal stenosis tend to produce backache, or vague leg pain above the knee, rather than sharper neurological pain. The tricky part is that, in many cases, more than one problem exists. In addition to this, severe muscle spasm can hurt horrifically until it has had a chance to settle down, making it difficult to distinguish types of pain.

The Neurological Exam

By this time, however, your physician should have a sense of what is going on. At this point he or she will begin the specific neurological examination to determine if any nerves have been affected, if there has been any loss of sensation or muscle atrophy, or loss of motor function — all specific neurological signs.

To start with, you will be asked once again to stand so that the functioning of the S1 nerve can be tested; this is the nerve that runs down the back of your calf into your heel, supplying power to the muscles of the calf along the way. To do this, you raise one foot several inches off the floor and then move up and down on the toes of the opposite foot, repeating the exercise ten times. Then you switch feet and do it again. If you can only go up once instead of ten times — that is, if you get up on your toes once and are simply too weak to continue — your physician will have a pretty good idea that the S1 nerve root is involved. But even if it is true that your S1 nerve is not supplying enough power to the muscles of your calf to allow you to perform this test, the cause is not always conclusive. The culprit could be a disc. Or an osteophyte could be pinching the nerve. An experienced diagnostician can get a pretty good idea of which it is, but before recommending surgery, your doctor will want to see a correlation between what shows up clinically and a CT scan or MRI. The clinical evidence is what makes you a candidate for a high-tech test.

Your ankle reflexes will generally be tested next. Most physicians will have you kneel on the seat of a chair with your toes pointing toward the floor and your back toward the examiner. Then your ankle will be tapped with a reflex hammer. If the S1 nerve is conducting messages properly, the foot will respond by involuntarily jerking backward. If the nerve is not conducting properly, there will either be no response or a reduced response. Your physician will also look for subtle differences between your left and right reflexes.

Next, you will be asked to sit on the chair so that your knee reflex can be tested with the same hammer. If this reflex is absent, the L4 nerve, which emerges from between the fourth and fifth lumbar vertebrae, is probably involved. However, this happens only rarely.

To test the L5 nerve root (which is involved more often than L4 but less often than S1), your physician will test the power of the dorsal flexor muscles in your foot. These are the muscles you use to elevate your toes and move your foot from side to side. First you will be asked to elevate the big toe of each foot against the downward pressure that the examiner applies, then the other toes. Then, you will be asked to **evert** (turn out) each foot, and finally to **invert** (turn in) each foot. Most doctors like to do this test while you are sitting rather than lying down, because they find it easier to detect subtle differences in strength between one foot and the other.

At the back of the knee, your sciatic nerve runs close to the surface. For this reason, your physician will palpate the back of your knee to see if it is tender. (But don't forget, a number of nerves combine to make up the sciatic nerve.) Often, there is tenderness in the muscles on the outside of the leg as well. If the muscles on the inside of the leg are tender, it is likely that the L5 nerve root is involved; weakness in the muscles higher up in the leg generally indicate a problem with the second, third, and fourth lumbar nerve roots, which, as I've already mentioned, is very rare.

While you are still sitting, you will next be asked to pull each leg back in toward the chair, once again against the force applied by the examiner. What your doctor is looking for is weakness in the hamstring muscles. This points to a problem with the most commonly affected nerve, S1.

The final part of the examination will be conducted while you are lying down.

First, while you are lying **supine**, or face up, you will be given the **straight leg raising (SLR) test**, which will indicate whether any of the nerves that merge at the hip to form the sciatic nerve are being irritated, most likely by a disc. With your legs straight, your doctor will first raise one leg to a 90-degree angle, then raise the other one slowly. This stretches your sciatic nerve. If you feel severe pain between 35 and 70 degrees, then most likely there is a nerve problem. (Pain between 70 degrees and 90 degrees, however, usually indicates a joint problem — either a facet joint, hip joint, or sacroiliac (SI) joint problem.

Next, while you are still supine, the **Babinski Sign test** will be performed: stroking the soles of your feet with the pointed end of a reflex hammer. Normally, this will cause your toes to curl downward. If they spread upward and outward, it is a sign that your spinal cord is being compressed, or that you are suffering from another neurological disease such as multiple sclerosis.

Next you will lie on your side and your doctor will test for sacroiliac (SI) joint problems by pressing down on each hip; the idea is to see if putting stress on the sacroiliac joints causes pain.

Finally, you will be asked to lie **prone**, or face down, while several tests are performed. One is the prone knee-bending test, which stretches the femoral nerve. If either the L3 or L4 nerve roots are the source of your problem, this test will cause pain. The second test, which is for the L5 nerve root, is the contracting of the gluteus maximus muscles of the buttocks. What your doctor wants to see is if one side is flatter than the other, as well as if there is the same amount of muscle tension on each side.

If you are a male and over the age of forty-five, your doctor will likely also perform a rectal examination to check your prostate gland for swelling, or a tumor.

That's about it. If you're like me, at this point you're probably reeling from the amount of data you've been trying to jam into your poor brain. Just remember that your physician may be reeling as well, not because he or she is confused by the findings but because it's so tough to find a way to make something so complex sound logical to you. If there is evidence of a neurological deficit, your physician will probably order some diagnostic tests. The most frequently used test is the CT scan, although sometimes it's better to have an MRI if possible.

Even if this is the case, a trial of conservative treatment will probably be prescribed. For reasons only Mother Nature can explain, many back pain patients who are awaiting their date with the surgeon get better as a result of conservative treatment. It's also good to keep in mind that, even with the best technician and an unequivocal diagnosis, surgery is not the perfect solution. A back that has been operated on will never be totally normal again.

But as I said at the beginning, it is likely that no neurological problems will be found. Rather, like the vast majority of back pain sufferers, you will fall into one or more of the five categories discussed in the beginning of Chapter 2. You sometimes have to ask the right questions, however, in order to find this out. For instance, if after the clinical examination your doctor tells you that nothing is wrong, be direct. Ask if there is really nothing wrong, or if there is simply nothing wrong that makes you a good surgical candidate. If you have had plain X-rays taken, ask if there are any visible degenerative changes. If the answer is yes, have your physician point them out.

The Living-Room Diagnosis

One final note on back pain diagnosis — don't underestimate the contribution of the person who knows your back best of all: you. You can often take at least the first step in figuring out which category of problem is causing your back pain right in your own living room, by paying attention to what kind of movement brings on (or increases) your pain.

Your back can move in three ways: **flexion** (bending forward), **extension** (arching backward), and **rotation** (twisting). (See Figure 3.1.)

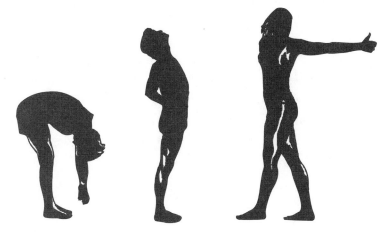

Figure 3.1 The Three Postures: Flexion, Extension, and Rotation

Strains and Sprains

If you have a strain or sprain, then positions that demand extreme ranges of motion, particularly rotation, will increase your pain. So will any kind of jarring move. Strains and sprains usually begin to hurt fairly soon after the injury that caused them.

Disc Problems

With a disc problem, flexion, and rotation toward one side (whichever way the disc is bulging or herniated), usually causes the most pain. Occasionally, however, a disc may bulge or herniate centrally, so the pain isn't always one-sided.

Spinal Stenosis

Prolonged extension aggravates spinal stenosis. The type of pain associated with this problem tends to be chronic rather than acute.

Facet Joint Problems

Prolonged extension also tends to increase facet joint problems, which also tend to cause chronic pain. People who do experience an acute flare-up in a facet joint usually find rotation increases their pain dramatically.

Osteoarthritis

This kind of pain, like that from strains and sprains, is generally increased by extreme ranges of motion. It will also increase, however, from vibration and compression — for example, jumping up and down. Osteoarthritis pain also tends to develop more slowly, in some cases not until the next day.

4

Diagnostic Testing

I still find it hard to believe that, just over a decade ago, the CT scanner was a new, revolutionary tool for diagnosing back pain. In 1985, there were fewer than a hundred CT scan machines across Canada. Today, even a medium-sized hospital can't function without one. Perhaps even more amazing is the fact that, just a few years after the CT scanner made its debut, an even more sophisticated diagnostic test appeared on the scene: magnetic resonance imaging (MRI).

HIGH TECH — WHO NEEDS IT?

Radiologists can now examine tiny segments of the spine (and other parts of the body, such as the brain) in ways that boggle the mind. Yet medical science's ability to diagnose the majority of back problems has not changed very much. Yes, many difficult-to-pin-down problems involving nerve damage can now be solved with the help of a CT scan or an MRI. These high-tech tests can also help confirm a clinical diagnosis and provide an excellent "road map" for surgery without the need for invasive, painful tests such as the myelogram (described later in this chapter).

However, for the vast majority of back pain sufferers, these high-tech tests generally add very little to what can be learned from the clinical exam.

Many people have wondered why the invention of these miraculous machines did not provide us with the answers we expected and prayed for. The question is a fair one and, in my opinion, it has to do with the evolution of back pain in terms of both cause and treatment. But in order to understand this evolution, you have to wade through a bit of history.

At the beginning of the century, most health-care professionals believed that severe, lingering back pain — especially pain that radiated into the buttock or leg — was caused by sacroiliac (SI) joint strain. Then, in the 1930s, two American surgeons concluded that bulging, or herniated, discs were the most common cause of serious back pain and sacroiliac (SI) joints fell out of fashion.

Shortly after disc problems became the favored diagnosis, surgery began to be used to remove discs. In most cases, the joints above and below the disc were fused to provide stability. Precision diagnosis increased in importance, since a surgeon had to know which disc was the culprit before beginning the operation; one couldn't very well open up a patient's back and *then* start looking for problems. In the early years, a diagnostic test called a myelogram was used to pinpoint the abnormal disc.

If you have read even a little about the evolution of treatment, you already know that many of these early back surgeries were less than successful. In some cases, because of scarring and/or other problems caused by the surgery itself, patients ended up in worse shape after surgery than before. Obviously, these failures caused some amount of skepticism.

They also stimulated new research. Some surgeons began to look for less radical surgical procedures. Eventually, it became more common to remove a disc without fusing the joints. Techniques such as microsurgery were ultimately developed. Other researchers turned away from discs to look toward other causes of back pain. For a short time during the 1970s, a lot of attention was focused on facet joints.

But a great number of researchers bent their heads to the challenge of finding the perfect way to diagnose back pain. Over the years, a kind of philosophy emerged: if back problems could only be pinpointed, better solutions would be within our grasp. That attitude was at the forefront of medical thinking when the 1980s arrived — the decade of high technology.

You probably recall the excitement of those years. It seemed as though back pain was constantly being written about in the lay press, with high-tech tests front and center. The mystery of the back pain diagnosis seemed on the verge of being decloaked.

But, of course, that's not what happened.

By the beginning of the 1990s, a group of world-class **radiologists** (physicians who specialize in X-rays) realized that, once again, not all that much had changed. Back problems, in fact, were on the increase, and pinning them down was still the health-care professional's nightmare. They set out to do more research and further reflection.

The first thing these radiologists did was to gather together thousands of the early CT scans and MRIs, which they meticulously re-analyzed; in most cases, more than one person's opinion was sought. Next, they performed a number of CT scans and MRIs on a number of pain-free people in the name of research. The results were startling:

- In studies of people who had never felt a twinge of back pain in their lives, abnormal findings, or false positives, showed up routinely on CT scans and MRIs. In one study, a third of the X-rays actually showed a herniated disc! In another, 20 percent of pain-free people over the age of sixty had clear signs of spinal stenosis.
- Other studies showed that the interpretation of CT scans and MRIs differed substantially among professionals.
- Yet another study showed that more than one abnormal finding frequently showed up in many cases. Often it was impossible to say which — if any — of the findings was causing the patient's pain.
- Further studies indicated that performing a high-tech test soon after a patient developed back pain led, in some cases, to unnecessary surgery. This happened when the decision to operate was based on the results of the high-tech test, rather than the clinical exam.
- At least in Canada, many back pain patients had to wait months for a CT scan or an MRI. In the meantime, they were sent to physiotherapy,

but many of them didn't put in much effort because they were afraid of causing themselves further damage. The upshot was that, when the test date finally rolled around and showed nothing, their general fitness level had declined to the point where recovery was much harder to achieve.

At first, these results seemed pretty depressing to a lot of people. If all the fancy technology in the world wasn't going to help us make sense out of back pain, they asked, where should we go from here? But, in fact, once researchers took the time to think about it, they realized that all this new knowledge had actually allowed them to look at the diagnosis of back pain in a far more creative way.

More studies were done. Some showed that pain is a very poor diagnostic clue when it comes to backs. Sometimes a very slight injury can cause a lot of pain; other times, a very severe problem will cause very little pain. This was not a new concept, but the findings did cause researchers to think about psychological factors in a much more serious way than they had in the past.

A lot of attention was focused on stress and how it affects a person's ability to deal with *any* illness or injury. Soon studies began to show that, with back pain, the stress factor is disproportionately large. Chronic back pain has so much to do with a person's lifestyle and emotional well-being that it's often hard to separate these issues from the physical findings.

Finally, after decades of looking at the diagnosis of back pain in a rather narrow-minded manner, we came full circle and the clinical exam regained its former reputation as the gold standard for diagnosing the majority of back problems. Nevertheless, it feels as though we've come a long way!

CT SCANNING AND MRI

Despite all I've just said, I still find something magical about high-tech diagnostic imaging. If you're like every other back pain patient I've ever met, you will still wish in your heart that you could have a CT scan or an MRI. So be it. We're human. I myself have had several CT scans over the years and I too am fascinated by it and the MRI. Even if you never have either, you may find how they work intriguing.

The CT Scan
Like the older myelogram test, a **CT scan** (the letters stand for "**computerized tomography**," but the full term is almost never used) can confirm a clinical diagnosis of a pinched nerve, and help pinpoint the problem. Sometimes, a CT scan is done after a myelogram; the dye used for the myelogram produces a sharper picture.

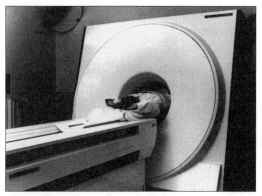

Figure 4.1 The CT Scanner

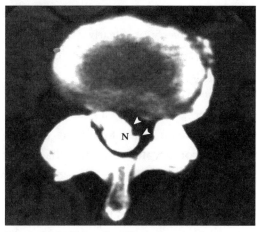

Figure 4.2 An X-Ray of a CT scan showing a herniated disc impinging on a nerve (N)

The patient is positioned on his or her back, then literally slid through the CT scanner's donut-shaped gantry into the machine (see Figure 4.1). X-rays are taken of tiny "slices" of the spine, then analyzed by a computer program to produce views almost beyond belief (see Figure 4.2).

Describing how this is done is like trying to explain an Einstein theory! Cross-sections of the spine, called **transaxial slices**, are able to show an area no more than one-fifth of an inch thick. From their appearance you might think that, to get them, it was necessary to slice up the spinal column the way a lumberjack slices up a fallen tree. If you had a stacked-up deck of cards, and you pulled one from the middle then held it up to study its face, you'd be looking at the kind of image a CT scan shows. All this is accomplished with less radiation than is used to take about five plain X-rays.

In Canada, a state-of-the-art CT scanner costs between $500,000 and $1.5 million; one test costs about $350.

Magnetic Resonance Imaging (MRI)

The **MRI** machine also takes a detailed picture of your insides, but instead of radiation, it relies on a huge magnet, radio waves, and the hydrogen molecules found in many of the cells in our bodies. (Nerve cells, for instance, are surrounded by a sheath of fatty tissue and fat that happens to contain a lot of hydrogen. Bone cells contain very little of this.)

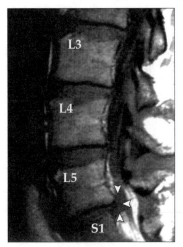

Figure 4.3 An MRI X-Ray, Lateral View

In some cases, an MRI will provide a better picture than a CT scan because it shows nerves more clearly. (Bone, on the other hand, shows up more clearly on a CT scan.)

The machine itself looks a bit like a CT scanner. As with the CT scanner, the patient is slid through a donut-shaped gantry.

The workings of MRI are even more complicated to explain than those of a CT scan, but here goes. Basically, the huge magnet I mentioned affects **protons** (tiny, positively charged particles) in hydrogen cells. Next the MRI machine sends out radio waves and these waves hit the protons. An instant later, to put it very unscientifically, the protons boot the radio waves out — that's nature's way of trying to get back to normal! These booted-out waves are sent to the MRI's computer, which analyzes them and produces a picture. The image can be a lateral view, as shown in Figure 4.3, or a cross-sectional view, as in Figure 4.4. In the pictures of a

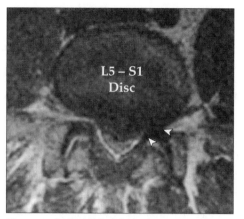

L5 – S1
Disc

Figure 4.4 An MRI X-Ray, Cross-Sectional View

herniated disc shown here, bone appears as black and fat is white, but that can be reversed by the computer operator if desired.

A state-of-the-art MRI machine costs $2.5 to $3 million to buy and install. One test costs about $1,200. At the time of writing, there were thirty-four MRI machines in Canada.

OTHER DIAGNOSTIC TESTS

Besides these two high-tech superstars, doctors have a range of less glamorous tests at their disposal for diagnosing back pain. It would take at least a dozen pages to describe them all in detail, but this brief overview should give you an idea.

The Myelogram

A **myelogram** is performed when there is reason to believe that surgery will be necessary to decompress a nerve that's being pinched by a herniated disc or by bone, for example a bone spur. The test can also point to spinal stenosis, for which surgery is sometimes performed if the case is very severe. The purpose of a myelogram is to confirm the clinical diagnosis. It can also provide a "road map" for surgery, since it's sometimes tough to know from the clinical exam just which disc, or which bit of bone, is the culprit. In the case of stenosis, a myelogram can show how much narrowing has occurred.

For a myelogram, the patient is positioned face down on a table that can be tilted. Radiopaque dye, which blocks X-rays, is injected into the spinal canal. Next, the table is tilted back and forth, causing the dye to flow slowly up and down the canal, filling the space around each nerve root, while X-rays are taken from various angles, creating pictures like the one in Figure 4.5.

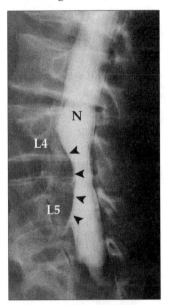

Figure 4.5 A Myelogram X-Ray

The nerve sac on the X-rays appears as a white mass. Discs and bone appear as shades of gray. If a nerve is being compressed, it will show up as a dark blotch impinging on the white nerve sac. If the patient is suffering from spinal stenosis, the canal will appear abnormally narrow.

After a myelogram, the patient should take it easy for a day to decrease the chance of headache.

Because it is an invasive test that can sometimes be very uncomfortable, the myelogram has largely been replaced by the CT scan and the MRI. However, a myelogram can provide an extremely clear picture, and for this reason some physicians like to have one done in certain cases. As well, myelograms are sometimes performed before a CT scan because the scan will produce a clearer picture as a result of the radiopaque dye that will still be inside the spinal canal. (The CT scan shown in Figure 4.2 was taken after a myelogram.)

The Plain X-Ray

Plain X-rays, which show bone but not soft tissue such as discs, are used mostly to rule out the possibility of a fractured vertebra or a tumor; they generally indicate what's *not* wrong. They can also be used to indicate the presence of osteophytes and osteoporosis, in an area where the patient feels no pain at all! Plain X-rays will also show when the space between two vertebrae is narrower than normal, but this does not necessarily indicate a herniated or bulging disc; it's simply a picture of a space. The patient may have been born with the abnormality.

Blood Tests

These tests are sometimes used to rule out or detect infections, cancerous or noncancerous tumors, and diseases such as rheumatoid arthritis.

For instance, if a blood sample reveals a white blood cell count that is higher than normal, there is a good possibility that the patient has an infection. A hemoglobin test can point toward one of several types of cancer. If the blood reveals what is called a rheumatoid factor, the patient will be tested further for rheumatoid arthritis. As well, certain tests that examine the amount of calcium, phosphorus, and particular enzymes in the blood can point to certain types of cancer or systemic diseases.

Urinalysis

An infection or other malfunction of the kidneys can sometimes produce back pain. If a clinical exam indicates that the kidneys could be involved, a simple urine test — called **urinalysis** — will be ordered. This can confirm, or rule out, the presence of an infection.

The Bone Scan

A **bone scan** is performed when a tumor is suspected. Radioactive "tracers" are first injected into the bloodstream. These are absorbed by bone cells and, several hours later, a special machine takes an image, which looks similar to a plain X-ray. If there is a tumor, which is a rare cause of back pain, it will show up as a "hot spot" because the cells in tumors divide more quickly than normal cells. Remember, however, that not all tumors are cancerous. If a tumor is found, it will be biopsied to determine if it is malignant or benign. Most tumors, in fact, are benign.

The Discogram

It's a good thing **discograms** are rarely performed these days, since they hurt like the dickens. Dye is injected into a suspected herniated disc. If there is, indeed, a herniation, the dye will leak out through the rupture in the disc. It will then hit the nerve root and reproduce the pain, thus confirming the diagnosis.

Electromyography

Neurologists may use **electromyography (EMG)** when they suspect that a nerve is being compressed. They study the reaction of a certain muscle when it is stimulated by the nerve that brings messages to it. This test can be uncomfortable for two reasons: fine needles must be inserted into the leg, then hooked up to a machine; and the nerve in question must be stimulated by an electrical shock.

Nerve Conduction Study

A **nerve conduction study** uses the same machine as an EMG test. In this case, the objective is to see whether muscle contractions and nerve impulses are normal — in other words, is the nerve able to transmit signals properly?

Surface Electromyography

A way to assess the impact of a soft-tissue injury on a muscle is through **surface electromyography (SEMG),** which measures the muscle's ability to function. No needles are used. Instead, electrodes placed on the skin measure the amount of electrical activity that the muscle is generating.

111

PAIN

5

Pain 101

Pain of one kind or another is a fact of life. Yet somehow back pain looms larger than any other kind, at least in the North American worldview. Just look at our language — how often do you hear phrases like "Get off my back!" and "Back off!" and "He's got no backbone!" Then there's "a pain in the neck" and of course the perennial favorite "a pain in the butt" — which just goes to show you that both ends of the spine have made it into our idiomatic lexicon! I've never heard anyone say, "My boss is a pain in the knee," although knees can cause excruciating pain.

Maybe it's because back pain seems to be such a metaphor for life that I have a hard time finding the right words to write about my own back pain. Nevertheless, if I expect you to read a 400-page book full of my own opinions about back problems, I think it's fair for you to expect me to at least try to explain what back pain has meant to my life.

MY OWN EXPERIENCE

It began quite suddenly in 1975. I was only twenty-six, but I was writing feature articles for most of Canada's national magazines. I also wrote a weekly restaurant column for the *Toronto Star*. All in all, life was pretty grand.

Then one spring morning I woke up looking more like a clock set at 6:10 than a restaurant critic. Frankly, I simply couldn't believe that back pain, which I'd never heard of in a young, healthy human being, could strike me down. When my friends called I made a joke of being bent over. I assumed that, like a head cold, this nonsense would quickly disappear and I'd get on with my insanely busy life. In fact, my life had been more insane than busy for months and my stress level was approaching infinity. I knew I'd wrenched my back while wrestling with my young nephew; I had no idea that, during a less stressful time, such an injury would probably have subsided within a few days.

Well, by the time the weekend rolled around I did manage, with the help of warm baths and hot packs, to restore my standing posture to vertical. But my back still hurt like hell. I did my best to deny it, but by the end of the summer my right leg hurt as well, and *this* kind of pain was impossible to ignore. I tried to sit up straight — although in 1975 I didn't have the foggiest idea what good sitting posture meant. I certainly didn't know that sitting all day was torture on my back.

I also exercised with a vengeance. (If ten minutes are good, I thought, two hours must be better!) I chose all the wrong exercises for the category my back problem fell into, and I did most of them incorrectly to boot.

I'm embarrassed to admit that, once a week, I also took a painkiller, then played tennis — in a daze! My rationale was that bashing at tennis balls did wonders for my battered psyche. Looking back, I wish someone had recommended bicycling or walking for a few months to replace an activity that added insult to injury.

Somehow I kept my *Star* column going, although it just about did me in. My contributions to other publications dwindled, then ceased altogether. Plus I started to play possum: lest my editor discover that I was a washout as a specimen of humanity, I sent my reviews down to the office in a cab. I was a self-employed freelancer; my bank balance was moving in the wrong direction and I was discovering stress levels that I had never known existed.

By mid-fall I had consulted a variety of health-care professionals. Each had a different idea about what was wrong and what I should do. Every time I conformed to a new person's philosophy, I felt like an amoeba changing its shape. It was beginning to dawn on me that many health-care professionals didn't care about *my* needs. Few of them wanted me to be involved in any decision-making processes about my own body. Thank God not too much more time had to pass before I could get angry, because in the end I believe that rage helped me survive.

Little did I know how important psychological factors were to chronic pain like mine. Today, their contribution is common knowledge, but in 1975, only one health-care professional I consulted even mentioned this theme. This is not to minimize my physical problem; I did have significant degenerative changes and mild spinal stenosis. But what was wrong should not have been causing such agony.

I would like to describe my feelings during this bleak period. My back Pain — I started to think of it with a capital letter, as if it were a living entity — had taken on a life of its own. It was as if it had a heart and a brain and an agenda over which I had no control. Worse, this Pain also possessed a soul — one that was much tougher than mine. My lumbar spine hurt all over, my leg still ached off and on, and deep in the left side of my buttocks was a spot the size of a loonie where my Pain gnawed at me like a ferret, sapping what little energy I had left. Today, the skin over that spot still feels like old leather from my rubbing at it day after day. Sometimes, I would actually dig my nails into it while I was sleeping. I know this because, when I woke up, the skin would be raw.

So what happened? Why, a couple of years later, did this intolerable Pain begin to subside into the dull roar I now cope with quite nicely? I'm not sure of the precise answer, but I know that it has something to do with finding an outlet for my frustration and anger. I made an unselfish decision to found the Back Association of Canada (BAC) and discovered that my decision served a selfish need as well: It left me without a moment to focus on my own back. A bonus was that health-care professionals had to be respectful to me; otherwise, I might write nasty things about them in the association's journal, *Back to Back*. But the best part was that my life gained some value and some meaning over which I had some control.

I should explain that, by this time, I was still doing remedial stretching and strengthening exercises. Thankfully, I'd learned a few things about technique by now. I'd also hung up my tennis racquet. Instead, I gardened and walked whenever I could. As I began to feel better, I exercised more faithfully because I felt good. Being active (in a way that didn't increase the strain) helped my anxiety to subside, which, in turn, caused the psychogenic part of my pain to diminish as well. Once a ray of hope was rekindled within my universe, my anxiety declined further.

Of course I see all this in retrospect.

At the time, the climb back to normal functioning took place in such small increments that, for the most part, I didn't notice each tiny success. Plus, I wasn't always successful; some weeks I'd slide backward and feel depressed. But over the course of about eight months, I was beginning to spiral up.

Still, since 1975, I've never had a day without back pain. I consider this very bad luck, but more in theory than in reality. I no longer consider myself disabled. I love gardening and walking far more than I ever loved tennis. Somehow the noncompetitive aspect of these activities feels . . . mature! Best of all, I no longer *worry* very much about my back. Even when I'm in the middle of an acute flare-up, I'm never scared that my Pain is back for good. And I believe that this fact is what has taken the life out of my back pain and given me back my own.

That's my story. I've never shared it before — you, my readers, are the first! I included it here so I could share with you a few pearls of wisdom that I've picked up along the way.

To begin with, I believe I inherited a lousy attitude toward pain — particularly chronic pain. The consequences of this were disastrous when I had to cope with it for the first time. For openers, like most people I was raised with the philosophy that all pain is unacceptable and should be eradicated, completely and immediately, at any cost. I now know that chronic pain simply does not disappear overnight. It endures over time, although there are certainly ups and downs.

The second pearl of wisdom is that coping with chronic back pain involves a lot of juggling — and even the best jugglers sometimes fumble their pins. It also means juggling in different ways at different times.

When I'm at a meeting, for instance, I disassociate myself from my back pain using a kind of self-hypnosis. I can't do this for too long because it uses up a lot of energy. And I never do it when I'm exercising, having a massage, or trying to assess my progress, because at times like these, I need to be in touch with my back. At still other times I do what I want to do, and my back be damned! Every May, for example, I garden all day, although I know perfectly well that my limit is one hour. Of course, I pay for this cavalier attitude for the next day or two. But from my point of view, it's worth it.

The toughest part of juggling is being a writer. I sit for hours every day, just as I'm doing right now. When I turn out a good piece of work, my back usually feels terrible, and each time I finish a book, I'm sure I've gone insane! On the other hand, when I don't work I miss the pleasure of feeling productive.

The last pearl of wisdom is that chronic back pain is worse than any other kind of chronic pain. You can tar me and feather me and run me out of town on a pole with yogurt on my head . . . BUT I WILL NEVER RECANT!

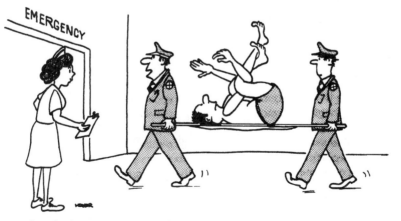

"His back pain is gone. He is in complete harmony with the world. But he's also in a reef knot!"

WHAT EXACTLY *IS* PAIN ANYWAY?

Besides the unfathomable personal cost to the sufferers, pain costs our society a fortune, and the largest portion of the bill is for back pain. According to some studies, the tab in North America comes to a whopping $100 *billion* a year when compensation costs are included along with treatment. Researchers estimate that something like 80 million North Americans currently suffer from chronic pain. And yet, until the last couple of decades, only a very few researchers devoted their careers to its study.

Luckily for all of us, one of the first researchers was an American physician named Dr. John Bonica, whose most important contribution was founding the International Association for the Study of Pain. Dr. Bonica died in 1995, but his legacy lives on.

Dr. Bonica's first task was to bend his head to the job of finding out what his fellow physicians knew about the subject of pain. After surveying 22,000 pages from standard medical textbooks, he came up with a grand total of fifty-four references to pain. "It was an extraordinary revelation," he said at the time. "No wonder so many doctors feel uncomfortable dealing with chronic pain patients."

Just explaining what pain is can be difficult. In fact, a number of world-class researchers agree that pain — particularly back pain — is the most mysterious aspect of medicine. Only over the past few decades have we come to understand some of the basics about it. Most professionals generally start off by describing the two different categories: acute pain and chronic pain.

Acute Pain

The sharp, immediate pain you feel from, for example, a toothache or a burn, is fairly easy to understand. By nature **acute pain** is short-lived, even when it is severe. You usually have a sense of what's causing it as well as when it will end, and that knowledge provides you with at least some comfort.

Acute pain also usually occurs for a good reason, which is to signal your body that something is wrong so that you can take appropriate measures.

For example, if you have an infection, the pain alerts you to the fact that medication may be required. If the pain is caused by an injury such as strained back muscles, your natural reaction is to avoid making further movements that could make the injury worse.

Acute pain also sometimes prevents an injury from occurring in the first place by producing a lightning-fast reflex action. For example, you will usually remove your thumb from a hot stove before any serious damage can take place.

In all these examples, the pain has a source — a physical source that you can point your finger at. Physicians call this kind of pain **organic**, meaning that it originates in an organ, even though we don't generally think of muscles as organs in the same way as livers or hearts. Sometimes, acute pain occurs for a reason that modern medicine can't explain. In a situation like this, doctors scratch their heads and point out that pain is one of the most complex subjects known (or should I say unknown!) to mankind.

Chronic Pain

The second category, **chronic pain**, is very different from acute pain. Chronic pain can go on and on, sometimes for months or even years. Unlike acute pain, chronic pain serves no useful purpose.

In some cases, such pain is organic. But the fact that health-care professionals know which part of your body is causing it doesn't mean they know how to stop the misery. In other cases, the pain continues long after an injury has healed; what was once acute pain turns into chronic pain. We are not completely sure why, although new research indicates that some injuries do not heal 100 percent. In such cases, a person's ability to function may be restored while the pain, or at least some of it, still lingers. This appears to be connected to the way individual cells heal, and to the fact that gentle stretching exercises during the healing process work better than bed rest. (See Chapters 12 and 13.)

Finally, in some cases, there never was an injury in the first place. Just what caused the pain to begin is a mystery.

In all these cases, however, doctors have an idea that at least part of the pain's cause is usually related to stress. Sometimes this portion is very large; other times it's very small. In either case, the stress-related portion of chronic pain is called **psychogenic pain**. This is the scientist's way of saying that the pain is psychological rather than physical. Psychological pain starts in the psyche, rather than coming from a **pathology** — an illness or injury in an organ. But psychogenic pain is very real; make no mistake about that.

Chronic pain has another quality: trying to cope with it can take over your life. While acute pain can get you down, it is not depressing in the same way as chronic pain. Acute pain can make you cry out for relief, but it does not change your personality or your view of the world. On the other hand, people who live with chronic pain day after day, year after year, sometimes lose the will to carry on. And, in many instances, chronic pain causes fear, anxiety, or depression . . . any of which, in turn, can increase the pain. It's a vicious cycle.

Your state of mind can also change the nature of your chronic pain. Let's say, for example, that you have a minor back injury, which nevertheless stops you from working because lifting is part of your job. After a while, you may start to feel useless. Eventually — as if to justify this state of inactivity — your brain may actually increase the pain. The result is that a minor injury ends up causing far more pain than it ought to.

Here's another example: Let's say you've been in a car accident and are waiting to hear about compensation. You may find that the pain increases just before the adjudicator is about to render his or her decision.

Finally, here's a third example, one which insurance companies have been studying over the past number of years. Let's say that you have genuinely injured yourself at work but your manager has dismissed what you have said. First of all, you probably feel that you are being treated unfairly, and this may also cause you to question the severity of your injury. Again, in the interests of self-justification, your brain may actually increase your pain.

In all of these cases, the pain is REAL. I cannot stress this too often. No informed professional should ever try to make you feel that you are "faking it," or that you're making a mountain out of a molehill, or that it's your fault.

Note, too, that in all three of these examples, if your situation improves (a desk job opens up; the adjudicator rules in your favor; your boss experiences an attack of back pain and becomes sympathetic), your pain may decrease.

Toward a Precise Definition

It is one thing to differentiate between acute pain and chronic pain, but early researchers also felt that it was important to come up with a definition that would cover both. The one that seems to work best was proposed by a psychiatrist from London, Ontario — Dr. Harold Merskey.

Dr. Merskey defined **pain** as "an unpleasant sensory and emotional experience associated with actual or potential tissue damage, or described in terms of such damage." While its use of the word "unpleasant" seems rather undramatic, this definition has two important strengths. First of all, it allows for a loose association between the degree of injury and the amount of pain. This is important because, in certain circumstances, a small injury will produce a lot of pain, while in other circumstances, a severe injury will produce very little pain. Even the mere memory of pain, with no new injury whatsoever, can cause excruciating pain for reasons that no one understands. Second of all, Dr. Merskey's definition recognizes the emotional dimension of pain. Pain hurts, but it also conjures up fear, feelings of desperation, bad memories, and a whole host of other emotions that can make it seem a lot worse.

THE GATE-CONTROL THEORY OF PAIN

While Dr. Merskey can be credited for defining pain, another Canadian — McGill University professor of psychology Dr. Ronald Melzack — was responsible for changing medical science's entire concept of it. In 1965, he and a British professor of anatomy, Dr. Patrick Wall, proposed the **gate-control theory of pain**. Up until this time, scientists believed that X amount of injury produced X amount of pain — that the ratio was one-to-one. Melzack and Wall proposed that the amount of pain "input" at the site of an injury need not be equal to the amount of pain that is felt when the message finally arrives at the brain.

For example, just because X amount of pain is received by your big toe at the point where it makes contact with a big rock does not necessarily mean that your brain will perceive X amount of pain. Pain, said Melzack and Wall, is often modified on its way from the toe to the brain. On one occasion, your brain might perceive more pain than would ordinarily be expected from such an impact. On another occasion, such as during a moment of distraction, less pain might be perceived.

In other words, by the time a pain message runs along a nerve fiber to the spinal cord, then up the cord to the thalamus, then farther along in the brain to the cerebral cortex, where things like emotions are added, the original message may become altered. The agent that alters the pain Melzack and Wall called a "pain gate"; hence the name of the theory.

If the pain gate is completely open, the theory goes, pain messages can breeze through to the brain with the speed of Mercury. When the pain gate is partly open, pain sensations of a diminished quality get through. If the pain gate is closed, however, no pain messages at all will find their way up to the brain and no pain will be felt.

Long before the gate-control theory was proposed, researchers knew that soldiers in battle, or players in the middle of a crucial game, could suffer tremendous injuries without feeling any pain. But researchers lacked a theory to explain how this was possible. That's what Melzack and Wall offered. The soldier feels no pain because his pain gate is shut.

ANATOMY OF A PAIN MESSAGE

It's not very difficult to understand the basics of how a pain message is transmitted from your toe to your brain, or how that message can change en route. Physicians who work with chronic pain patients almost always take the time to explain these mechanisms because, in almost all cases, understanding what's going on is the first step toward learning to cope with it.

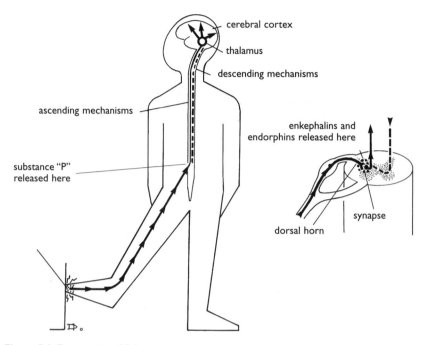

cerebral cortex

thalamus

descending mechanisms

ascending mechanisms

enkephalins and
endorphins released here

substance "P"
released here

synapse

dorsal horn

Figure 5.1 Transmission of Pain

Let's return to the example of the big toe that has made contact with the big rock (Figure 5.1). At the turn of the century, researchers had the notion that pain messages from the toe were transmitted to the brain in an uninterrupted fashion. You stubbed your toe, and presto! The message zoomed along a nerve fiber to the spinal cord, then up the cord to the cerebral cortex, where it was perceived as mild or severe depending upon the quality of the altercation with the rock.

Now we know that this concept is faulty. Pain messages do not travel to the brain like a non-stop airplane flight. When they get as far as the **dorsal horn**, which runs the entire length of the spinal cord, they encounter a gap in the nerve fiber called a **synapse** (see Figure 5.1).

If a message is going to get to the brain, it must bridge this synapse. It can do this only if a chemical called a **neurotransmitter** is produced within the fiber and is excreted at the synapse end. There it acts like a biochemical ferry, transmitting the message to the next nerve fiber.

From here the message travels up the spinal cord to the **thalamus**, a center of the brain where it encounters a second synapse. If this synapse is crossed, we respond with what are called **reflex reactions**. These are black and white, all-or-nothing, unemotional responses, such as withdrawing the injured toe with the speed of lightning.

But this is not the end of the message's journey. From here, it must bridge a third synapse in order to arrive at the **cerebral cortex**, where the location of the sensation, as well as its intensity, are consciously perceived. The cortex also adds information about the kind of pain — often called "color" — to the picture and makes decisions about the appropriate response. Taking into account present emotional states and past experiences with pain, it consults its roster of possible replies and picks one or more.

For example, the cortex might decide in one set of circumstances that the appropriate reaction is to scream, or cry out, or wring your hands in woe. In other situations, however, it may decide that it is more important to get on with the war, or winning the game. In the second case no response will occur because no pain will be felt.

Other examples: If you are afraid of pain, perhaps because of a bad experience that your memory has stored for decades, your cerebral cortex may actually intensify the painful sensation. Anxiety about the impact this pain is going to have on your life can do the same thing. As well, we all learn pain responses from our parents; in some cultures, people learn to tolerate quite high amounts of pain with little response, while in other cultures people are very vocal about every little ache. Studies have shown that Jews, for example, tend to be concerned with the meaning of pain; if they can understand its mechanisms, they can often tolerate it much better. (Since this is my own cultural heritage, I have to smile. Look at the lengths I've gone to in order to give meaning to pain!) On the other hand, some cultural groups seem to be more interested in immediate relief, cause being of less consequence than making the pain go away. And in still other cultures, being able to cope with pain is part and parcel of ceremonial rituals. For example, in parts of India, hooks are embedded in the flesh of the back during some ceremonies, but they cause no pain at all!

Positive thoughts or emotions can also reduce the amount of pain that is perceived. The anticipation of a meeting with an old friend, or a large cheque waiting in the mailbox at the end of the path, are reasons why the cerebral cortex may not perceive the altercation with the rock as severe. These decisions, however, are not made consciously. They are within the realm of the subconscious, that vast, largely unexplored recess that is more complex than any human-built computer.

When Melzack and Wall first proposed their gate-control theory, they thought the pain gate was located at the first synapse at the dorsal horn. We now know, as I've just explained, that there are several places along the route where a pain message can be altered on its way to the cerebral cortex. In addition, no physical "gate" has ever been found. Today, researchers realize that the mechanisms of pain are far more complex than Melzack and Wall first proposed.

The Journey from a Chemical Standpoint

To understand just how a pain message can be altered, we have to look at its journey in chemical terms. If chemistry isn't your bag, however, don't feel obliged; just skip to the next section.

If you cut the nerve that serves the big toe cross-sectionally, then examine it under a microscope, you'll become aware of some interesting things. First of all, you'll see many bundles, each of which contains huge numbers of nerve fibers. There are many different types and sizes of these. Large fibers carry sensory messages, such as touch, heat, and cold. Small fibers carry pain messages. At the toe end of all fibers are various **receptors**, which receive these incoming messages.

During a normal walk down a normal path (seconds before the now-infamous collision with the rock) these receptors are busy picking up sensations from the world. They are also "firing," which simply means that the messages they pick up travel along the nerve fibers at a normal rate.

Only a certain amount of information can be processed by the nervous system to be consciously perceived by the brain at any one time. Normally, the large fibers fire at a higher rate than the small fibers, so the sensations coming in from them (such as soft earth and a warm breeze) prevail. The relatively few sensations traveling along the small pain fibers are ignored by the body.

Things change very rapidly, however, when the toe bangs into the rock. Very quickly, a number of potent chemicals are produced at the point of contact. One is called **bradykinin**. It sensitizes the small pain fibers and their firing rate increases.

Other chemicals, called **prostaglandins**, also increase the firing rate of the small pain fibers, but they have another job as well. They increase circulation to the big toe, causing swelling, or inflammation. This attracts infection-fighting white blood cells to the area to reduce the inflammation and fight any bacteria that have wandered in through broken skin. Meanwhile, a powerful neurotransmitter is being produced inside the fibers. It is called **substance "P."** Yes, the P stands for "pain."

By now, the situation in the dorsal horn will have changed. Far more messages will be coursing along the small, pain-conducting fibers than along the large sensory fibers. This is where the gate-control theory comes into play. Since only a certain amount of information can be perceived at any time, a choice must be made. Will the messages from the large or small fibers prevail? Before the big toe's close encounter with the big rock, there was no contest. Now, however, in Melzack and Wall's terms, the pain gate is open. Perceptions of soft earth and a warm breeze fall by the wayside. The small fibers have a monopoly on the situation and the predominant message — the one that is perceived — is PAIN.

Up the dorsal horn these messages go. If they are strong enough, they bridge the second synapse at the thalamus. Here pain is first perceived, although, as I've explained earlier, this kind of pain is as colorless as a November sky. If and when these messages bridge the next synapse and arrive at the cerebral cortex, however, they will develop in a qualitative sense. Sometimes, these qualities are very different from what one would expect.

For instance, as I've already mentioned, very little pain might be felt because you're in a hurry to get home to see a friend. The physiology of how exactly pain is modified in such a case is far from completely understood, but basically, scientists believe that there are two ways that this pain can happen. Either the impulses that are coursing along the small pain fibers can be inhibited, or decreased, or, the input into the large fibers can be facilitated, or increased. The latter occurrence can override the input into the small fibers, preventing or at least reducing its transmission.

Rubbing the sore toe, for example, will result in increased firing of the large fibers, which conduct the sensations of touch and warmth. A hot pack can accomplish the same thing. According to the gate-control theory, if you rub the toe hard enough, the messages in the large fibers will override the messages in the small fibers, thus opening the large fiber gate and closing the small. The electrical stimulation of a TENS machine (see Chapter 15) is thought to work on this principle, and some researchers suggest that spinal manipulation may also accomplish this feat.

Decreasing the firing rate of the small pain fibers can achieve the same end. When you take an ASA tablet, for example, the production of prostaglandins is inhibited and the firing rate of the small fibers is reduced. Other painkilling drugs, such as morphine, will also reduce the firing rate of the small fibers, although they work on the brain rather than at the site of the injury.

THE LEGACY OF MELZACK AND WALL

Research into the anatomy and physiology of pain blossomed during the late 1960s and 1970s. As more information emerged, many researchers abandoned some of Melzack and Wall's original conclusions. But these two researchers get the credit for a lot of what followed. Because of these two men, new concepts illustrating that pain is a much more complex phenomenon than we originally thought have gained ground. Most researchers have stopped thinking of the "gate" as a physical entity; rather, it has become a metaphor, a symbol of the fact that the body can modify pain messages quite dramatically.

Endorphins and Enkephalins

The next major breakthrough occurred when a group of American researchers established how morphine and other opiates work. They had been convinced for some time that morphine killed pain because of the existence of special **opiate receptors** throughout the nervous system. In 1975, these receptors were found.

But this discovery begged a question: Why would the human body have developed opiate receptors? People don't, after all, go around ingesting morphine on a daily basis. The answer to this question was discovered by University of Aberdeen pharmacologists John Hughes and Hans Kosterlitz.

Hughes and Kosterlitz postulated that the purpose of the opiate receptors was to receive powerful, painkilling, opiate-like chemicals that the human body itself produced, and that's what they began to look for. They found two kinds of them, and called them **endorphins** and **enkephalins**. Enkephalins were found in the pituitary gland of the brain, endorphins in the brain and the spinal cord itself. For their efforts, Hughes and Kosterlitz won the Nobel Prize and broadened the dimensions of pain research.

Finding these chemicals changed the way scientists thought about pain yet again. Not only was it possible for messages on the way up to the brain to be altered (by stimulation of the large fibers, for example), but, if natural painkilling chemicals were being produced up top, there must be mechanisms that could alter pain messages on the way back down as well.

Some researchers talked about the endorphin discovery in terms of a kind of sequel to Melzack and Wall's gate-control theory. They postulated that the stimulation of large nerve fibers was causing endorphins to be produced. Once produced, endorphins would stop the production of bradykinin and prostaglandins, which would in turn decrease the firing rate of the small pain fibers.

Other researchers, however, believed that endorphins provided an alternative, rather than a sequel, to the gate-control theory of pain. These scientists also realized that the mechanisms controlling pain are so complex that more questions were arising than were being answered.

A few years later, several other opiates and some non-opiate pain-altering chemicals were discovered, and the mechanism of pain blurred again. The entire field has turned out to be far more complicated than anyone ever dreamed possible, and the final answers are not yet in sight.

But the research continues — and into a reassuring variety of topics. Some scientists are searching for analgesics that can be received by the body's opiate receptors but are not addictive like morphine. Other researchers are looking for drugs that may activate other systems. According to very new research, **adenosine triphosphate** or **ATP**, the chemical that provides us with the power to tense our muscles, also appears to play a role in pain reduction by sending electrical signals to the brain. At least several years will probably pass before there is another major breakthrough.

While this search continues, still other researchers are looking for drug-less answers to dealing with chronic pain. Dr. Bonica always spoke about the day when people will look to their own innate mental powers to relieve themselves of pain: "I don't think it takes too much scientific licence to say that we will discover mental activities that can produce specific analgesia," he said back in 1965. "In ten or fifteen years, perhaps we can begin to teach people to control their own pain."

Well, this has clearly not happened yet. However, a number of studies have shed at least some light on the issue of chronic pain, and we are moving forward in baby steps.

For example, research suggests that people whose backs have healed but who continue nevertheless to suffer from pain may be deficient in their ability to produce endorphins and other pain-decreasing chemicals. Those who advocate acupuncture, for example, theorize that in some instances, the treatment may kick a faulty endorphin system back into gear, so to speak. Indeed, experiments conducted at the University of Toronto on the brain cells of cats have shown that acupuncture can cause endorphins to be produced. Unfortunately, when the treatment was first introduced to North America, it took the lay press by storm and many people expected it to act like snake oil. When that unrealistic expectation didn't come to pass, the pendulum swung full force the other way. A few excellent researchers are still doing work in this area but whether or not acupuncture will ever emerge as a major treatment for chronic pain is anyone's guess. (For more on acupuncture, see the end of this chapter.)

Other research is clearer. For instance, many people whose lives have been dominated by pain for a long time become depressed and, quite often, they suffer not from vegetative depression but from atypical depression, whose main feature is anxiety. Some studies indicate that depression also causes endorphin production to decrease. As well, antidepressant medication has been found to be effective as a pain reliever for some chronic pain sufferers, although the mechanisms are not well understood. (For more details on drug therapies, see Chapter 8.)

Studies have also shown that chronic pain can cause the small nerve fibers to become "sensitized." Whereas in normal circumstances, a certain amount of painful stimuli are necessary to provoke the perception of pain, much less is required once a small fiber has become sensitive. This means that a smaller amount of stimulation than normal will trigger the perception of pain.

Still other studies have associated the efficacy of **placebo** pills with endorphins. *Placebo* is Latin for "I will please." Doctors have found that when patients are given placebo pills — usually they contain nothing but sugar — their pain is decreased about a third of the time. Researchers at the University of California in San Francisco have shown that placebo pills can stimulate the body's endorphin system.

Some of the most recent work indicates that aerobic exercise also stimulates the production of endorphins. These days, a general fitness program is almost always part and parcel of treatment for chronic pain. (See Chapter 13.)

Still other studies have shown that laughter (and, in fact, any kind of activity that you find relaxing) can stimulate your body to produce these natural painkilling chemicals.

From all of this research a philosophy has emerged: our main goal should be to discover very early on who is likely to become a *chronic* back pain sufferer. The answer to this question is not as obvious as it may first appear and it is certainly, in most cases, unrelated to the severity of the physical problem. Researchers began to look for answers other than physical findings when studies showed that, while 80 percent of the population suffers from back pain at some point during their lives, the major part of the cost of back pain to our society is due to the very few people, relatively speaking, who become chronic: about 80 percent of health-care dollars for back pain (treatment, rehabilitation costs, etc.) is spent on less than 20 percent of the people who experience an acute episode. The vast majority of people get better within six weeks no matter what we do. More get better by the end of three months. But after six months, the curve changes.

Pain clinics are finding better methods of treating these people and how they work is what I'll be describing next. But if we could only identify which people are likely to become chronic sufferers and why, more money than you or I have ever dreamed of could be saved.

Researchers are trying to isolate what are called **psychosocial predictors**. In plain English, these are the things that cause a person to become disabled. Some researchers believe that, at least with work-related injuries, how satisfied a person is with his or her job is the key. (See Chapter 20 for more on this topic.)

The studies that look at this issue tend to ask acute back pain sufferers far more basic questions. For instance: How do you rate your pain on a scale of one to ten? What kind of impact, on a scale of one to ten, is your back problem having on your life? How would you rate your health on a scale of one to ten? In all these examples, the higher the number, the greater the likelihood that a person who is suffering from acute back pain will go on to become a chronic sufferer — regardless of the severity of the back problem from a pathological sense.

Other predictors can be measured in different ways. For instance, people who fear pain have a greater risk of becoming chronic sufferers than people who take pain in stride. As I've already explained in this chapter, these kinds of reactions are often cultural.

Other studies indicate that, if a person is told by a health-care professional that he or she "will get better in four weeks" and that prediction proves to be untrue, anxiety may cause the problem to become chronic. How a patient's family reacts to the problem and how supportive they are is also important. What's amazing to me is that, in some cases, a very supportive, coddling type of family is more of a hindrance than a help. (See Chapter 7.)

If I had to come up with a bottom line — and I think, if you've read the story of my own introduction to chronic back pain, you'll agree that I have a right to an opinion — it would be this: Back pain, as I have said, is a metaphor for life. Therefore, the ways one's life develops during an acute bout of back pain, combined with one's self-image, determines to a large extent one's future. These sorts of factors matter as much as the actual injury.

Frankly, all this has been pretty obvious to me for many years! I truly don't understand why it took medical science so long to wake up and smell the coffee.

PAIN CLINICS

The concept of the multidisciplinary pain clinic was pioneered in the early 1960s by Dr. Bonica. From his experiences in dealing with wounded World War II combat soldiers, he realized that, if we were going to learn how to manage chronic pain successfully, we would need to rely on the input and perspective of professionals from many different disciplines. Dr. Bonica honed his theories at the University of Washington Medical Center's Clinical Pain Service in Seattle; most large North American cities now have more than one such facility. Sometimes, pain clinics are housed in teaching hospitals. But more often they are operated as small, freestanding clinics.

To become a patient, a chronic pain sufferer must have a referral from a general practitioner. Often there is a waiting time of several months.

The majority of pain clinic patients suffer from chronic back pain. In most cases, the sole criterion for becoming a patient is having pain for at least six months, although the average patient has been suffering much longer than that by the time he or she arrives.

Most pain clinics focus on teaching patients how to *manage* their pain as opposed to how to get rid of it. A variety of health-care practitioners from different disciplines offer their input according to the specific needs of the individual chronic pain patients. These professionals usually include a social worker, a clinical psychologist, a nurse, appropriate physicians who act as consultants, a chiropractor, a physiotherapist and/or an occupational therapist, an ergonomist or kinesiologist, a massage therapist, and an exercise therapist. In recent years, pain clinics have put far more emphasis on physical fitness than in the past.

The main goal of a pain clinic is to teach sufferers how to minimize the disruptive effects of chronic pain without necessarily expecting it to go away completely. Self-reliance is the key. Patients who are able to accept responsibility for much of their own progress — who can take an active, as opposed to a passive, role — almost invariably do best.

The first appointment at a pain clinic is coordinated by one of the team members, often a psychologist or nurse. Unless the reports from the family physician are up to date and very comprehensive, a physician will take a medical history and conduct a clinical exam. Any other diagnostic tests that are necessary will then be ordered.

Medications will be reviewed. But here is where the similarity to the regular health-care system ends. At a multidisciplinary pain clinic, patients see a psychologist, psychiatrist, or social worker, and it is this professional's job to assess the psychogenic aspects of the patient's chronic pain. In many cases, family members are interviewed as well. When the information has been collected, the team meets and forms a plan. At many centers, patients are encouraged to attend this conference so that they can begin to take control right from the start.

In some centers, four groups are used to "type" patients. The first group, into which only 10 to 20 percent of chronic pain patients fit, is the "organic" group. For these people, the source of the pain is obvious, although not always curable. While there may be emotional and psychological overtones to the pain, they are minimal. In the fourth group is the very small (1 to 2 percent) proportion of individuals who actually feel no pain, and they themselves are aware of this fact. While this is a much rarer phenomenon than was thought in the past, there exist some malingerers who are simply lying about their condition for one reason or another.

The great majority of chronic pain sufferers fall into the other two groups. Their pain has an organic source but there are also psychogenic aspects to it. In some cases, the ratio is about half and half; in other cases, the organic source is minimal while the psychogenic proportion is very large.

Part and parcel of the treatment plan at a typical pain clinic is the contract that the patient, the patient's spouse if there is one, and the treatment coordinator all sign. Several specific goals are sought: working toward managing the pain without pain-killing drugs; recognizing and adjusting to the limitations of the pain; decreasing the importance of the pain relative to the rest of the person's life; and being able to accept an occasional increase in pain without becoming frightened that the pain is going to take control.

Some programs last for a couple of weeks. Others go on for several months. Some are conducted on an in-patient basis, but most people continue to live at home.

Patients attend educational sessions, relaxation training sessions, and physiotherapy sessions in which better posture and exercises are learned. As I've already mentioned, exercise, including aerobics, is considered far more important nowadays than it was in the past. There are also a lot of group sessions so that people can share their experiences with others in similar circumstances. It is also essential for people to learn which activities provoke pain, how long a flare-up usually lasts, and what techniques work for them.

Learning techniques to help control stress are always part of a back pain control program. Sometimes, massage, TENS machines (see Chapter 15), or acupuncture are also used. But the most important goal of a pain clinic program is to change people's attitudes toward pain. It's important for people to learn how to conquer the intimidating aspects of pain. Just as stress and tension can exacerbate pain, decreasing tension can work the opposite way.

Above all, patients who have previously been sitting around focusing on their pain are kept busy. Each day has a purpose, and at the end of it they can usually get a good night's sleep. It is clear that people who are busy and diverted feel less pain than those who focus on it — based on the same principle behind the wounded soldier's lack of pain.

Some studies show that about two-thirds of pain clinic patients have significant pain relief as a result of their experience. Follow-up studies also show that about 75 percent of patients have maintained their gains a year down the road. People with large amounts of organic pain and small amounts of psychogenic pain make the most gains.

There is an account of a chronic back pain sufferer's pain clinic experience in Chapter 17.

SELF-HELP GROUPS

Self-help groups, such as the North American Chronic Pain Association of Canada, also exist for chronic pain sufferers. Among other things, these groups help people to focus on what they *can* do rather than on what they can't. Says Diane Cachia, president of the association, "Support systems can make a big difference. They teach people how to take some responsibility for their own well-being as well as how to become active and involved." Helping others is certainly a good therapeutic technique for many, many people.*

NATURAL STIMULATION PAIN TREATMENTS

Acupuncture

How **acupuncture** treats pain is to stimulate the body to heal itself. The acupuncturist inserts needles one to three inches long into the skin of the patient and twirls them by hand into the appropriate branch of a nerve root near the point where it exits the spinal canal.

Acupuncture has been used to treat chronic pain in China for some 4,000 years. The classical Chinese approach divides the body into meridians, or pathways, along which are about 800 points where energy and

---

* For more information about the association or about chronic pain, write to the North American Chronic Pain Association of Canada, 150 Central Park Drive, Suite 105, Brampton, Ontario, L6T 2T9.

blood are supposed to converge. Western clinicians began taking an interest in acupuncture in the 1970s. The realization that virtually all of the Chinese meridians and points corresponded to neural structures led to the development of a "Western" method based on anatomy rather than ancient tradition. Since then acupuncture has slowly been gaining acceptance in Canada.*

The treatments are not especially painful. Patients feel a pinprick as the needles, which are very fine and have rounded tips, go in and are twirled, and may experience a dull ache or "tight" sensation while the needles remain in place.

Patients typically receive weekly treatments, and usually see results — decreased pain — within seven or eight visits. Some find their pain stops completely or improves to an acceptable level; others find they need periodic treatments to remain free of pain.

How does it work? Current theory is that acupuncture alleviates pain by sending signals to the brain to stimulate the production of the body's own pain-deadening substances, endorphins, which are sent via the nervous system to the precise site of the injury, where they "turn off" the pain. Research to date has not, however, explained all aspects of the procedure.

Acupuncture-Derivative Therapies

In **electro-acupuncture**, instead of twirling the acupuncture needles by hand, an electrical stimulator is hooked up to the needles. Different currents or intensities can be used with this device, which provides uniform stimulation. The procedure does not hurt but simply gives a pulsating feeling.

Laser acupuncture has been used in Europe for forty years and in Canada for at least twelve years. The procedure is less invasive than conventional acupuncture and more acceptable to those who feel uncomfortable about the use of needles. A cold laser is used to biologically stimulate the body (versus a hot laser, which destroys tissue). A metal probe about the length of a pencil, attached by a cord to a machine, is

---

* The Acupuncture Foundation of Canada provides training to doctors and physiotherapists in the procedure. The Foundation is located in Toronto and can be reached at (416) 752-3988.

applied against the skin. An infrared ray is used for deep pain while a helium neon beam is used for more superficial pain.

The therapy is believed by some to stimulate or activate the human body's electrical system, causing cellular changes. Sometimes conventional and laser acupuncture are combined together to treat back pain.

Intramuscular Stimulation (IMS)

This type of stimulation is similar to acupuncture in the sense that dry needles are used to stimulate areas of the body. The theory behind the technique and the points of insertion used are, however, different. **Intramuscular stimulation** focuses on muscles. Research performed in Vancouver in the early 1970s indicates that nerve root irritation, which can be caused by stress, tension, poor lifting techniques, or poor posture, leads to prolonged muscle spasm. The spasms strain the tendons and joints, affecting the alignment of the back. Poor alignment leads to wear and tear on the joints and other problems, resulting in further nerve root irritation, which causes chronic pain. IMS aims to treat these chronic muscle spasms directly, dealing with the muscle.

A needle is inserted into the muscle itself, so the procedure can be quite painful. It may require more needles than acupuncture. They are used in conjunction with a Japanese plunger-type needle holder, which prevents the needle from becoming contaminated and allows it to be reused during the treatment.

The points chosen for needling are located along the taut tender bands of the muscle. Because muscles are made of bundles, more than one point must be needled to release the entire spasm.

Spinal Cord Stimulation

For **spinal cord stimulation**, two electrodes and lead wires are implanted under the skin near the spine. The wires run under the skin to a disc-shaped receiver situated either below the collar bone or in the abdominal area. The external portion of the system consists of a stimulation transmitter, which can be worn on a belt, and an antenna. When the wearer activates the transmitter, it sends signals through the skin, which are then picked up by the receiver, converted into tiny electrical impulses, and sent to the spinal cord. The implant is performed at only a few teaching hospitals.

The average patient activates the stimulator for about ten minutes each hour. Researchers can't explain why these electrical impulses seem to short-circuit pain messages so that some patients are able to better manage their pain. Various models of spinal cord stimulator available include Itrel 3, X-trel, Mattrix, and Synchromed.

CHEMICALLY STIMULATED PAIN TREATMENTS

Epidural Injections

Although **epidural injections** have been around for ninety years, much controversy surrounds their use. The therapy is sometimes used in especially difficult cases of lower back pain that have not responded to conservative methods and seem unlikely to respond to surgery. The procedure takes about twenty minutes and is similar to the epidural used for pain control during childbirth. An anesthetic solution is inserted into the **epidural space** (the space that lies between the dura mater, which is the outer membrane that surrounds the spinal cord, and the outer bony edge of the spinal canal) by means of a long syringe.

Some doctors insist that this procedure be performed in hospitals; some do it in their offices. The solutions used can differ. A procaine/saline solution, sometimes with cortisone, is the most common, however, occasionally morphine or cocaine is used. The usual routine is to perform the procedure three times at one-week intervals. Another approach, rarely used, is to insert a slow drip tap that gives a constant dose of solution.

Proponents of the treatment believe it blocks the transmission of pain messages from the site of the injury to the brain. It is not understood, however, why the effects do not wear off in a few hours as in the case of epidurals used for women in labor. The effects for back pain appear to benefit the patient for months or even years. One of the known side effects, however, is temporary retention of water when cortisone is included in the injection solution. As well, some experts believe the cortisone causes more pain than the inflammation.

Nerve Root Blocks

A **nerve root block (NRB)** is similar to the epidural injection but less invasive. Using a long syringe, the anasthetic novocaine is injected, but the needle is only inserted as far as the nerve root at the point where it emerges versus into the spinal canal itself. NRB therapy is thought to relieve pain caused by adhesions that sometimes form at the site of an injury (see Chapter 2). Medical professionals vary in their opinions as to when and why epidural or NRB injections work, but they generally agree that neither are useful in cases of herniated discs or mechanical wear and tear problems.

6

The Contribution
of Stress

T he word "stress" has come to have a negative connotation these days, but in fact, stress is normal and essential to your life. Without stress, you wouldn't get out of bed, make changes, meet deadlines, or break records. The problem is that sometimes your coping skills are challenged beyond your capabilities; that's when you become "stressed out."

Dealing with stress is a hot topic. It seems that every time I pick up a magazine, I find an article on how to deal with "stressors," which is the new buzzword for negative kinds of stress. Every year, employers spend millions of dollars on courses put on by stress-management professionals who promise to teach coping skills to their employees. They don't do this simply because they are nice guys; they do it because they believe that, in the long run, it will save billions of dollars on illnesses that are either caused by, or made worse by, stress. Back pain is high on the list of such ailments.

Certainly it is true that stress can make a back problem worse. And dealing with back pain can itself be very stressful, resulting in a kind of vicious circle. Both of these concepts are now generally accepted by health-care professionals and back pain sufferers alike. What we don't understand nearly as well is why some people find their backs act up in response to stress while other people don't — and what can be done to help those who do.

As we have studied the connections between the mind and the body over the past couple of decades, we have come to understand how complex the relationship is. Our increased knowledge has produced answers, but it has also produced questions. Do stressed-out back pain sufferers hurt more because of a change in the way they *perceive* pain? Or does stress cause overly sensitive muscles to tense up even more? Are the chemicals that have to do with our emotions also involved in back pain? Not that long ago, few people even asked these questions. Now that we are asking them, we realize how little we know.

Some of the basic aspects of stress, however, have been understood for decades. For instance, the "fight or flight" reaction to stress relates to the human instinct to survive. This response was organized by evolution thousands of years ago when dealing with physical danger was the norm. It works like this: When you become aware of danger, your pituitary gland (which is attached to the base of your brain) releases a hormone called **ACTH**. ACTH causes your adrenal glands to release other hormones. (I'm sure you've heard of adrenaline, which is one of them.)

These chemicals prepare your body to either fight or flee. Your pulse quickens. Your muscles tense up and your blood pressure increases. Blood is directed away from your stomach toward your limbs, and chemicals for quick energy are released into the bloodstream. Other chemicals that help the blood to clot are also released — just in case.

When a lion has an eye on your best goat, these are excellent reactions. They can also be useful when your car skids off the road. However, when your in-laws get on your case and you know this is likely to happen every Sunday for the next two decades, such responses are not very appropriate; you can't fight or flee.

Some people — I don't know any! — can laugh off such stressors as needling in-laws. They let it go into one ear, as they say, then out the other. Other people get angry; among this group, some people hold their anger in, while others yell and scream — usually at some innocent bystander who ends up becoming stressed-out as well. Still others start to get anxious about Sunday dinner when they wake up on Sunday morning; by noon, they feel restless, jittery, and irritable. Others get depressed in the sense of feeling sad, or melancholy; when *they* open their eyes on Sunday morning, they feel like sticking their heads under the pillow and pulling the covers back up. Still others — and I'm one of them — develop back pain.

While different stressors do sometimes produce different effects on the same person, most of us tend to react in more or less the same way most of the time. Why is that? Some researchers believe that we learn certain ways of responding to stress from our role models; our parents react in a certain way, which becomes our way. This makes a lot of common sense. Others believe that chemistry plays an important role; I can also see the logic behind this theory. Probably both have some merit, and how we react is a combination of both environment and genetic predisposition.

LESSONS FROM DEPRESSION

When it comes to back pain and stress, a lot has been learned from research on depression. Some studies, for example, show that stress can trigger a bout of depression in a person who is prone to it. We also know that antidepressants will sometimes relieve, or reduce, back pain in depression patients who happen to suffer from back pain as well. What we don't understand is exactly why the medication works. And no wonder — the brain is a complicated animal, containing over ninety chemicals.

There are theories, however. For example Dr. Ranga Krishnan, a psychiatrist who teaches at Duke University in North Carolina, has come up with some interesting findings. For instance, in some cases, antidepressants appear to enhance the effect of painkillers that are prescribed at the same time. In other cases, however, there is no need for the patient to take pain medication — the antidepressants themselves do the trick. What's really interesting is that, on average, it takes about three weeks for antidepressants to build up to levels high enough to affect depression. Yet in many cases, the patient's pain decreases after just a week or two. Again, why this happens is not really understood.

There are two types of depression: vegetative depression, which is the most common, and atypical depression. Interestingly, when back pain sufferers become depressed, they tend to develop atypical depression.

Vegetative depression is what you probably think of whenever you hear of someone being depressed. The people who suffer from it have no energy. They can't see the point of getting out of bed.

Those with **atypical depression** — and I'm a classic example — develop symptoms of anxiety as well. They are depressed in the sense of feeling sad, but rather than taking to their beds, they become irritable and extremely worried. Often they are too nervous to concentrate on one thing for very long. "Jittery" is the word they often use to describe how they feel.

Some of Dr. Krishnan's research has been on this kind of depression. One of the interesting things he has found is that people who suffer from atypical depression are more likely to develop back pain or another physical ailment than people who tend toward vegetative depression. This tendency seems to apply to less severe levels of emotion as well. Those of us who get anxious when we feel blue (but not so blue that you could label it as depression) often react by developing back pain.

"If you are under a lot of stress and you have a tendency to worry a lot, then anxiety will probably be a part of the way you react," says Dr. Krishnan. This anxiety manifests itself in some people as an emotional response, while others develop physical problems such as back pain. The first type is called **psychic anxiety** (from the Greek word *psyche*, which means "mind"). The second type is called **somatic anxiety** (from the Greek word *soma*, which means "body").

People who are under a lot of stress can suffer from both psychic and somatic anxiety, but one form is usually dominant. If you ask how they are feeling, they will complain about the angst in their life or their back pain, but probably not both.

When anxiety is expressed through back pain, Dr. Krishnan feels that at least part of the pain is linked to muscle tension. Keep in mind that pain from muscle tension is now believed to be chemically driven, just like the pain from a broken leg, or for that matter from a broken heart when someone we love dies. In my opinion, thinking about stress-related back pain in this way seems to make it, well, more respectable. Let's hope these chemical links will someday be better understood.

WHAT CAN YOU DO?

In the meantime, on a practical level, the first step for those who suffer from stress-related back pain is to recognize when the cycle is starting to happen *before* it gets out of hand, which is not all that easy to do. The next step is to learn some coping skills — and these are not the same for everyone.

To begin with, you may be only vaguely aware of what sorts of stressors set you off. In addition, so many of us lead such hectic, high-stress lives that we no longer remember what it feels like to be relaxed. "Normal" has come to mean a state of chronic tension, which continues until things get so bad that it takes a physical problem like back pain to force us to take stock. By this time, of course, our ability to learn new coping techniques is a lot less.

On the other hand, convincing people to take the time to learn about stress management when their lives are going fairly well is a tough sell — who wants to buy umbrellas on a sunny day? Prevention is great in theory, but it usually takes a crisis to get someone really motivated, which is a pity because learning to deal with stress isn't as difficult as you might think. While stress management has become a big business, it's not really all that complicated. First you need to know a few basics: stressors can be broken down into three main categories; stress produces three kinds of symptoms; and there are three basic ways of coping with a stressful situation.

To help us do this better, professionals have developed quite a number of clever techniques, some physical and some mental. At least a few of them will feel right and work for you.

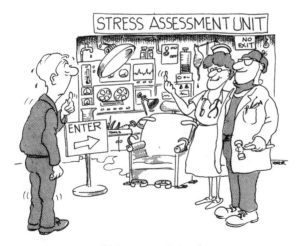

"Take a seat. Relax."

Three Kinds of Stress

*Inter*personal stress has to do with the relationships you have with other people: a boss who drives you crazy, a spouse who sets your teeth on edge by finishing your sentences for you.

*Intra*personal stress has to do with the demands you place on yourself. For instance, if, like a lot of people, you have unrealistically high expectations, you will feel increased stress whenever you do a less-than-perfect job (which, by definition, is most of the time). We usually know this stress by its common name: guilt.

Environmental stress has to do with external stressors: noise (the kid next door who plays his drums every Sunday morning) or physical discomfort (having to sit all day in a lousy chair).

Three Sorts of Symptoms

As I mentioned at the beginning of this chapter, the human body reacts to stress the same way it did 30,000 years ago, with the "fight or flight" response. In our modern-day society, however, physical responses such as increased adrenaline and muscle tension often make matters worse rather than better. Eventually, something has to give.

In some cases, stress is transformed into emotional symptoms: anger, irritability, depression, burn-out, or anxiety.

In other cases, the symptoms are mental: You think the blackest thoughts. You start to see everything as a matter of life or death; or you focus on failures, and/or dwell on a stressful event over and over again, even after it's been solved. (Health-care professionals call this **catastrophizing**.)

The third type of symptom is physical: a stomach ache, fatigue, tension headaches, or back pain. As I've already mentioned, those of us who, under stress, tend to become anxious rather than depressed in the vegetative sense, also tend to develop physical symptoms.

Three Ways to Cope

Sometimes, it makes sense to deal with stress by taking on the stressors directly. If you change jobs, you don't have to deal with your quirky boss. If you convince your company to buy you an ergonomically designed chair, the strain on your back will decrease. (On the other hand, changing jobs can have its own stress, and these days, there aren't many jobs to change *to*. In each case, the pros and cons must be weighed.)

Other times, it's a good idea to take a break from a stressful situation for a while. So in spite of the fact that you have seventeen deadlines looming, you have dinner with a friend, or go for a walk.

The third way of dealing with stress is the indirect way: you change how you perceive and/or react to a stressful situation when the problem itself can't be changed. If you can't get another job, you must learn to let the quirks of your boss go in one ear and out the other, with no smoldering in between. For many of us, this is the toughest challenge of all.

STRESS BUSTERS

So much for the overview. How can you translate this into day-to-day techniques for coping with stress? Well, you can read one of several dozen books, take a course, buy a tape, or consult a stress management professional. (Don't know how to find one? Just look in the *Yellow Pages!*)

Many people, however, can manage without professional help. First you need to start recognizing "cues for wellness" — signs that your stress level is rising: fighting with your mate, a twinge in your back, a little guilty voice in the back of your head. . . . Then try out some coping techniques and find a few that work for you.

I've outlined some of the more popular ones below; you may come across the same ideas, with fancier names, in many books and seminars. Some of them work best when you want to deal with stress directly; others are suited for the indirect approach. Some prevent stress, while others — especially the physical techniques — help to eliminate built-up stress. But there's a huge amount of overlap in these categories.*

---

* An excellent publication is *The Relaxation and Stress Reduction Workbook*, 4th ed., by Martha Davis and M. McKay (Oakland, Calif.: New Harbinger Publications, 1995). It describes the techniques mentioned and gives instructions for mastering them. To order a copy, contact Raincoast Books at 1-800-561-8583.

Body Awareness

You can't reduce unnecessary muscle tension in your body if you're not aware of it. That's pretty logical. By learning to focus on one part of your body at a time, you begin to recognize where you "store" your stress. By keeping a stress awareness diary, you can learn which stressors cause which symptoms.

Progressive Relaxation

Practice tensing a muscle, then relaxing it, and learning to tell the difference. Then use this knowledge to start consciously relaxing in your "real" life. For instance, do you really have to tense up your left shoulder when you type? If you're late for a meeting, does it really do you much good to be a tensed-up, physical wreck when you finally do arrive?

Deep Breathing

Along with certain postures, breathing is the basis of yoga. When people learn to deep breathe, they are shocked by how little air they have been used to taking in. The benefits? Increased oxygen does wonders for reducing muscle tension and anxiety.

Meditation

Does this sound too hokey for you? Try this little exercise: Count slowly from one to four without letting a single thought come into your head. Each time a thought does drift into your mind, go back to one. Tough, huh? How many thousands of thoughts roar around your brain everyday? Wouldn't it be nice to be able to turn them off when you want to? When you think of meditation this way, it doesn't seem so weird after all. . . .

Imagination (also called Visualization or Guided Imagery)

Imagine that your back pain is a jagged block of ice stabbing your spine. Try to actually see it in your mind's eye. Now imagine that the sun is slowly melting the ice and, as the ice melts, your back pain slowly fades away. Learning to do this takes time and practice. Don't give up because it doesn't get rid of all your pain right away.

Self-Hypnosis

I'm sure you've heard of it. There is a narrowing of consciousness, much like when you sleep. But with hypnosis, you never lose your awareness completely. With self-hypnosis you can learn to improve your ability to sleep, reduce your perception of pain, and reduce muscle tension and anxiety.

Autogenic Training (AT)

There are twelve basic AT physical exercises. Their purpose is to reverse the physical effects of the "fight or flight" response. (There are also AT exercises that are meditative rather than physical.) Each exercise, which you practice for a week, has a theme. For instance, "heaviness" is the theme of week 1. For a couple of minutes, half a dozen times a day, you get into a comfortable position and repeat the formula: "My right arm is heavy. My left arm is heavy. Both of my arms are heavy." By learning the art of passive concentration, you can actually reduce muscle tension, blood pressure, pain, anxiety, etc.

Thought Stopping

It may sound crazy, but it works, especially as a technique to reduce anxiety. As soon as you become aware that you are catastrophizing, going over a stressful situation again and again for no good reason, you shout "STOP!" Out loud! An alternative, which some professionals feel isn't strong enough for an obsessive type, is to visualize a relaxing scene in your mind's eye. (Here's a suggestion for times when it would be inappropriate to shout "Stop!": Put an elastic band around your wrist, and when you find yourself catastrophizing, snap it. Hard!)

Refuting Irrational Ideas

With this technique, you learn to change your inner dialogue — the silent conversation that goes on in your mind all day long. If your "self-talk" is accurate, you tend to do well in life. If your self-talk is untrue, your stress level goes up, along with your back pain. For example: "This time, I've done it! My back will *never* get better no matter what I do!" is neither logical nor true. A better bit of self-talk would go like this: "I've done it again! My back is killing me. But I've been through this many times before and it's always gotten better, so this time it will get better too." Learning this technique involves homework: written exercises, focusing on tiny negative habits, and not expecting your back pain to go away completely, right off the bat.

Coping Skills Training

The concept is simple: just because you are in a stressful situation does not mean that you must *feel* anxious or upset. These are responses that we have learned, and therefore they can be unlearned. For example, your back may hurt but you don't have to be a wreck about it, since that will increase muscle tension, which increases pain. The coping skills exercises teach you to change the way you think about a stressful situation, as well as your opinion about how the stress will affect your life.

Assertiveness Training

Most techniques take days, or weeks, to learn. This one takes longer. But in the end, you reduce stress by learning to stand up for your rights without bullying others or letting them bully you.

Biofeedback

Biofeedback uses a special machine to help you become aware of things that you don't usually notice: muscle tension, brain wave activity, heart rate. Once you are aware of them, the next step is to use the biofeedback machine to control them. It's impossible to explain exactly how this happens. But it does work for many people.

Massage

The benefits of massage, which are discussed in detail in Chapter 18, have to do with touch and relaxing tense muscles. Some studies show that being touched can actually reduce pain. Others show that, when tensed-up muscles relax, oxygen and nutrients can get into muscle cells, and waste products can get out.

Nutrition

If your diet is poor — especially in calcium and B vitamins — then your ability to cope with stress is reduced.

One more thing — whatever works best for you, combining it with exercise will make it work better.

Five Points for Exercise!

To put it bluntly, fit people are better able to deal with stress, both physical and emotional, than people who are in lousy shape. And since fitness also plays such an important role in controlling back pain in general, putting in the effort to get fit (and stay fit) is doubly important if you must also cope with chronic back pain. The trouble is, most of us have a tendency to slack off on exercise when our stress level goes up — just when we should be exercising more!

Need convincing? I thought you might. That's why I asked Linda Woodhouse, an exercise specialist, researcher, and physiotherapist (you may recall her comments on diagnosis from Chapter 3), to come up with five good reasons why you can't get off the hook.

1. Chemistry

Whether you are undergoing physical stress (moving boxes) or emotional stress (having an argument with your mate), many of your body's responses are the same: your heart rate increases, your muscles tense up, blood flows toward your limbs, and fat and other fuels are broken down so that they can be released into the bloodstream. If you remember that these responses are all chemical changes, it will make sense that, to get your body back to normal, these chemicals must return to pre-stress levels. After a heated argument, it helps to meditate, or breathe deeply. However, Mother Nature built your body in such a way that regular physical activity, which helps the body return to normal faster, is the best way to get the job done. Ignoring this can increase your risk of developing stress-related ailments such as heart disease . . . or back pain.

2. Prevention

From the point of view of prevention, physical activity is also essential. The fitter you are, the more it takes before stress gets to you. Translated into real life terms, this means that as you get more fit, it may take moving 150 boxes (rather than 100) for your heart rate to reach 140. Or you might have to argue for an hour rather than twenty minutes before your blood pressure rises.

3. Muscle Tension

Sufferers of stress-related back pain, take note. If you exercise regularly, your muscles will get bigger. And stronger. They will also develop more capillaries, which are the tiny blood vessels that deliver nutrients and oxygen to muscle fibers and get rid of waste products. The advantage of this? Very simple. It will take more stress for those muscles to go into spasm. You can sit longer. Move boxes longer. And cope with a whole lot more aggravation before your back and neck muscles give you grief.

4. Endorphins

Remember these from Chapter 5? They're the natural painkillers produced by the human brain. Endorphins are also responsible for "runner's high" — that feeling of extreme well-being that athletes experience after a hard workout. Studies have shown that, if you exercise regularly, your body will produce more endorphins. It's that simple.

5. Self-Esteem

Studies also show that people who exercise feel better about themselves — more confident, less anxious — and that it's more than just a simple matter of liking how they look. How can this be? That part we don't exactly understand. So just do it!

To reap the full benefits of exercise, however, choose an activity that doesn't put your self-esteem on the line. In other words, playing tennis isn't your best choice if losing means that your day is ruined. Solo aerobic activities — biking, skiing — tend to work better. However, even they can be a problem if you're one of those highly competitive types who gets upset if a buddy beats you to the bottom of the hill. The point of physical activity is to do it in moderation and to have fun — *that's* good for your self-esteem.

STEP RIGHT UP . . . TEST YOUR STRESS

As I have mentioned, research indicates that people who respond to stress by becoming anxious (rather than typically depressed) are far more likely to develop stress-related physical symptoms such as back pain. If you're not sure whether this sounds like you, try this little stress test.*

Rate all of the following statements with (a) almost always; (b) often; (c) seldom; or (d) never.

When I'm stressed out I . . .

1. tend to imagine all of the terrible things that could possibly happen to me rather than just concerning myself with the stressful situation at hand.
2. stop what I'm doing and devote all my energy toward fixing the problem immediately. (I might as well do this because, if I don't, I will just drive myself crazy with worry.)
3. relive my latest crisis in my mind over and over again, even after it's been solved.
4. actually picture the stressful situation in my mind's eye, as well as picturing the worst possible outcome.

---

* Adapted from *Controlling Stress and Tension: A Holistic Approach* by Daniel Girdano and George S. Everly Jr. (Englewood Cliffs, N.J.: Prentice-Hall, 1986).

5. get the feeling that I'm losing control over everything.
6. feel a sinking feeling in my stomach, my mouth getting dry, my heart pounding, or my neck and shoulder muscles tightening up.
7. have trouble falling asleep at night, or wake up in the middle of the night.
8. tend to make mountains out of molehills. (I sort of know I'm doing this but can't stop myself.)
9. have difficulty speaking or notice my hands and/or fingers trembling.
10. notice my thoughts racing.

Now add up your score. For every (a) answer, give yourself 4 points; for each (b), 3 points; for each (c), 2 points; and for each (d), 1 point.

If you scored between 25 and 40, you're way up there among the anxious types. (Don't be embarrassed; I scored 25!) A score of 20 to 24 is average. Below 20 means that anxiety is not your issue.

If you found yourself on the high side, remember that most people are not like us. Anxiety is part of life, yes. But most people experience an anxious moment and then it quickly ends once the "stressor" has been removed. We are the catastrophizors, eking out the anxiety for long periods.

Many professionals have found that one of the most successful techniques for dealing with anxiety is thought stopping, which is described earlier in this chapter as a "stress buster."

7

Chronic Back Pain: A Family Affair

H alf a century ago, a daring American physician by the name of Henry Richardson wrote a book called *Patients Have Families*. Today, you might scratch your head and wonder why a world-class researcher would dedicate himself to such an obvious theme. In 1945, however, Richardson's ideas were considered radical. "Patients," he suggested, "have families: hospitals have patients: therefore hospitals have something to do with families."

PATIENTS HAVE FAMILIES

Today, it's pretty well universally accepted that medical ailments, particularly ongoing problems like chronic back pain, have an important impact on the families of those who suffer — in some instances, as much as on the patients themselves. Needless to say, this impact is usually negative. Consider the following research findings:

- A higher-than-normal percentage of children who grow up in households where a parent suffers from chronic pain end up suffering from chronic pain themselves when they reach adulthood.

- High numbers of men and women who are married to chronic back pain sufferers eventually develop chronic ailments; these spouses also tend to suffer from depression, anxiety, and fatigue more often than normal.

- Divorce rates in "chronic pain families" are significantly higher than the national average. To boot, health-care professionals who counsel such families say that many couples who do stay together only do so because of strong cultural and/or religious beliefs. They live as husband and wife in the technical sense, but their relationship no longer provides the love and support both partners were expecting when they took their marriage vows. Chronic pain is like a wall that has come between them.

This picture is certainly a sad one. However, many studies indicate that counseling frequently helps chronic pain families find better ways to cope, especially when the therapy involves not just the pain sufferer but also the spouse and, when appropriate, the children. But there is little agreement about what type of therapy is most effective; in the real world, social workers and psychologists rely on experience, gut feelings, and a variety of techniques, depending on the needs and circumstances of the family they are dealing with at the time.

After five decades of research and soul-searching by caring, intelligent professionals, there are still no clear-cut solutions. The most obvious reason is that families are enormously complicated. They operate as systems, and, as is true of every system, any action on the part of one member affects every other member. After a while, there can be so many actions and reactions that it's incredibly hard, even for a trained therapist, to distinguish between cause and effect.

In some instances, chronic pain is like a crutch that enables families to hide from other problems. In a situation like this, a therapist is faced with the proverbial question: "Which came first, the chicken or the egg?" In other words, which problems existed before chronic pain descended upon the family? Were family members actually part of the reason why someone's acute pain turned into a chronic problem? Or did most of the problems begin as a result of one member's chronic pain?

To predict the best way of helping a particular patient learn to cope with something as stressful as chronic pain is tough enough; add to the pot the needs and personalities of several other family members, and the challenge can sometimes feel like *Mission Impossible*.

How families cope depends on how well their members are able, among other skills, to communicate, solve problems, and change roles — roles that, in many cases, have been established for years. In turn, these sorts of skills depend on so many other factors that it would be impossible to list them all, let alone unravel the "fabric" they create. A few examples are: family members' own experiences with pain; cultural heritage; support from outside sources; a sense of control — or victimhood.

But there is another, even more complex, aspect to consider. This has to do with the difference between acute pain, which is time-limited, and chronic pain, which goes on and on (see Chapter 5). It is almost always true that back pain sufferers — and their families — start out believing that a back problem is temporary. It is only when, months later, the pain has not subsided, that reality starts to sink in: There may never be a total cure. More often than not this realization takes place slowly over a confusing period of time.

During this time it is common — and, indeed, reasonable — for people to feel frustrated, vulnerable, and angry. As well, not all of the members of a family will come to terms with reality at the same time. Sometimes one person is able to face up to the grim truth, while others are still in what professionals call **denial**, refusing to admit there is a problem. While some members begin to look for positive ways of adapting, others devote their time and energy to the search for a nonexistent cure.

When different people are at different stages, communication typically flies out the window. When they don't know what to do, or what to say, some people say nothing. Others yell and scream. In still other families, communication continues, but it is so indirect that no one knows what the others really mean, or feel. Everyone walks on eggshells. Perhaps they even know that they are doing this but have no idea how to change.

Take, as an example, the wife of a chronic back pain sufferer who is wondering whether it would be a good idea to encourage her husband to resume some of his old chores. Maybe it's pretty clear to her that, when he mopes around the house doing nothing, he just becomes more depressed. On the other hand, if she pushes him to take out the garbage or shovel the walk, the effort may cause his pain to increase. If it does, will he blame her? At the same time, not participating in the marriage as an equal partener is terrible for his sense of self-esteem. In the end, she may feel that it's easier (just this once!) to put out the garbage herself. But of course, this solicitous gesture solves nothing.

It's also a sad fact that, when it comes to chronic pain, modern medicine can sometimes be part of the problem, rather than part of the solution.

When we are ill or injured, we expect a health-care professional to make a diagnosis and prescribe a treatment that will return us to the state we were in before the problem reared its ugly head. That's what health-care professionals generally expect to happen as well.

During the recovery period, the patient's job is to follow doctor's orders and tough it out; the family's role is to pick up, for the short haul, the extra burden the ailment has placed in their paths. When it's successful, this model is a fine one; in most cases, families find ways of pulling together, and sometimes they even end up feeling closer for having shared a difficult experience.

The trouble is, this model doesn't always work. A classic example of a situation where it breaks down is when back pain becomes chronic. For one thing, even coming to the realization that this is their situation is tough for most families. When is the right time for patients and their families to set aside their hopes for a total cure? Whose job is it to deliver such depressing news? In most cases, there is no obvious moment. Rather, the transition occurs over a period of time.

It would be helpful if the family physician could sit them all down and explain — as gently, but as clearly, as possible — what's happening. Some health-care professionals, however, feel uncomfortable about being the messenger of such news; they see it as their personal failure. Unfortunately, teaching future doctors how to handle these sorts of issues is not a high priority at our medical schools.

On the positive side, many chronic pain families who are having trouble do seek help and find solutions. Ironically, in many cases, when a family learns new ways of coping, the intensity of the pain also begins to decrease — the vicious cycle is broken.

It is also true that chronic back pain sufferers who are married tend to function better, and suffer less from depression, than those whose marriages fall apart. That fact alone is good enough reason to take up the challenge and run with it. Okay, walk with it! To help you along, I've included some practical advice from experienced therapists Louise Koepfler and Barry Brown.

Can a Family Help Too Much?
LOUISE KOEPFLER

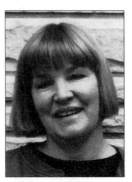

Louise Koepfler,
Psychologist, Scarborough
Health Recovery Clinic

In some families, it's the norm to rally around a member who is suffering from back pain. No one even thinks of questioning the extent of the injury, or suggests that being anything but 100 percent supportive is the right way to act. Now, in some situations — for instance, when someone is going through a bout of acute pain — this kind of unconditional support is really helpful. But when it comes to chronic pain, unconditional support can sometimes do more harm than good.

Let me give you an example. Recently, I was seeing a woman who had been involved in a minor car accident. Three years later, she was depressed and suicidal. She couldn't sleep. She was in extreme pain and she was exhibiting what therapists call "pain behavior" — a lot of moaning, groaning, and grimacing. To put it bluntly, she was a real basket case.

She came to talk to me quite a number of times. After a while, I came to see that she was really a lovely lady. She was in her late fifties with grown-up kids. She lived in one half of a duplex and one of her daughters occupied the other part. She had raised her kids successfully as a single parent, worked hard, and managed on her own in a culture where this was unusual for a woman. Then she had this minor accident and everything fell apart.

When she had had this injury, her kids had said to each other, "Hey! Mom took care of us all these years. Now it's our turn." To a certain extent, the mother had also embraced the idea that it was the kids' turn. On the surface this made good sense. But finally, I had tell to them, "Look! You're killing her with kindness." With the very best of intentions, they had taken away everything — her independence, all her little jobs, her activities — and along with it, her self-esteem. Then, after three years of inactivity, doing anything increased her pain — and her complaints.

When I suggested they could help more by helping less, intellectually, her kids could understand what I was talking about. But it was very difficult for them to learn how to say, "I know it hurts but do it, it's good for you." On top of it all, I couldn't assure them that, if they supported what I was suggesting, their mom would get rid of her pain. All I could say was that she wouldn't be so limited, and wouldn't feel so useless — and that in many cases, being active and feeling valuable causes pain to decrease.

In order to be able to make these kinds of demands on a chronic pain sufferer — and to understand when not to — families need to have some knowledge. People are afraid, especially when it comes to back pain, that if they demand activity it may injure the patient more. But backs really are resilient; the majority of people are not at risk when they do normal, everyday things. Their pain may increase at first, but eventually the downward spiral will usually begin to reverse itself.

There's another thing. If you suffer from chronic pain, it's not helpful to moan and groan. First of all, it causes you to focus on your pain. This makes you look disabled, which, in turn, causes the people around you to respond to you as an invalid. Studies also show that constantly talking about pain, and exhibiting pain behaviors, causes the human body to gear up physically. Heart rate and muscle tension increase. The brain thinks you are under siege, and reacts by producing pain — real pain — as a warning.

You can try this and see for yourself. Sit back in your chair and think about the most painful experience you've ever had — say, at the dentist. You will probably feel yourself tensing up as your brain relives the memory.

I've also dealt with the opposite scenario: people who hate to complain and so say nothing even when they are miserable. One woman I counseled talked about going out for dinner with her husband and sitting for two hours having a terrible time. On top of it, she said "yes" when he asked her if she would go to hear a jazz band after supper. She hated jazz! Eventually, she learned that she could give her husband information about how she was feeling without necessarily complaining — and that it was possible to arrive at a mutually satisfactory middle ground.

When people are flexible, they can change roles and still keep their self-esteem. By doing this, families can stay bonded. Rigid families, on the other hand, tend to get into ruts.

Helping the Whole Family
BARRY BROWN

It's embarrassing to think how little we do for chronic pain families. We are supposed to be an evolved society. Counseling is not a new thing. We have put men on the moon. And yet, we don't automatically teach people how to listen to family members, understand how they feel, and respond to those feelings in a calm and thoughtful fashion — particularly when a

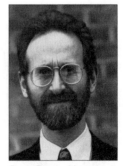

Barry Brown, Marriage Counselor and Chronic Pain Therapist, Toronto

family has the added stress of trying to cope with chronic pain.

Sometimes, when I'm trying to illustrate how families work — all families, not just those with a member who suffers from chronic pain — I use the example of a mobile. Each family member is one of the pieces, and if you touch one piece, all of them move. It's a system.

If one member of a family changes significantly after six months of chronic back pain, other family members will feel the effects of his change and react to it. It's a reciprocal process. And it can get very complicated.

Here's an example: I suffer from chronic back pain. I've had the whole day to sit around feeling useless and think about nothing except my pain and how everyone else has a life and a purpose. My wife walks in at suppertime and asks me how my day went and I bark at her, "How the hell do you think it went?" She's had a hard day and she yells back. I get doubly upset and yell even louder. The point is, once a downward spiral like this gets started, it's difficult to put a stop to it. And it's even more difficult if, for instance, my wife has no idea whether she did something to upset me, or if I yelled because of the pain. My family can't read my mind.

This sort of thing happens more often than you'd think. If an individual who is in pain for a prolonged period of time doesn't understand what's happening to her (say it's a her — it could be anyone, of course), and is beginning to wonder if there will ever be an end to it, she's likely to become what professionals call "egocentric." It makes sense. She's frustrated, fed up, embarrassed, not very aware of what's going on around her, and probably not all that interested. She is focused almost entirely on herself.

As time goes on, her ability to cope with stress — any kind of stress — decreases. Her sense of hope becomes eroded along with her dignity; in its place is shame. She's worried sick and she's angry. And, quite unintentionally, she hurts the people she cares about most.

Unfortunately, teaching people how to vent their frustration in a way that's appropriate, rather than hurtful, is not part of what our health-care system automatically offers. As a therapist, I try to fill that gap.

To even begin to deal with this kind of problem, first, and foremost, people need a calm, safe forum. It can be their own home, but many families find it easier to address problems in a counselor's office. It's more difficult to be emotionally explosive when you're in a professional setting!

Generally, I start by talking to the chronic pain sufferer. I need to find out how he or she feels as an individual, as a spouse, and as a parent. Then I generally like to talk to the family members — sometimes together, sometimes separately. What I'm trying to get a sense of is what has changed.

Sometimes, I learn that the family is more or less coping, at least to some degree. But more often, the spouse — say the wife — feels like she's married to someone she doesn't know anymore. Her husband doesn't go to work, is withdrawn, doesn't communicate, no longer pursues hobbies, doesn't participate in anything with her. There is little intellectual or emotional expression to let her know he cares. Sexual intimacy is too often sporadic at best. To put it bluntly, they are living parallel lives.

This guy has to ask himself if his family deserves what he is dishing out, and if there's a better way. Yes, he has a right to be frustrated and angry; he didn't ask for this pain. But the point is, if he can look at his life and estimate the value of it — say, out of ten — he will have to conclude that, while he is down three parts, he still has seven out of ten left.

The question is, what is he going to do with that seven? He can continue to vent his frustration onto his family, reduce what he's got left to five and maybe lose them in the process — or he can accept his losses, refocus, and learn to adapt. I'm not saying that accepting and refocusing is easy. I'm just saying that the alternative is worse.

I try to explain to couples that marriage is like a three-legged race. If one hurts the other, that partner will fall; but the one causing the hurt will also stumble. I try to provide "mental tools" one can use to reduce anxiety.

At the same time, the family members of chronic pain patients need to know, and accept, that they are people too. They have rights and they have to take care of their own needs. It's essential for them to understand the nature of the chronic pain problem, as well as what kinds of activities will actually cause harm as opposed to a temporary increase in pain. They also have to learn to encourage and reward what therapists call "well behavior."

People must also understand the difference between being in pain and being disabled. Chronic pain sufferers can still function, even if it's not at the same level as before. And just about all of them find that they feel better when they do.

GOT THE GIFT OF THE GAB?

If the relationship between two adults in a family is strong and loving, there's a good chance that the family will work well as a whole. It's also a good bet that the family will be able to find ways of coping successfully with one member's chronic back pain.

On the other hand, some couples discover that they are living in different worlds. One partner is extremely dissatisfied with the relationship, while the other partner is not even aware that a problem exists. In these families, chronic pain can be the straw that breaks the camel's back.

How well do you and your partner communicate? Are you both satisfied? A number of years ago, Dr. David Olson, a family social science professor at the University of Minnesota, realized that many couples weren't sure — especially when it came to the happiness of their better half.

To help them find out, he developed several questionnaires. The one provided here has been adapted for couples where one member suffers from chronic back pain. Try our questionnaire, one person at a time. (If you're going second, no peeking at the responses of your partner!)

It's normal for partners to have different scores; no two people, after all, think exactly alike. However, if one partner's score is 29 or less, or if both scores are 34 or less, it should be taken as a signal that something is amiss.

How Well Do You Communicate?

RESPONSE CHOICES				
1 Definitely false	**2** Usually false	**3** Neither true nor false	**4** Usually true	**5** Definitely true

PARTNER A		PARTNER B
_____	1. It's very easy for me to express my true feelings about back pain to my partner.	_____
_____	2. When we are having a problem, my partner often gives me the silent treatment.	_____
_____	3. My partner sometimes makes comments that put me down.	_____
_____	4. Sometimes I am afraid to ask my partner for what I want.	_____
_____	5. I wish my partner were more willing to share his/her feelings with me.	_____
_____	6. Sometimes I have trouble believing everything my partner tells me.	_____
_____	7. Often, I don't tell my partner how my back is feeling because he/she should just know. (or: Often my partner doesn't tell me.)	_____
	8. I am very satisfied with how my partner and I talk with each other.	
_____	9. I don't always share negative feelings I have about my partner because I'm afraid he/she will get angry.	_____
_____	10. My partner is always a good listener.	_____

SCORING		
A. _____	Add your choices for items 1, 8 & 10 – insert the total on line A.	_____ A.
B. +42	Add 42	+42 B.
C. _____	Subtotal – add lines A & B.	_____ C.
D. _____	Add your choices for items 2, 3, 4, 5, 6, 7 & 9 – insert total on line D.	_____ D.
E. _____	Subtract line D from line C to get your final score.	_____ E.

FINAL SCORES
40 or more: You feel understood and are able to share your feelings with your partner.
35 – 40: You feel generally understood and can share most of your feelings with your partner.
30 – 34: You are not comfortable sharing many of your feelings with your partner.
29 or less: You do not feel your partner understands you and you rarely share your feelings with him/her.

This questionnaire is reproduced with the kind permission of Dr. David Olson.

8

Medication for Pain

Before I get down to the sad facts about drugs and back pain, I'd like to share an amusing but extremely embarrassing story of what happened to me a few years ago due to a side effect of a painkiller that I was taking. I've decided to 'fess up because the story illustrates how even a knowledgeable back pain sufferer — that's me! — will sometimes ignore a label.

DO AS I SAY, NOT AS I DO!

Here's the background. I had just spent three days shoveling eight cubic yards of Triple Mix into my garden. To put it mildly, I was in agony.

Generally, I try to stay away from painkillers. (If you suffer from chronic back pain, you can't go taking drugs all the time. They simply stop working unless you keep upping the dose, as I'll discuss later in this chapter.) This time, however, because I had to go to Montreal to interview a couple of people, I had appealed to my family physician and he had prescribed a relatively new brand of analgesic that would kill the pain without making me drowsy.

So, here I am in Montreal. My first interview has been a great success and I am at a lovely little Algerian restaurant relaxing over a lamb couscous and a glass of white wine. With me is Karla Minello, my sophisticated colleague from Whitehall-Robins, the Back Association of Canada's (BAC's) stalwart corporate supporter. The restaurant, which is owned by a refugee from Algeria, has a total of eight tables — a good thing, since this guy is a one-man band: chef, maître d', waiter, bus boy, and . . . well, you'll see.

All of a sudden — *tout à coup* — a crown that has been covering the stump of my knocked-out front tooth for twenty years plummets onto my plate. And it does so in French, *merde alors*, since *français* is the language of the evening. (Mine, you could say, is passable.)

Suddenly I have a fuzzy memory of the label on my pill vial. Dimly, I recall the gist of it: *deux vers de vin* will feel like *quatre vers de vin* while I'm taking this drug, and I have just finished my second glass of Chardonnay. The fact is, I am tipsy. Quite tipsy. And the up-till-now dull ache in my back is definitely reacting to this stressful situation. It is very quickly picking up steam.

What to do? I clamp my hand over my mouth and, in my best ventriloquist's voice, I tell Karla, "Ah . . . *j'ai un problème avec un de mes dents. Je m'excuse . . . pour un instant."* I get up and lurch off to the loo. Only I make a mistake — the first of several, as you will soon come to understand.

I go into the men's washroom.

I stand in front of the mirror and gaze at my fuzzy features. Then I try to figure out how to stick my crown — *ma couronne* — back into place until I can get some Crazy Glue to tide me over until I fly home. I'm wiggling the darn thing into position, and the whole time I am saying to myself: "Self! Whatever you do, don't drop this bloody $500 *couronne* down the drain."

Thunk.

My crown is now in the S-trap of a Montreal drain. The only positive thing I can think of is that my last French lesson was based on the bathroom; at least I know the French word for sink (*lavabo*) and for drain (*tuyau*).

By this time it has also hit me that no medication on earth could be a match for such stress. My lumbar spine is killing me!

Well, I can laugh or I can cry, right? I choose the former and go back to the table giggling like a lunatic. I explain the problem to Karla, we call over the chef/maître d', and, somehow, I describe my predicament. The diners at the next table prick up their ears.

It seems that I am in luck. *"Pas de problème!"* says the chef. "Before I was a refugee, I was an ENGINEER! I can rescue your *couronne* . . . but you'll have to wait until I cook the couscous for the next table!"

With a flourish, he hangs an "Out of Order" sign on the door of the men's room, then heads back to his kitchen. I reach for the bottle of wine.

Ten minutes later, he emerges with a pair of pliers that look more like tweezers. He regards them forlornly, admitting, "I think this may not do the trick. But," he adds, "I can go to the hardware store. They open at ten in the morning."

I shake my head vigorously. No way. My second interview is at NINE the next morning. And I am in total agony.

It is now midnight. Karla hauls out the *Yellow Pages* and we start calling plumbers.

At 12:30 we find one who is not sleeping or drinking wine. For $103, he will come to Chez Berber and fish out my *couronne*. In two seconds flat, I am as sober as a judge. I promise to pay. Karla and I count up our cash. Between us we have $110.

At 12:50 *le plombier* arrives. He goes to work and, in less than a minute, hands me my precious crown. I go back to the loo — the ladies' loo — where I wash the thing out and arrange a temporary fitting. He and Karla finish the Chardonnay.

As for me, I grab a cab, go back to my hotel, crawl into bed, and take another pill. Maybe two.

But let this be a lesson to you! If you are taking medication for an acute bout of back pain, it's your responsibility to find out what side effects may be looming in the wings. Do as I say . . . not as I do!

THE POSSIBILITY OF DEPENDENCE

At a meeting of the Canadian Medical Association way back in 1981, doctors were asked which problems they found most difficult to treat. Almost without exception, they mentioned drug dependency. Physicians whose practices included a lot of patients with chronic back pain talked specifically about painkillers.

Today, a decade and a half later, medical science has learned an amazing amount about analgesics, which is the medical term for painkillers. We understand a lot more about the effects these drugs have on the human brain. We are also more knowledgeable about nondrug therapies such as acupuncture, massage, biofeedback, and the various relaxation techniques that decrease muscle tension. And yet, the situation has not really improved. Drug dependency is still the family physician's nightmare, and a recent study conducted at the University of Toronto confirms that at least half of the people these physicians prescribe drugs for don't take them as directed. (The study also estimates that this lack of compliance costs the Canadian health-care system $9 billion a year!)

Dr. Jan Dowsling is the medical consultant at Toronto's Jean Tweed Centre, a facility that helps women who are trying to kick a drug habit. Many of Dr. Dowsling's clients are dependent upon alcohol or illegal drugs such as cocaine. Over the years she has also treated many people who have become dependent on the drugs they take for chronic pain.

"These people," she says, "are the most difficult to help. They start taking drugs — *legal* drugs — for legitimate reasons. Then the amount gets out of control. You can take away the medication and you can help them go through the physical symptoms of withdrawal. And, like patients who are dependent on other types of drugs, they will recover from that. But they are still left with the problem that drove them to take the drug in the first place: chronic pain. It's a terrible dilemma for both physicians and patients."

If you take an analgesic for chronic pain, the amount can easily get out of control. This is because, over time, human beings develop what is called **tolerance**. This means that the normal dose no longer does the trick. In order to suppress the pain, you need to increase the dose, and then increase it again.

Dr. Dowsling recalls one patient who was suffering from severe arthritis. She had been taking Demerol, a strong painkiller, for months. Generally, for an acute bout of pain, the maximum daily dose of Demerol is four tablets, and the drug is not usually prescribed for more than ten days. But in order to get any relief at all, this woman had to take eight or ten pills per day, and even this enormous amount was no longer completely effective.

But concern about what seventy pills a week might be doing to her body and soul was not what drove her to seek help. Nor was it the loss of a method of pain relief that she used to be able to count on for particularly bad days. What happened was that her doctor refused to increase her prescription.

"Supply problems are the number one reason why drug abusers of any kind finally seek help," says Dr. Dowsling, adding that most people who take painkillers do not turn to the street when their doctors finally refuse to increase their prescription.

How and why human beings develop tolerance to drugs is a fascinating subject. As is true of most physical reactions, the survival instinct plays a role.

Dr. Harold Kalant, who does research in this area at the University of Toronto, explains the mechanism. "When people use a drug — any drug — they do it because it makes them feel better. Either it relieves something distressful, such as pain or anxiety, or it gives them a sense of well-being. When a particular substance produces a good feeling — medical science uses the term "reward" — the chances that the person will repeat the behavior increase. Particular chemicals that are produced in the brain are responsible for this phenomenon."

In most cases, it is a good thing that your body has a built-in reward system. Because food is rewarding, you are driven to seek it out, and as a result, you don't starve. The fact that sex is pleasurable ensures that mankind survives, and that *your* offspring are a part of it.

Painkillers touch off the same reward system. In this case it is the reduction of pain, which feels awfully good when you are suffering from a bad back. However, where painkillers are concerned, another survival mechanism tends to gum up the works.

Your body usually produces pain for a very good reason. Pain tells us that something is wrong, or dangerous. You put your finger on a hot stove, and pain causes you to withdraw your finger even before you are aware of it. (See Chapter 5.) Likewise, when a certain movement causes your back to hurt, the pain is a warning sign. It tells you to take a break from the activity so that your back can have a chance to heal.

And what has all this to do with tolerance? "When an analgesic causes a nerve cell to become less sensitive to pain," explains Dr. Kalant, "the nerve cell tries to do something about it, since it thinks it is producing pain for a good reason. What it does is compensate by increasing its sensitivity. The result is that it takes a higher dose to suppress the same amount of pain."

Let's use as an example a woman who has a bulging disc. After a couple of hours of gardening, her back will start to hurt. But she loves to garden and so, at the end of May, she starts taking a couple of painkillers — say Tylenol 1 with codeine — at around noon. For a while, these pills do the trick; she can garden until mid-afternoon without much discomfort. But by July, the pills are about as useful as the water she takes them with. And so she ups the dose to three. By August, four tablets do nothing for her back pain, not to mention the fact that all this codeine is making her constipated. The trouble is, when she cuts down, her back hurts even more than it did before. She has developed both tolerance and physical dependence.

But just because your body develops tolerance to a drug in a physical sense does not necessarily mean that you are addicted. **Addiction** involves both physical dependence and psychological need.

Most people don't realize this. When we think about drug addicts, we imagine people who get the shakes when they stop taking illegal drugs, or huge quantities of alcohol. "That's a popular misconception," says Dr. Kalant, "because, in fact, the essence of addiction is behavioral as much as it is physical."

In other words, addiction has to do with how a person acts because of a drug — how the drug actually controls that person's behavior. Yes, addiction is physical; addicted people can have violent physical reactions when their drugs are taken away. But addiction also has to do with being obsessed: people who are addicted do things they wouldn't ordinarily do in order to get more of the drug they crave. "You can't separate the two concepts," says Dr. Kalant.

Say a man is in hospital after a serious car accident, and he is given injections of the painkiller morphine. If the pain lasts long enough, he may become physically dependent on the drug, and his body will have developed tolerance. But this does not mean he is addicted.

"When the drug is withdrawn," explains Dr. Kalant, "he will feel lousy. He may also suffer through the symptoms that are associated with physical dependency — chills, stomach upset, general malaise. But he will wait until these symptoms subside rather than going out to find more morphine. In order to be addicted, you have to play an *active* role in the taking of the drug. The body's reward system must be stimulated by a behavior that you yourself perform."

The key to addiction is the link between a certain behavior (taking a drug) and a certain feeling (the stimulation of the body's reward system). Back in the 1940s a group of American researchers at the U.S. Public Health Service Hospital first discovered the power of this link. They were working with heroin addicts who had been given the option to either kick their habit or go to jail. They chose the former, and so the motivation to stay off drugs was very high. After a couple of years, both the patients and their physicians believed that the program had been successful. The former addicts were normal in the physical sense and they said that they had no desire to go back to their old ways.

And yet, many of those who returned to their former environments took up the drug again, often within a few hours. When they met their old cronies and found themselves in the same doorway where they used to take drugs, they felt the same old urge to repeat the behavior — even after two years. They were like Pavlov's dogs, who salivated every time their trainer rang the bell.

As Dr. Dowsling explained at the beginning of this chapter, the same can be said for chronic pain patients who are hooked on painkillers. Even after someone breaks the physical dependence, the pain is still there, ringing that bell. And when the bell rings, people tend to reach for the bottle of painkillers. There is an emotional link between the two.

The best solution, of course, is prevention. But many drug-dependent chronic pain sufferers do get off the drugs they are dependent upon and turn their lives around.

"They somehow learn ways of walking through their pain," says Dr. Dowsling. "They learn to use nondrug alternatives to help them live alongside of their pain rather than in it. It's a tough concept to explain. It has to do with learning how to externalize pain. You feel the pain and it hurts; the difference is that it doesn't drive you around the bend."

Unfortunately, family physicians who prescribe most of the analgesics that chronic pain sufferers take do not get a lot of training in these areas. "Doctors come through medical school and, if they are lucky, they probably spend a month in a pain clinic," says Dr. Dowsling. As well, working on these concepts with patients takes time. It's difficult for a doctor who has fifteen patients in the waiting room to spend an hour talking to a person who is suffering from chronic pain. Nor does the health-care system compensate doctors adequately for taking this kind of time.

"I think that is why a lot of the nonmedical folks are starting to work in this area," says Dr. Dowsling. Let's hope this means that, for those of us who suffer from chronic back pain, the gap will soon be filled.

Kicking the Painkiller Habit

Strong painkillers taken on a regular basis are not the answer for people who suffer from chronic back pain. For one thing, painkillers are addictive. As well, there is a lot of evidence that, for many people, the pills they pop don't even provide much relief. Some studies show that placebos (fake pills) work just as well.

And yet, many chronic back pain patients do take prescription painkillers for years. Eventually, they end up with two problems: a back problem and a drug dependency problem. In many cases, the second problem is as bad as, or worse than, the first.

But what is the best way to kick a drug habit? This is the big question that researchers have been trying to answer for a long time.

A number of years ago, Dr. Harold Gottlieb, a psychologist from the Casa Colina Hospital for Rehabilitative Medicine in Pomona, California, tried a new approach with a group of chronic back pain sufferers who were in his rehabilitation program. The men and women in the study were all addicted to painkillers. In order to help them kick their habit, he put them in charge of their own medication: the patients themselves had to decide how much medication they'd take, and when. The idea was to see if people could reduce their dependency on drugs if they played an active role in their own treatment. And it worked!

First, the patients were taught about drugs: how they work, why they are addictive, and how drugs can change a person's emotional state. In addition, they were taught nondrug ways of coping with pain and reducing stress. These methods included self-hypnosis and biofeedback.

At the beginning of the week, the patients were given all the medication they generally took for seven days. They were asked to keep a strict record of what pills they took and when. In addition, they were encouraged to talk to their fellow patients. Within a few weeks, most of them learned that taking fewer drugs, less often, worked better than they thought.

In fact, after six months, almost 70 percent of the patients were taking no prescription painkillers at all, just the occasional over-the-counter ASA or acetaminophin tablet. Even more encouraging was that, a year after the program had ended, less than 6 percent had increased their drug use once again. And most of them were back on the job.

Who were these patients? When they entered the program, more than 90 percent of them were unemployed. On the average, they had been disabled for four and a half years! Many were suffering from depression and anxiety. They were not a group of people for whom success would have been predicted.

Dr. Gottlieb believes that the method works because it takes control away from the health-care professional and gives it back to the patient, with whom it belongs.

"When the patients were in control, they felt less helpless and less angry about their situation," he explains. "They also felt less like victims, and this gave them the confidence to succeed."

At the end of five years, Dr. Gottlieb contacted most of the patients who had been in the original group. "We expected that some of them would have gone back to using medications. But very few had." In fact, approximately 65 percent of the people were still off strong painkillers. They continued to use nondrug methods to control their pain. And they were still employed.*

---

*   Dr. Gottlieb's study, which was called "Self-Management for Medication Reduction in Chronic Low Back Pain," was published in the June 1988 issue of Archives of Physical Medicine Rehabilitation.

DRUG DEPENDENCE — COULD IT HAPPEN TO YOU?

When used properly and appropriately, medication saves lives, decreases pain and increases the well-being of mankind. It's not my intention to focus only on the negative aspects of medication. But the possibility of dependence should be taken seriously. If you take medication for your back pain on a regular basis, have a look at the questions that follow. If you must answer "yes" to any of them, it's time to do some serious thinking. Consult your doctor if you even suspect you may be heading toward dependence.

- Have you ever lied to your doctor in order to get your prescription renewed a bit sooner? Example: "My purse was stolen along with my medication."
- Have you ever spent time thinking up schemes to get another prescription? Example: Your family physician is out of town, so you use the opportunity to call your specialist.
- Do you sometimes take pain medication because you are feeling lousy in general, rather than because your back really hurts?
- Have you ever increased your dose (just this once!) with the excuse that your pain is doubly bad?
- Do you sometimes drink alcohol while you are on medication, even

though you are aware that alcohol increases the effects of pain-killing drugs?

- Have you ever promised that you will cut down on the amount, or frequency of a drug, in the future — but not now because at this particular moment, you are under a lot of stress?
- Do you sometimes suspend your judgment for the few seconds it takes to swallow a pill? (Not sure what this means? Think of the "not totally there" feeling you experience when you put your brain on hold, then eat a piece of chocolate cake.)

DRUG BASICS

Now that we've discussed all the dangers of taking drugs, let me stress once again that they can play a valuable role in controlling back pain if used safely under the supervision of a good physician.

More than a hundred different kinds of medication exist for back pain — I certainly can't tell you everything about all of them here. But I've outlined the four major categories of drugs prescribed for back pain sufferers below, along with a discussion of some important concerns. For more detailed information about specific drugs, see the chart on pages C1–C6.

Main Types of Medication

Analgesics primarily relieve pain. They may be classified as **narcotics**, which act on the brain to reduce the perception of pain (and therefore pose a risk of tolerance and dependence), and **non-narcotics**, which act at the site of the pain to reduce the stimulation of the nerve endings. The two types are sometimes combined. Some analgesics also decrease inflammation.

Non-steroidal anti-inflammatory drugs (NSAIDs) relieve pain, stiff-ness, and inflammation in bones, muscles, and joints. They do not cure the problem, but provide relief from symptoms by blocking chemicals called prostaglandins that are released at the site of an injury.

Always take NSAIDs with food or water, and avoid lying down for fifteen minutes afterward so the drug can reach your stomach. Be aware that long-term use of NSAIDs can increase the risk of gastrointestinal problems. They may also increase or prolong bleeding, so discuss their use with your doctor if you are expecting to undergo surgery. Discuss any allergies you may have to ASA or other NSAIDs with your doctor before taking them.

If you have been taking NSAIDs for more than three weeks, do not stop suddenly — consult your doctor. Also call your doctor immediately if, while on NSAIDs, you encounter black or blood-stained stools, unexplained wheezing, or breathlessness. Note that steroids, such as cortisone, Prednisone, and dexamethasone are prescribed for back pain in rare cases.

Muscle relaxants reduce spasm and tension in muscles as well as pain. They are sometimes combined with analgesics. Most work by slowing down the signals from the brain that cause muscles to contract. In the same category are **anti-anxiety drugs** (minor tranquilizers), which can also be used to relax muscles. Most have a strong sedative effect.

Antidepressants are sometimes taken in low doses to relax muscles, reduce pain, and aid sleep. Monoamine oxydase inhibitors (MAOIs) may help people who are anxious as well as depressed, but they are rarely used these days because of their side effects.

Things to Watch Out For

If you do take medication, or are considering a treatment that includes drug therapy, it's important to understand a few concerns.

All drugs produce certain reactions. That's why we take them! Most drugs also produce other, unwanted, symptoms as well; these are commonly called side effects. Some side effects occur in a large number of patients who take a certain drug; others occur very rarely. Examples of common side effects include dizziness, an upset stomach, or a rash. Side effects often increase for patients over the age of sixty.

Some factors may make it risky for you to take a certain drug. These factors are known as **contraindications** (*contra* means "against.") For example, if you have a heart condition, it may be risky for you to take a particular type of NSAID. It's important for your doctor to know your medical history so he or she is aware of any possible contraindications.

The drug chart on pages C1–C6 alerts you to the major side effects and contraindications associated with specific back pain drugs.

Another concern to be aware of is that if you take a drug over a period of time, you may develop tolerance. Tolerence and addiction are discussed in detail earlier in this chapter.

If you have any questions about any of these concerns and how they relate to your medication, be sure to bring them up with your doctor.

IV

HELPING YOURSELF: POSTURE, FITNESS, AND EXERCISE

9

The Sitting Back

If you're like most people I know, lousy posture is the last thing you want to hear about when you're in the middle of an acute bout of back pain. Of course you know that good posture is better for your back than bad posture. Who doesn't? You probably even know that sitting (particularly in a poorly designed chair) strains the discs of your lower back — far more, in fact, than standing. But if I were to insist that something as seemingly innocuous as posture is ultimately responsible for the agony you are in, you'd probably think I'd gone mad.

Well, I haven't gone mad. According to many health-care professionals, poor posture *does* cause most back pain in that it hastens the normal degeneration process. What's more, a growing number of researchers are starting to produce an impressive amount of information to support this opinion. When they talk about posture, however, these scientists are referring to something a lot more complex than you probably imagine. In fact, in order to grasp the essence of it, I had to change my concept of what posture means, as well as how it affects human backs, almost entirely.

A few years ago, my definition of good posture went something like this: keeping your spine in its natural position (neither increasing nor decreasing its normal curves) when you are sitting, standing, or lying down. On a thoughtful day, I might have thrown in a sentence or two about the best posture to be in when you lift. But that would have been about it.

Now that I've been educated, I see the whole issue in quite a different light. Yes, posture has to do with the demands you place on your body when it is in various stationary positions. But how you use your body when *in motion* is as important a part of good posture as how you use it when you are still. Furthermore, our bodies — and, in particular, our spines — do not like to remain in one position for very long. While they hate to be thrown about, or wrenched beyond the normal range of their muscles, joints, and ligaments, human bodies do prefer to change positions frequently.

With those ideas in mind, here's my current definition of **good posture**: putting the least amount of stress on your body while it remains in, and moves through, thousands of positions and motions during the course of a day — in fact, during the course of your entire life. If you do this in stressful rather than efficient ways, the extra strain will hasten the normal degeneration process.

In this chapter, I will deal with various aspects of **static posture** — stationary positions, such as sitting or standing still. **Dynamic posture** involves the positions your body assumes whenever you're on the move; Chapter 10 is devoted to this topic.

YOU NEED A HORSE!

Before I get to the nuts and bolts of the chapter, though, I can't resist sharing an amusing story that took place while I was in the middle of sorting out my thoughts on this issue. (As you must have begun to realize by now, a lot of amusing things happen to me!) It all started when I came across a fascinating study performed in 1981 by a Swedish researcher, Dr. A. C. Mandal. Among other things, he had investigated the posture that people assume while they are riding a horse.

Have I got your attention?

Dr. Mandal pointed out what has been known — at least by some people — for decades: horseback riding is the perfect sitting posture from the standpoint of the human spine. Because the hip joints only bend to a 45-degree angle when you are sitting in the saddle (as opposed to a 90-degree angle in a regular chair), your low back can maintain its natural lordotic curve, almost effortlessly. The result is that, while you ride, there is far less strain on the discs of your lumbar spine.

But that's not the whole of it. Because of the way horses move when they walk, your back is also treated to a kind of gentle, rhythmic stretching motion that increases the mobility of your lumbar spine in every direction. As well, riding is a great way to stretch out tight hamstring muscles, which are a common problem among low back pain sufferers. This is important because it's virtually impossible to maintain your lumbar curve if your hamstrings are tight.

To put it mildly, I was intrigued by Dr. Mandal's research. For the next few days I talked "horse talk" to anyone who would listen. Well, you know how it is; soon stories about horseback riding and back pain started emerging from the woodwork.

For instance, I learned that horseback riding is an accepted form of therapy for people with certain kinds of disabilities, including multiple sclerosis. These patients suffer from severe **low back spasticity**, which is a condition that goes hand in hand with a flat lumbar spine — i.e., a lumbar spine that lacks its normal curve. After riding a horse, a great many of these people find that their spasticity has decreased and that the curve in their lumbar region has increased. What's more, this effect seems to last for a couple of days.

My horse obsession continued. Early one morning, I got a phone call from a guy in Gander, Newfoundland. He had a back problem and he was at his wit's end. His story went like this: Because of the nature of his work, and the fact that his "territory" spanned a large rural area, he was obliged to drive around for most of the day. Therefore, just for openers, he was sitting far more than was good for his back. He had no particular complaints about his vehicle — a Chevrolet Caprice — but the majority of the roads he drove on were unpaved and deeply rutted. From his description it seemed that the best suspension system on the planet wouldn't have helped his situation very much. The vibration was terrible, he said, but it was not as bad as the pain that coursed through his spine each time his car hit a bump. The image of him bouncing up and down was enough to send my own back into spasms of sympathy. But when he told me he was an officer for the Royal Canadian Mounted Police, something in my brain must have snapped!

"You're a Mountie!" I shrieked at him. "And you *drive* up and down unpaved, pot-holed roads in a *car*?" I took a moment to calm my voice, which had gone up several octaves. Then I read him the Riot Act: "What you need, *Sir*, is a horse!"

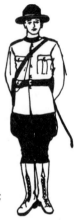

Well, not half bad one-liners notwithstanding, what this RCMP officer needed was a lot more than a horse. For one thing, Mounties — like all police officers — have more problems than most people who spend their days behind a wheel. To begin with, they pack a helluva lot of equipment: side arm; baton; radio; pepper spray; extra bullets; etc. It all hangs from a thick black belt and weighs about fifteen pounds. To make matters worse, police officers do paperwork and run a computer while sitting in their mobile "offices" — a setup that leaves them little option but to twist while they type. Furthermore, each time they get in and out of the car (which they do more often than most drivers) they twist — to the same side — again. Mounties in cars are crying out for their vehicles to have a better ergonomic design. But they can't take their belts off; nor are there many options for changing the location of the equipment they need.

How do I know all this? Because not too long after this guy from Gander called me, I got another call from the RCMP. This time it was Dr. Jeremy Brown, chief of the force's occupational health division. He was on the line to tell me that the RCMP was in the process of putting together a back injury prevention program for its 17,000 members; would the Back Association of Canada like to be involved? To make a long story short, I said we'd love to consult on an ad hoc basis, and, without so much as a handshake, a relationship was born.

Because the RCMP is a federal organization, it does not come under the jurisdiction of any of Canada's provincial health-care plans or workers' compensation boards. This, in my opinion, gives them two advantages over companies that must tow provincial lines! My bet is that their back injury prevention program will ultimately become a model for other employers. Ask me in a couple of years.

The Bambach Saddle Seat

In the midst of my horse obsession, a large envelope arrived from Steve Reinecke, the Vermont ergonomist who designed an amazing backrest called the BackCycler (see Chapter 11). I ripped it open with great gusto — and the photograph reproduced in Figure 9.1 fell out.

At first I thought Steve Reinecke had used some fancy software program to create this picture just to make me laugh. But it turns out that this chair actually exists. A number of years ago, an Australian occupational therapist named Mary Gale did some horseback riding work with several disabled patients. She was amazed that many of them could not sit unsupported in a regular chair but could ride a horse. From this experience, she asked herself an interesting question: if riding is so beneficial for the low back, might it be a good idea to make a saddle into a chair that ordinary back pain sufferers could use at their desks? Eventually, she joined forces with an engineer, built a model, and conducted a couple of small studies, with very positive results.

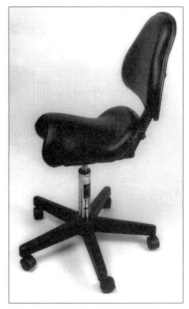

Figure 9.1 The Bambach Saddle Seat

In 1988, she presented her findings in Beijing, China, where she was attending an international ergonomics conference. An American occupational therapist was so impressed that she ordered ten chairs on the spot! That was enough to convince Mary Gale to start manufacturing and selling the Bambach Saddle Seat which, unfortunately, has not taken off as a money-making enterprise. Part of the problem is its hefty price tag: $720 (U.S.) (Mary faces the proverbial chicken-and-egg problem of small-volume sales and high prices.) As well, in order to use a saddle seat, you have to adjust your work station upward by several inches, which puts some people off. Nevertheless, Mary Gale continues to persevere, and the moment this book makes the bestseller list, I intend to become one of her customers!

For information on the Bambach Saddle Seat, write to: Andrew Smith, Customer Service, The Bambach Saddle Seat Pty. Limited, 752 Pittwater Road, Brookvale, NSW 2100, Australia.

Why Sit?

More and more studies are showing that sitting, especially for long periods of time, causes as much back pain as lifting or falls. Not very long ago, hardly anyone had heard of the science of designing products to fit the physical needs of the human body rather than the other way around. Today, **ergonomics** is a buzzword of the modern office.

Companies that sell ergonomic seating products (such as Steelcase Canada Inc., which made my ergonomic chair — Bob Taylor, Steelcase's director of seating, is my personal professor of ergonomics) claim that their seats can reduce back pain caused by poor sitting posture, which is certainly true. However, with regard to our backs, there is no perfect chair, and there never will be, because Mother Nature did not design human spines to sit still.

Sitting, and especially sitting in the same position for hours on end, is generally harder on your back than lying down, standing, and even lifting, assuming you lift wisely. One glance at a group of children at play makes it instantly obvious that, given the choice, human beings do not opt to sit. On the contrary, they prefer to change positions gently, fluidly, and constantly. The trouble is, we have built ourselves a world in which a huge number of tasks (entering data into a computer, writing this book, eating dinner) are done sitting down.

A well-designed chair is certainly a thousand times better for your back than a lousy one. But the bottom line is that, eventually, back pain tends to creep up on most people who sit a great deal of the time, no matter what they sit on.

The news gets worse before it gets better! Researchers have known about the evils of sitting for a long time. And yet, as a society, we are sitting more rather than less. Studies in the United States indicate that almost half of today's workforce is made up of people who sit for a large chunk of the work day. (It's a good bet that most of them also sit in cars, or buses, on their way to and from work.) This percentage is a lot higher than it was just a few decades ago, and the numbers are going up rather than down. Many back experts believe that the huge increase in back problems in recent years is related, at least in part, to this trend. (More on this at the end of this chapter.)

Why, if it's so hard on our backs, did we start sitting in the first place? There are several good reasons. For one thing, sitting is less demanding than standing in terms of aerobic energy. For another, when you sit, you take a load off your feet and legs. But the main attraction of the chair is that human bodies are more stable when they are sitting than when they are standing. Try threading a needle while you're on your feet and you'll quickly realize that vertical bodies have a tendency to sway.

For these reasons, sitting makes good sense. The trouble is, rather than striking a balance, it seems that mankind created the chair, then pounced on it as if it were the best invention since the wheel. Sitting has become a huge part of our culture, our language, and even our work ethic — as in, "Sit down and get to work!" In many situations, being productive is thought to go hand in hand with sitting still. When they fidget in their seats, students are accused of being inattentive. When they lean back in their chairs — a change that is, in fact, great for the back — many workers worry that their bosses will think they are goofing off. In addition, computers have increased back ailments. In the good old days, you had to get up from your chair every few minutes to get a file from the cabinet. Now you push a button and continue to sit still.

Why is sitting so hard on your back? The answer has to do with what happens to your spine when you change from a standing to a sitting posture.

If you stand sideways and look into a mirror, you can see the natural curve of your lower back — you probably know by now that this is called a lordosis, or lordotic curve. During the mid-1970s, many experts advised back pain sufferers to flatten this curve by doing a pelvic tilt while they were standing, and even while they were walking around. Now we know much more about human biomechanics and we realize that it's almost always better to maintain this curve than to exaggerate or decrease it. In this natural position, the structures that support your spine — your muscles, ligaments, and discs — can do their job with the least amount of strain.

When you sit down, your muscles have to work harder to keep you upright and stable. Chair backs are meant to provide support for your back. For many reasons, however, many people tend not to use their chair backs most of the time; I'm embarrassed to admit that I'm one of them!

Why don't people use their chair backs for support? Sometimes, it's simply because the chair backs are poorly designed in terms of shape or height. Other times, people simply sit on the edge of their chairs out of habit, which is what I tend to do. (Since my Steelcase chair is one of the best desk chairs in the world, this is a great pity.)

But if your back is not supported, your muscles get very tired, very quickly. When this happens, you slouch (we all do) in an attempt to give those tired muscles a break. Unfortunately, slouching causes a number of negative things to happen: First of all, your center of gravity shifts forward. This causes your pelvis to rotate backward, as shown in Figure 9.2. I personally find this tough to picture in my mind's eye and even tougher to explain. But the only thing that's essential to grasp is that, when this happens, your normal lumbar lordosis decreases; in other words, your lower back flattens out.

Without this normal lordosis, your lumbar discs must bear the weight of your upper body unevenly. Poor sitting posture is one of the main

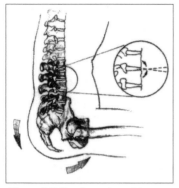

Figure 9.2 Slouch causing pelvic rotation

reasons why so many people end up with bulging and/or herniated discs. As well, as I've explained in Chapter 3, the job of keeping your body upright will be pawned off onto your ligaments, which were not designed for such a task. Over time, strained ligaments will stretch and, once this happens, they will no longer be able to provide your spine with the kind of support it needs — which means that the job will be sloughed off onto your muscles. By now you must be getting a picture of the vicious cycle this creates!

Even if your back is supported, however, and your posture is perfect, your spine will suffer from sitting in the same position for long periods of time. Luckily for me, the reason why is fairly easy to explain.

In order to function, your back muscles require nutrients; they also produce waste products. (The harder they work, the more nutrients they need and the more waste products they produce.) When you're on the move, this is not a problem: The heart increases its pumping action, the blood circulates faster, nutrients move in, and waste products move out. When you sit still, however, this system doesn't work nearly as effectively. Your discs must also absorb nutrients and get rid of waste products. And, like muscles, they do this far more efficiently when you're moving than when you're sitting in one place.

Choosing a Chair

The aim of an ergonomically designed chair is to minimize the effects described above as much as possible.

To put it in a nutshell, your chair should:

- provide support for your back so it can maintain its natural lower lumbar curve;

- give you the freedom to change your position easily and often, without the loss of either comfort or support; and
- promote comfort by distributing your weight evenly (for instance, a poorly designed seat pan can place a lot of pressure on the backs of your thighs).

What type of chair you need depends on your size and what you do while you're in it. (As well, the experts point out, you really should try a chair for at least a week before making a final decision, although, in practice, following this advice is easier said than done.) How your work station is arranged is equally important. This includes things like the height of your monitor; where you place your keyboard; lighting; etc. (See Chapter 19 for more on computer ergonomics.)

It would be impossible, in a single chapter, to describe everything you need to know about choosing a chair. But I can give you a few tips to spark your interest.

First of all, decide whether you need a chair designed for people whose jobs involve performing many different kinds of tasks, or one for people whose jobs require them to perform one task for a longer period of time.

Chairs for Multi-Task Work

Just for openers, be thankful. If your job requires you to do a lot of different tasks, your back will suffer less than if you had a job that required you to do the same thing over and over, for instance, entering data into a computer. If, during the course of a day, you work on a computer, talk on the phone, read, write, reach for files, etc., you will change your posture without even having to think about it.

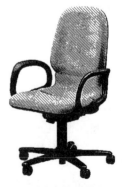

In this case, what you need is a chair whose backrest is at the right height to support *your* back. (For example, if you're very tall, you'd be unlikely to choose the same chair as your very short colleague.)

Your chair should also be flexible enough to

Figure 9.3 A Multi-Task Chair

allow you to move easily. For instance, you should be able to recline (lean back) without having to sacrifice back support. When you recline, the angle between your trunk and your legs should increase so that your normal lordosis can increase as well — a change that's as good as a rest! Figure 9.3 on the previous page shows a fine multitask chair made by Steelcase.

Chairs for Dedicated-Task Work

The corporate "pecking order" is often the underlying problem behind workers' backaches for the simple reason that companies tend to spend less

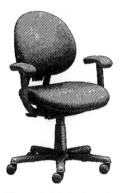

money on chairs for people who work at repetitive tasks than on chairs for executives. This is a pity, since ergonomic seating is far more important for people who do dedicated-task work all day long.

The most common dedicated task is working at a computer's video display terminal (VDT) for hours. If you have a job such as this, you must sit in one particular position almost all day. To add insult to injury, your arms and head must remain in a certain position as well.

Figure 9.4 A Dedicated-Task Chair

This calls for an adjustable chair that allows you to select a position, then lock into it quickly and without too much effort. Being able to change positions with ease is important as well. For example, while waiting for data to be stored by the computer, a VDT operator should be able to lean back for a few seconds.

When it comes to adjustments, the following are important: backrest height, tilt and lock; seat tilt, height, and depth; and armrest height and width. Figure 9.4 shows a good dedicated-task chair for VDT work.

Not everyone's idea of comfort is the same. For instance, when working at a VDT, you may prefer to sit totally upright, while another person may choose to lean forward slightly. Still others prefer to lean back if their work stations are set up in a way that will permit such a posture. In fact, when given the opportunity, some people will actually set up flexible work stations so that they can change from a sitting to a standing position with very little effort.

GETTING THE BEST FROM YOUR CHAIR

Many people who own a comfortable, ergonomic chair don't use it properly. To begin with, they don't take the time to read the manual, which means that they (or their bosses) are often paying for wonderful features that are never enjoyed.

For instance, the "tilt tension" on a good ergonomic chair is adjustable. But if you have it set for someone who weighs 180 pounds while you weigh in at 125, the ability to change positions easily will be lost to you.

The point is, getting the best out of an excellent chair takes time and effort. First, you must ensure that you have set it up properly in terms of your height and weight. Second, you must put its features to use. While I believe that companies are responsible for providing their employees with excellent seating, it's the employee's responsibility to use that chair to its best advantage. But I wish I had a boss to get on my case!

SIT MUCH? WELL, HOW MUCH?

In 1972, an American researcher, Dr. Alexander Magora, published a study linking back pain to the occupations of approximately 3,300 people. He asked how much of each person's day was spent doing three kinds of tasks: those that required them to sit; those that required them to stand; and those that required them to lift.

In the case of sitting and standing, the workers were asked to choose "often" if they sat for more than four hours of each working day; "sometimes" if they sat for between two and four hours each day, on average; and "rarely or never," if they sat for less than two hours a day. (In the case of lifting, the categories were a bit different, since the weight of the object also had to be considered.) Figure 9.5 shows his results.

Here's what Dr. Magora learned with respect to sitting: only 3 percent of the people who suffered from back pain sat "sometimes." On the other hand, approximately 54 percent of the people who suffered from back

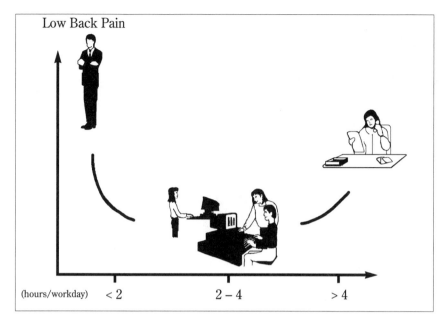

Figure 9.5 Relationship between back pain and sitting.

pain sat "rarely or never," and 42 percent of the people who suffered from back pain sat "often."

"Both too much sitting, and too little sitting," Dr. Magora concluded, "seem to be related to low back pain." People, it seems, are far less likely to suffer from back pain if their jobs require them to do a variety of tasks — some sitting, some standing, some lifting — during the course of a working day.

It will require a commitment from management if jobs are to accommodate this finding on a large scale. In the meantime, however, you could probably change some of your work habits to some degree, if you made this a priority. For instance, if you have three hours of typing and two hours of filing to do, why not alternate tasks every half hour or so? At the very least, it wouldn't do your back any harm.

10

Dynamic Posture

A s I mentioned in the last chapter, how you use your body when you're on the move is as important as how you use it when you are stationary. Think about what sorts of demands you place on your body when you stand up — not, that is, while you *are* standing, but during the time it takes you to get out of your chair and become vertical. Do you move efficiently, or do you, like many people, wrench yourself up, mainly using the muscles of your back rather than the much stronger muscles of your legs? Do you have a habit — acquired who knows when or why — of tilting your head to one side, thereby increasing the strain on the muscles, ligaments, tendons and joints of your neck? What kind of cumulative effect might such tendencies have on your back?

These are the kinds of questions that researchers who are interested in posture — and particularly dynamic posture — have been asking.

MAN IN MOTION

The term "dynamic posture" was actually coined decades ago. In 1946, an American physician, Beckett Howorth, wrote about it in the *Journal of the*

American Medical Association. Dr. Howorth talked about how posture develops. (The spines of newborns, for example, have neither lordotic nor kyphotic curves.) He discussed static postures: lying down, sitting, and standing. And then he went on to describe the best way to run, climb, jump, and lift. By "best," he meant the most efficient way of performing these dynamic activities from the point of view of the human spine.

For example, Dr. Howorth explained how to walk in a way that expends as little energy — and creates as little stress — as possible, taking into consideration center of gravity, body angle, timing, balance, and rhythm. Unfortunately, Dr. Howorth was unable to be precise about the effects of dynamic posture because his measuring tools were far less sophisticated than the ones that exist today.

"We've come a long way," says Lina Santaguida, a Toronto physical therapist who has been doing research in this area for several years. "But, even today, a lot of what we're talking about is theory rather than fact. We're pretty sure there is a 'best' way to walk but we're not totally sure what it is."

If you want to create a picture in your mind's eye of the impact poor dynamic posture can have on your back, imagine a letter carrier. Let's call her Laura. Say she works for Canada Post, and to make the example more interesting, let's also say that her psoas muscles are tight. (Don't worry about why these muscles are tight; just picture them running from Laura's lumbar vertebrae and through her pelvis, where they attach to the top of her upper leg bone, or femur; look back at Figure 1.9.)

The point is, because her psoas muscles are tight, Laura cannot extend her body fully when she walks around delivering mail. Rather, she must walk with her trunk slightly flexed, or bent forward. Bear in mind that the trunk is the heaviest part of the human body, so even if Laura's trunk is overflexed just slightly, her body balance will be affected.

By now I'm sure you're starting to get the picture: Laura's lumbar discs have to bear a lot of extra weight. Certain muscles will be forced to work constantly just to keep her from toppling forward. Laura also carries a heavy bag over her right shoulder day after day, year after year, which, of course, makes her even more unbalanced. In turn, this further increases the strain on her already-strained muscles.

If her back feels tired at the end of the day, it's no wonder.

The human body, however, has an amazing ability to adapt. To help her cope with the discomfort, Laura's body will make some changes. These are called — logically enough — **adaptive changes**. Certain muscles will become chronically tight, while others will become chronically stretched, or lax. The trouble is that lax muscles are not very helpful when it comes to keeping a human spine stable.

Eventually, joints that were designed to work smoothly and effortlessly within a certain range will start operating beyond this range. Ultimately, a disc may bulge or a joint may become worn, and the resulting pain will alert Laura to the fact that she has a back problem which is more than just a matter of tired muscles. And poor posture — poor *dynamic* posture — is the underlying cause.

To shed more light on the spirit of dynamic posture, Lina Santaguida gave me a more subtle example — stretching your arm out to pick up a book. "When you reach out to pick a book up from a shelf," she told me, "the problem is not generally muscle power. Most of us are quite able to get the job done. However, *several* muscles are involved in this movement, and researchers are beginning to realize that sequence — that is, your body's ability to recruit these muscles in a particular order — is also extremely important."

This new way of thinking raises an important issue, especially when it comes to back pain. As children, most of us were not taught to move in a way that is mindful of these subtle aspects of good posture, so we developed poor habits. As well, we grew up in an era during which ramrod-straight spines were praised over postures which respect the fact that spinal structures work best when their natural curves are maintained.

To make matters worse, our western lifestyle does not promote moving in an easygoing way. We know that activity is good for us. But when we are active, many of us strain ourselves — our joints, our muscles — because we equate activity with winning, or achieving a goal. *Mea culpa!* As a kid I used to splash around the swimming pool for hours. Today, I generally try to cram twenty lengths into twenty minutes because I always seem to be in such a rush. To make matters worse for myself, that's twenty lengths of a less-than-perfect — i.e., not very well balanced — crawl.

"All of which brings us right back to the issue of the way our bodies adapt," Lina Santaguida put it to me. In other words, when you move in a way that produces stress — my unbalanced crawl stroke is a good example — your body does its best to compensate. At least it does over the short term. Over the long term, there's a hefty price to pay.

In an effort to understand these ideas and translate them into methods of improving dynamic posture, researchers are exploring a number of areas. Some people, like Lina Santaguida, are studying the fine points of dynamic posture from a biomechanical point of view: for instance, how *exactly* do tight psoas muscles affect particular joints?

Still others are looking at performing artists — dancers, for instance — who seem to grasp the principles of dynamic posture almost effortlessly.

Dr. Fadi Bejani, who is director of occupational/musculoskeletal diseases at the New Jersey Medical School in Newark, is one of these people. Over the years, he has treated hundreds of dancers and musicians whose main complaints are injuries of the feet and hands. But back trouble enters into the picture as well.

Using the example of a 120-pound ballet dancer who can lift (with apparent ease) a ballerina who is lighter by only twenty pounds, Dr. Bejani asks an interesting question. "How is this possible when, every day, I see muscle-bound, 200-pound workers who are unable to lift thirty pounds?"

Obviously, part of the answer is training. Another factor is that the ballerina is also in motion, which makes her easier to lift. But Dr. Bejani senses that there is more to it. "Maybe it has something to do with the music or the feeling of exultation that goes hand in hand with knowing how to use your body in such an extraordinary way," he mused.

What's heartening is that the people who are taking a keen interest in dynamic posture appear to be extremely open-minded. There is a sense of sharing information rather than the "guard your own turf" attitude that too often emerges when health-care professionals of different backgrounds delve into new vistas at the same time.

"The way I see it," says Lina Santaguida, "the thinking is starting to converge."

The way I see it, this means that over the next several years those of us who suffer from back pain are going to come out ahead. But even today, we can at least be aware of the concept of dynamic posture and the possible consequences of moving poorly.

TEN TIPS FOR SAFE LIFTING

Not very many years ago, back pain sufferers were advised to flatten the natural curve in their lumbar spine when they lifted even a moderately heavy object. Today, we believe that it's far better to maintain your natural lumbar lordosis when you lift. In fact, we know a lot of things about lifting now — so why does it seem that every brochure or article I come across simply focuses on bending your knees? Yes, it's important to bend your knees to ensure that your leg muscles (which are stronger than your back muscles) will bear most of the load. But lifting safely depends on many other things as well.

Say you are about to lift a forty-pound box. Even if you are in excellent physical shape, you should consider the following before you start:

- Are you going to lift the box from the floor onto a table right in front of you, or must you lift it onto a table to one side?
- Is the box rectangular or oddly shaped?
- Are you able to keep it close to your body, or (perhaps because it's dusty and you're wearing business clothes) must you lift it with your arms stretched out in front of you?
- Do you have to lift it higher than your shoulders?

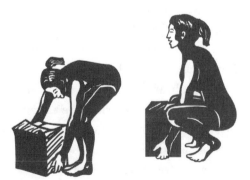

Figure 10.1 Lifting Techniques —
The Wrong Way (left) and the Right Way

- Do you have to lift it more than once?
- Are you able to lift it at a pace that suits you or must you lift it very quickly (or very slowly) to suit someone else's needs?

Does this sound complicated? It's really not. Learning safe lifting techniques is just a matter of expanding your thinking and planning your lifts in advance. The following tips can help you do exactly that. Figure 10.1 on the previous page illustrates safe and unsafe lifting techniques.

1. As I've already mentioned, your back is strongest when it's in its natural position — that is, when the normal curve in your lower back is neutral, rather than exaggerated or decreased. This is because your muscles are strongest when they are working at the middle of their range of motion. (They are weakest when stretched to their full length, or contracted.) What if you must lift while bending forward — for example when you have to take a dozen bags of groceries out of your trunk? The answer is simple: you can't lift as much! It's far better for your back to lift two bags at a time than to try to save time by yanking all of them out at once.

2. Not only are your leg muscles stronger than your back muscles, but they are also a lot stronger than the muscles in your arms. If you can keep your arms straight — straight down, that is, not straight out — your leg muscles will do most of the work. If you extend your arms, they will try to bear the load, but if they are too weak to manage the task, your back will have to take over.

3. It's much harder to lift something if you hold it away from, rather than close to, your body. For example, if you lift a ten-pound load that's fourteen inches in front of you, you will be lifting the equivalent of about 150 pounds.

4. Twisting while you lift puts enormous strain on your back. A better idea is to lift, then move your feet in order to turn your body. This may sound like more effort but it isn't. It just takes a moment longer. If you must twist while you are lifting a bunch of things, at least alternate sides.

5. The strain of lifting is cumulative; lifting a light object many times can cause as much strain as lifting a heavy object once.

6. Generally speaking, it's easier to lower something than lift it. But don't be fooled. Many back injuries occur because people think they can lower a heavy object, then get hurt when the object falls and they must lunge for it.

7. Speed matters, although it's difficult to describe why. The best rule of thumb is to lift at a moderate speed that feels comfortable: neither too fast nor too slow.

8. An odd-shaped box is a lot harder to lift than a box of the same weight that's rectangular. Why? Because, apart from the weight, your muscles have to keep you balanced. That's a job in itself.

9. If your upper body is in good shape, most lifting experts feel that it's okay to lift a box to shoulder level. However, it's best to split the lift into two parts. First lift it from ground level to waist level, then up to shoulder level.

10. Think ahead. Plan each lift *before* you begin, not after you get into trouble.

FEET: THE FOUNDATION

While researchers like Lina Santaguida focus on the trunk, others are directing their attention to the lowest part of the body: the feet. Specifically, they are interested in the **gait cycle**, which is basically the way you use your feet when you walk.

Studies performed over the past number of years have shown that the gait cycle of just about every chronic back pain patient is abnormal. What has been less clear is whether the abnormal gait causes back pain, or whether, because their backs hurt, people alter the way they walk to compensate. The most recent studies (performed by foot specialists, or **podiatrists**) seem to indicate that the feet, indeed, are the culprit, at least in some cases.

Like the spine, the feet are an amazing body part. There are twenty-six bones in each foot (that's a quarter of the body's bones!); nineteen muscles including the ones that attach to the lower leg (if you're still counting), and various tendons, as well as ligaments, arteries, veins, joints, and nerves. But what is really amazing is what they do. On approximately six to sixteen inches, the feet manage to support between a hundred and two hundred and fifty pounds — and in actual fact, the poundage supported per square inch is a lot larger, since the whole foot does not make contact with the ground.

Furthermore, the feet act as the body's main shock absorbers, the levers which propel it forward when walking and running and the mechanism by which the moving body adapts to different terrains.

If your feet, which are supposed to act as a foundation, are not level and solid, your entire body will be thrown out of kilter each time you take a stride. If, however, you correct the problem by wearing better shoes, or using specially made inserts called **orthotics**, the stresses on your lumbar spine will be a lot less.

The message is not that solving gait problems can put an end to back pain. Rather, it's that the feet — and how we use them when we walk and run — are now considered to be one more piece of the back pain equation. A very important piece.

New Hampshire podiatrist Howard Dananberg has been studying gait problems and back pain for a number of years. "We're not saying that, with an abnormal gait cycle, the back is placed under tremendous stress each time you take a step," he explains. "What we're talking about is the cumulative trauma caused by the tens of millions of steps you take over a lifetime." On average, we stride 2,500 times a day — on each leg! "Try to think of the problem in the same category as a repetitive motion injury," suggests Dr. Dananberg.

The Normal Gait Cycle

A short course on the mechanics of walking will clarify the relationship between your feet and your back.

Take a look at Figure 10.2. As you read the next few paragraphs, follow the man's right foot as it goes through a normal gait cycle.

A gait cycle has two main parts: the stance phase and the swing phase.

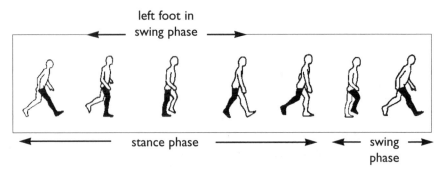

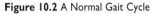

Figure 10.2 A Normal Gait Cycle

In the **stance phase**, the man puts his heel forward; this is called the heel strike. Next, the right foot goes through the mid-stance as the foot makes contact with the ground. Finally, the stance phase comes to an end as the right heel lifts up and the toe comes off the ground.

Next is the **swing phase**. The right foot is completely off the ground, which means it is bearing no weight at all. When the right heel strikes the ground, the cycle starts again. As one foot moves through the stance phase, the other foot moves through the swing phase.

So far so good. Most of us can understand this much by following the diagram. But the way our feet work — at least the way they are supposed to work — is more complicated. If you're fascinated by the biomechanics of walking, take a look at Figure 10.3. If not, skip it, and the next two paragraphs!

As the heel, mid-foot, and toe make contact with the ground, the foot rolls. First it rolls from the outside toward the inside; then it does the same thing in reverse. While this is happening, the distribution of the body's weight changes.

Specifically, during the first part of the stance phase, the foot should roll from the baby toe side toward the mid-

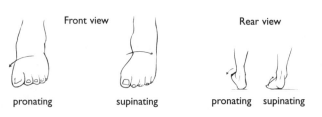

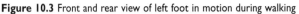

Figure 10.3 Front and rear view of left foot in motion during walking

line. This is called **pronating**. During the middle part of the phase, the foot should be in a neutral position. And, during the last part of the phase, the foot should move from the midline toward the baby toe. This is called **supinating**.

What Can Go Wrong?

Many things! One of your feet may pronate when it shouldn't. Or, it may pronate at the right time, but too much. It may also supinate at the wrong time, or too much.

Dr. Dananberg's research has also shown that, in some people, the joints between the toes and the foot, which act as a pivot while the toes lift off the ground, don't function properly. (You can feel these joints by pressing firmly on the fleshy ball of your foot; they're called the metatarso-phalangeal joints.) The point is, the result is always additional stress.

Muscles and tendons are strained. The way the body's weight is distributed is affected, which adds stress to the spine. Dr. Dananberg has found that many people with metatarso-phalangeal joint problems walk with their backs slightly flexed, rather than in a normal lordosis. Others have adapted by walking slightly twisted to one side, which puts a phenomenal amount of strain on the discs of the lumbar spine.

Strain of this nature can lead to inflamed, overly sensitive joints, bunions, corns, and calluses — which causes a vicious cycle to begin: in an attempt to reduce the discomfort, the gait becomes even more abnormal. And on it goes.

Solving Gait Problems

By watching someone walk, a skilled podiatrist can tell if a person's gait is abnormal, and can often pinpoint the cause. In fact, in recent years, modern computer technology has made gait analysis very precise. Electrodes are attached to a patient's feet, then hooked up to a minicomputer walking pack. As the patient walks, information is collected and the gait analysis is printed out. Even a subtle problem, such as faulty weight distribution, can be detected.

In many cases, the solution is as simple as a new pair of shoes that provide proper support. If that doesn't do the trick, or the problem is more complicated, over-the-counter or custom-built orthotic inserts can help many people. (Custom orthotic inserts can cost up to $400!) For a very few patients, foot surgery is necessary to correct a deformity.

"For some people with back pain, the back is not the area that needs to be treated," says Dr. Dananberg. "You have to look at the original cause."

THE LOWDOWN ON BEDDING DOWN

I can just hear you asking, "What in the world is she doing putting a section on sleeping into a chapter on dynamic posture?" Well, I once watched a time-lapse photography session of a couple sleeping in a double bed for eight hours. Condensed into about five minutes, this made an amusing short film. But it also confirmed my suspicion: most of us change our posture almost continuously while we sleep. Tossing and turning is the norm rather than the exception.

If you believe this, then much of the advice you've been given on the best posture to assume while getting your forty winks should be thrown out the window. I suspect that I've known this, at least subconsciously, for years. For instance, I've been advised to sleep on my side with a pillow between my knees more times than I can remember. I've tried it many times, but never once have I woken up in the morning with my knee-pillow in the right place. (Most of the time, it's on the floor beside my bed!)

The point is that, while health-care professionals have been doling out advice on sleeping postures for as long as mankind has been sleeping on beds, there is little if any evidence to back up what they have to say. It's more or less conjecture. For instance, for many years — and I'm sure you know this — it was considered anathema for back pain sufferers to sleep on their stomachs. Today, lying prone for at least part of the time is actually recommended during an acute bout of back pain!

There is even less evidence about the best type of bed for back pain.

What it boils down to is what feels comfortable, and about the only thing I can say with any certainty is that, for the vast majority of back pain sufferers, a comfortable mattress is one that is firm. The trouble is, my definition of firm is probably different than yours!

With that said, here are a few rules of thumb:

- If your bed is too soft, your spine will have to rely on its ligaments and muscles to maintain its normal curves.
- If, on the other hand, your bed is too hard — and particularly if you sleep on your side a good deal of the time — the same problem will occur. Think of your hips and shoulders as the towers of a suspension bridge, your spine being what is suspended between them. Because of the difference in both the weight and size of your shoulders and hips, a totally ungiving surface will not allow your spine to assume its natural shape much better than a saggy bed.
- If you have a saggy mattress, putting a plywood board under it won't help all that much. The board simply provides a hard base for the mattress to sag into.
- The most popular mattress is the spring coil, but be aware that their range of quality is very wide. For instance, a double mattress may contain anywhere from 252 to 630 springs; the thickness of each spring can vary from 13 to 16 gauge.
- If you prefer a foam mattress, make sure to buy high-density foam. (How do you tell? It's difficult, but if you push your finger into a foam mattress, then twist it, low-density foam will leave a mark.)
- King-size mattresses are great, especially for couples who both suffer from back pain and benefit from the extra room. But if you are thinking of buying a king-size mattress (eighty inches by eighty inches), make sure it is able to fit up your staircase and/or through the door to your bedroom; bending it can damage it permanently.
- The lifespan of a mattress is between seven and ten years — if you treat it properly, which means turning it at least three or four times a year so that it wears evenly.

- If you're in the market for a new bed, invest wisely. Think of your bed as the place where you spend approximately one-third of your life and budget accordingly, rather than trying to save a few bucks. Just as important is the retailer from whom you buy your bed. Pick one that will be around to honor your warranty rather than a fly-by-night operator who couldn't care less about you once the sale has been made.
- Waterbeds? The people who sell waterbeds insist that they are excellent for chronic back pain sufferers and that in many instances they can actually "cure" a bad back. (I especially love the waterbed brochure that features a smiling gentleman in a doctor suit on the cover!) On several occasions, I have asked these retailers for copies of the research studies on which these opinions are based, but none have ever arrived. The only research on waterbeds that I've been able to find suggests that they are helpful for burn victims and women who are pregnant.

    I do not mean to suggest, however, that waterbeds are *not* good for people who suffer from chronic back pain. Many people insist that the warmth of a heated waterbed is soothing for their backs. Only a few people that I've spoken to say that waterbeds make their backs feel worse. In trying to assess who is likely to benefit from a waterbed, I have observed that people whose back pain is better with activity seem to prefer waterbeds more often than those whose back pain responds to rest.

    If you're interested in a waterbed, buy it from a dealer who offers a money-back guarantee to customers who are not satisfied after thirty days. (Often it takes a month to get used to a new bed.) Be sure to read the fine print that goes with the guarantee; some companies require you to complain within seven days and give the company an opportunity to make adjustments to the bed's water level.

DYNAMIC POSTURE GURUS

Interestingly enough, dynamic posture is the basis for quite a number of "alternative" therapies that attract back pain patients. Unfortunately, the language they use — and the evidence they give to demonstrate their method's efficacy — is very different from the language that's used and the types of studies that are performed by health-care professionals trained in the scientific tradition. Therefore, there is less crossover than I think there should be.

But I also believe that, if you are interested in one of these disciplines, you'd be wise to bear in mind that these therapies tend to be holistic — they treat the whole body rather than specific symptoms and complaints. This can be disappointing if you arrive with the idea that your back pain (rather than your whole body) will be addressed. As well, trying to change your posture when you are in the middle of an acute bout of back pain can be very stressful.

With that said, I've heard all of these therapies being praised by dozens of back pain sufferers who would swear on the lives of their aged mothers that, mysterious though they may seem, they do work. Here's a very short — very inadequate — description of some of them. If they interest you, I suggest you check your library or bookstore for more comprehensive information.

The **Alexander technique** teaches people whose posture has become "disorganized" how to move freely. A typical lesson begins with the instructor guiding someone from a seated posture to a standing posture in a way that requires the least amount of strain. "By the time they become adults," explains one teacher, "most people just throw their bodies around."

The **Feldenkrais method**, which was developed by a Russian physicist, is based on the idea that human beings develop unique patterns of movement that become habits — in too many cases, bad habits that strain the body unnecessarily. Feldenkrais proponents believe that the body has the ability to learn better ways of moving if these ways are simply demonstrated. How? By the practitioner guiding the student through sequences of motion that make the body aware of a better way. Once it is aware of a better way, the body will adopt it.

Tai chi, which is actually a Chinese martial art, uses a twenty-minute sequence of slow, fluidly connected movements to correct poor dynamic posture. Proponents also believe that no other type of exercise is necessary.

Yoga, a 4,000-year-old system of postures developed by sages and mystics who observed the way animals stretch and move, improves dynamic posture by focusing on increased flexibility and improved breathing techniques. Done properly, yoga will also increase both strength and endurance.

The **Mezieres method** works on both dynamic and static postures by using a combination of gentle stretching exercises that focus on the spinal column, as well as improved breathing techniques. (Proponents believe that the breathing pattern becomes "blocked" because of a poorly functioning diaphragm.) Education is an important aspect of this method, which was developed in France. The idea is to provide people with tools that they can use to decrease their back pain whenever it flares up.

The **Sahrman exercises** were developed by an American physical therapist called Shirley Sahrman. The aim of this technique is to retrain your body to move in a balanced way, which sounds a lot like some of the Eastern therapies if you ask me.

11

Ergonomics: Designing Your World to Fit

O ver the past seventeen years, I've come to a sad conclusion: despite the efforts of the thousands of researchers and clinicians from dozens of disciplines, back pain is not destined to be wiped off the face of the earth like smallpox, or the plague. On a brighter note, I do believe that the number of people who suffer from back pain can be dramatically reduced, and that, if this happens, ergonomics will have played an important role. In other words, fewer backs will hurt once we have learned to pay more attention to the design needs of our backs rather than expecting spines to fit into whatever happens to be available. I hold this belief with great passion.

RISK FACTORS: ERGONOMICS COMES OF AGE

Ergonomically designed products have been around in some form since the first cro-magnon used a rock for a footrest. But ergonomics began to become a science only when back pain researchers changed their focus from trying to find *causes* to trying to identify risk factors, which turned out to be a far more productive area of study.

I discussed in Chapter 3 how difficult it can be to pinpoint the direct cause of a particular person's back pain. On the other hand, it can much more easily and accurately be shown that, of a large number of people, those who engage in certain behaviors or have certain environments develop back pain more than those who don't. Those behaviors or environments can then be identified as **risk factors**.

Once a risk factor has been pinpointed, it is possible — at least in theory — to eliminate, or at least reduce it. In effect, that will remove its harmful impact on the human back — even if the exact cause of that impact can't be pinned down.

How risk factors caught the interest of researchers, as well as how their study led to a sharp rise in the stock of ergonomics, is a wonderful story of human beings taking the best from basic science and then translating what they learned into products that have helped thousands of backs suffer a helluva lot less.

The science of ergonomics got its official start in the workplace. I hate to sound cynical, but the groundswell began when back pain started to cost industry and commerce — do forgive me just this once! — an arm and a leg. Looking for ways to bring down absenteeism and compensation costs, researchers started to focus on risk factors, and when they did, two main issues caught their attention. One was people's general fitness, which has a lot to do with lifestyle. The other was the particular risks that go hand in hand with certain jobs.

First, fitness. When you talk about fitness, you *have* to take lifestyle into consideration. Researchers very soon learned what seems today so obvious it is almost a truism: if you're an overweight couch potato — especially a potato with a physically demanding job — you have a greater risk of injuring your back than your buddy who rides his bike all summer and skis when the snow flies. (The importance of fitness in preventing back pain cannot be emphasized enough — I've devoted the next two chapters to the topic.) However, it's hard to pin down exactly *how much* your risk of developing back pain increases if you are in lousy shape.

When they began to assess the risk factors that accompany particular jobs, however, researchers discovered that they could be more specific.

For instance, as explained in Chapter 9, a job that requires you to sit for eight hours a day increases your risk of developing back pain; statistics can be used to measure, albeit imperfectly, the degree to which this is so, depending on a number of variables about the job. It's also possible to rate jobs for their potential for accidents such as falls. But without a doubt, one of the greatest risk factors for back pain is overexertion while lifting. Scientists have coined a far more sophisticated name for this every-day task: **manual materials handling**, or **MMH**. It is on this subject that the most interesting research has emerged.

In an effort to assess, and then reduce, the risk factors associated with MMH, researchers concentrated on three main areas. One was training people to lift properly. The second was job selection — mak-ing sure that people who are hired to do a certain job are physically capable of performing it. The third was job design — making jobs fit the needs of the people doing them, rather than the other way around. In other words, ergonomics.

All three approaches have their place when it comes to reducing risk factors for back pain in the workplace. But, as the results of the studies came in, researchers around the world arrived almost unanimously at the same conclusion: in most cases, ergonomics is the most important approach. (In part, this is because the two other areas are so hard to control.) Rather than placing the burden of strength and/or endurance on the worker, employers began to realize, it made more sense to design a job so that, in all but the most exceptional circumstances, the average worker could perform it without undue risk of injury. (A more contro-versial issue, which is discussed in Chapter 20, is whether jobs should be *redesigned* to meet the needs of people who are returning to work *after* they have been injured.)

It was these conclusions that transformed ergonomics, within a few short years, from a science that scarcely anyone could pronounce into one whose name rolls off the tongues of managers, back pain sufferers, and media watchers with great ease. In turn, this led to the development of literally hundreds of ergonomically designed products, which millions of back pain sufferers now use in their homes, gardens, and cars. Thank

God for the inventors who had the ingenuity to come up with the designs for these products, as well as the energy to produce and bring them to the marketplace.

SOME INVENTORS AND THEIR WONDERFUL MACHINES

While I was working on this chapter, I got stumped right at this point. I couldn't decide whether to mention a few dozen ergonomic products that have impressed me over the years, or to use the space to describe a few products in detail. The latter course, I finally concluded, was the better way to spark your interest in ergonomics, as well as to make you fall in love with the people who have the tenacity to become inventors. Once I had you hooked with a few great stories, I figured, I would provide a list of stores that specialize in such products and my readers could then write away for their catalogs and discover far more treasures than I could ever mention here. (This list is at the end of the chapter.)

But there was a second reason for my decision to concentrate on just a few inventors. Over the years I've seen many ergonomic products come and go. I've met with, and encouraged, literally dozens of inventors, all of whom had excellent ideas. And I'm sorry to say that, although they persevered — often beyond the bounds of reason — the majority of them lost their shirts. The most common story was that they spent all their money just to produce their products — which left them without a cent for advertising and promotion. Designing and developing an ergonomically designed product is a tough enough game when you're trying to accomplish the task on a shoestring, but getting that product to market and surviving until it takes hold is often a real nightmare when you don't have a million bucks. The truth is that the few who succeed usually do so because they are smitten and a tiny bit eccentric — which also helps make their tales more interesting than a long list!

So, what follows here are the stories of some of my favorite ergonomic inventions. I take my hat off to the people who invented these wonderful products and add the following caveat: If you think they live the life of

Riley, you'd do well to think again. If you want to get rich it's probably easier to win the lottery than to succeed as an inventor.

THE OBUSFORME: ERGONOMICS? NEVER HEARD OF IT

"Of all the machines which civilization has invented for the torture of mankind, there are few which perform their work more cruelly than the chair." This comment was made by an American researcher in 1879. Yet a century passed before ergonomic seating became an industry.

And had it not been for the efforts of a Toronto man called Frank Roberts, pictured with his invention in Figure 11.1, it may have taken even longer for ergonomic seating to become big-time.

When Frank Roberts designed his ObusForme backrest in 1980,

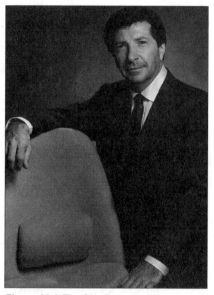

Figure 11.1 The ObusForme and Inventor Frank Roberts

he didn't have a clue what "ergonomics" meant. But because of him, countless numbers of people have woken up to the fact that, for years, they had been sitting in chairs that were murder on their backs — and that a better alternative existed. Frank Roberts's story is worth telling because it shows how a down-to-earth approach can sometimes be as effective as a high-tech operation.

It started in 1975, the year Frank almost had surgery on his back. But, as he says, he got lucky. A body cast did the trick instead. When the cast came off, Frank sliced it in half, then got a friend to help him lift it onto the front seat of his car to make driving more comfortable. It weighed sixty pounds and he used it for four years. By then, he had wrapped it in foam and covered it with numerous pillowcases, but the plaster was still crumbling into tiny pieces and making a mess of his upholstery.

Thoroughly disgusted, Frank got a guy who made fenders to fashion a fiberglass mold from the falling-to-pieces plaster cast. Frank then carried the mold into his garage and played around with foam and different fabrics. Eventually, he came up with a combination that worked, and the world's first ObusForme backrest was born.

A friend liked what he'd made, so Frank gave it to him as a gift. Every time he made a few more, the same thing happened. A short while after, Frank's brother gave him the gears: "You should be selling these backrests," he told Frank, "not giving them away." Frank thought about this advice, then hightailed it back to the garage, and began turning out fiberglass ObusFormes in quantity.

One of the first people whose back felt better because of an ObusForme was the late Toronto radio host Wally Crouter. Crouter liked the product so much that he convinced Frank to rent a small space downtown as a salesroom. Frank opened on a Monday with an inventory of a hundred ObusFormes. That same morning, Crouter talked the product up on his show, and by the end of the day, Frank was not only sold out, he had enough orders to keep him busy for six months — and a pretty good idea that a market for backrests existed!

Soon, Frank had to go to injection molding to keep up with the demand. The trouble was, his first polycarbonate mold, which took eight months to make at a cost of $28,000, didn't work. The ObusFormes that came off it were so rigid that they cracked. By the time the problem was fixed, Frank had spent about $40,000. Today, the same mold would cost several hundred thousand dollars — but today Frank Roberts could afford such a sum. ObusForme backrests are sold in twenty-six countries, and Frank has been involved in the development of more than half a dozen other products, including the ObusForme ergonomic chair, which is manufactured and distributed by a Canadian furniture company called Global. And today, Frank knows what "ergonomics" means.

THE BACKCYCLER: A CHANGE IS AS GOOD AS A REST!

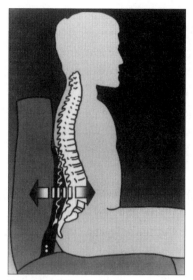

Figure 11.2 The BackCycler

The first time I met Steve Reinecke, he was a young, wonderful-looking scientist whose little office at the University of Vermont had been taken over by the craziest "chair" I'd ever seen. This was in 1990 during a visit to the Vermont Back Research Center at the university. (The center is the only back pain research center in the United States funded by the federal government; today, I'm the only Canadian member of their advisory board.)

At the time, there were about a dozen scientists there, each working on a particular assignment. Steve Reinecke's task was to study the effects of seating on the human back, and he had built this crazy-looking contraption for research. He was trying to figure out a way for people to cash in on the advantages of sitting *without* having to keep their backs still. Wow!

Two years later, I met Steve again in Montreal. (He was one of the people I was going to see when my crown fell into the couscous — see Chapter 8!) Nestled in the driver's seat of his car was the result of his years of labor: a neat-looking device called the BackCycler, pictured in Figure 11.2.

In a nutshell, the BackCycler is a "smart" backrest designed to be used in a car or truck. Inside this clever product is an air bladder and a computer. Like other backrests, the BackCycler provides support. But because the air bladder slowly inflates and deflates, the lower back of the person using it actually moves. The natural lordotic curve increases and decreases about once every minute, while the person drives. A similar version for use in office chairs is in the works.

As I've said, I've been writing about back pain for seventeen years. In all that time, I can count on the fingers of one hand the number of times

I've been bowled over by a product. This one did it to me. I predict that, among back pain sufferers, the BackCycler will become a household word.

The story of the BackCycler begins in 1986, when Steve Reinecke was at the Research Center doing research on the effects of different postures during sitting. He had tested a large number of subjects and was discovering that people do not find it comfortable to sit for very long. For instance, the average person is happy to sit in an upright position for sixty-seven minutes. But that same person will only last for six or seven minutes if you ask them to bend forward while they sit. And people are not comfortable sitting in any posture for hours at a time.

"What people needed," says Steve, "was a way to keep their spines moving while they sat. The solution came when Rowley Hazard, a physician who was working on other Research Center projects, showed me a contraption — a lumbar roll — he'd been using in his Le Car. He had been making a lot of trips to Cape Cod, and during the long drive he would use this lumbar roll in an unusual way. He'd drive for ten minutes, and when his back started to hurt, he'd stick the roll behind his lower back. Ten minutes later, his back would start aching again and he'd take the roll out. Ten minutes in, ten minutes out, all the way to Cape Cod. It wasn't a particular position that was helping as much as the change."

A while later, Rowley came up with an even better solution. He put an air-filled bag that he could inflate and deflate into his lumbar roll and used it to make the chair in his office more comfortable.

"It sounds crazy, but he actually took a bag from an old hospital kit that had been designed to reduce swelling in the end of a person's thigh after they'd had a leg amputation. It looked pretty bizarre and the pump was pretty noisy. But it was certainly interesting."

In fact, **continuous passive motion**, or **CPM**, had been used for a number of years on patients recovering from knee surgery. Moving the knee joint while it heals reduces stiffness and stimulates the healing process. Steve had actually designed a CPM device for knees back in 1981 while still in school.

On behalf of the Research Center, Rowley and Steve applied for and received a grant to find out whether a lumbar device that inflated and deflated would be helpful for people while they sat. Steve describes their first research thus:

"We built four prototype chairs with inflatable air bladders and measurement devices. We installed them at patients' workplaces and left them there for several weeks. At the end of three weeks, we were able to tell exactly how people used them. For instance, we found out that, on average, people preferred a sixty-three-second cycle for the air bladder changing its shape from empty to full. We also came up with the answers to many other design questions. This process took over two years.

"At this point, we had a device that we could use to conduct further research, although it certainly wasn't user friendly. We proceeded to test it. In the lab, we wanted to make sure we were actually doing what we said we were doing: changing the shape of people's spines. It took a year to build the tools that could measure the shape of someone's back and prove for certain that it did change when they used the device.

"The next step was to see how low back pain patients felt when they used it. We started with fifty people and, to our surprise, forty-seven of them said they felt more comfortable when they used the device than when they didn't use it. In fact, a few of them refused to give it back, which was a problem since we only had four!"

The big step from a research tool to a product began when, in 1990, Steve took a course called Transfer of Technology at the university and used the research device for his class project. His professor, Karel Samsom, was hooked! Soon the three of them — Rowley (a doctor), Karel (a business person), and Steve (a mechanical engineer) started a company called Ergomedics to transform the device into the BackCycler.

The technology transfer process didn't turn out to be as simple as the three had thought it would be. The young company faced challenges in both marketing and production.

"It's enough to say that these kinds of things taught us that there's a big difference between doing research and making a product for people!" admits Steve.

Finally, in the fall of 1993 the first production run of BackCyclers were ready to be distributed. Today, they are being built into cars, trucks, buses, airplanes, and even mattresses. The invention has been approved by the U.S. Food and Drug Administration and has won a prize given by the International Society for the Study of the Lumbar Spine. But making it all happen took a total of thirteen years!*

BackRelax: For the Love of His Life!

I've been billing Paul Waitzer as the world's most charming eclectic for nearly two decades. The man has sat on more boards than I've had hot dinners, and their diversity — Dylex and Toronto's Baycrest Geriatric Centre are but two examples — boggle my mind. Paul's company was the Back Association of Canada's (BAC's) first corporate supporter, winning him a place in my heart forever. He has supported BAC's efforts ever since.

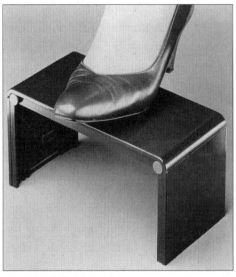

Figure 11.3 The BackRelax

But the accomplishment that really bowls me over is the one Paul Waitzer got hooked into because of his wife, a wonderful, outgoing woman named Valerie who has suffered from back pain for more than forty years. For Val, Paul created a portable footrest called the BackRelax (see Figure 11.3), adding "ergonomic inventor" to his curriculum vitae along with all his other successes.

The impetus was a smashed wicker purse that had been serving as Val's

---

* The BackCycler is available in Canada from Backworks. For more information about the product, write to: Ergomedics, Inc., Hillside Park, 276 East Allen Street, Winooski, Vermont, U.S.A., or telephone (802) 655-2225.

footrest during a family car vacation to the Maritimes in 1980. One morning, Paul accidently slammed the back seat of the station wagon down onto Val's wicker lifesaver. He promised to buy her a new one at the very next store, but he couldn't find a reasonable facsimile for love or money. So he assured his wife that he knew lots of people in the plastics industry, and that the second they got back to Toronto he'd get one of them to make a footrest that worked better than an old wicker purse.

In keeping his promise, Paul got far more than he bargained for. Within twelve months, he had spent more than $50,000 on patents, a design engineer, injection molding tools, packaging, and several hundred sample footrests — one of which was claimed by his wife. Val was thrilled, except for the fact that Paul started to spend a lot of time promoting his invention, both at health-care shows and to pharmacists.

Unfortunately, most of the druggists he convinced to buy a few knew very little about marketing ergonomic products; they stuck Paul's footrests on the shelf next to shaving cream and razor blades, where they languished. For a while the darn thing was costing, rather than making, him money. But Paul was moved by the letters that kept arriving from happy customers as far away as Europe. He felt he had a responsibility to back pain sufferers to keep his product on the market despite the thin sales.

In 1986, Paul licenced the footrest to a guy who paid him with a draft from a Swiss bank and promised to spend tons of time on marketing and promotion. Paul retained the patents and stipulated that if, for any reason, the footrest was not available in the marketplace, the licence would revert back to him.

For a couple of years everything seemed to go smoothly and Paul got involved in other things. Then, one afternoon in the spring of 1988, two young RCMP officers knocked on his door. It turned out that the guy with the Swiss bank account was not spending tons of time pushing footrests. Quite the contrary; he was using the Milburn BackEasers, as they were then called, to transport drugs! The RCMP had seized his entire inventory and stored it in a warehouse to be used as evidence at the man's trial.

Well, it took some time for Paul to get over the shock of the association, but eventually he set to work convincing the force to release the confiscated goods and canceling the arrested man's licence.

Paul Waitzer was back in the footrest business. To sever the dubious association completely, he changed the footrest's name to BackRelax. A short while later, he rented a booth at The National Home Health Care Exhibit in Atlanta, and to his delight, several U.S. companies purchased supplies of BackRelax and added the item to their mail-order catalogs. For a while, sales began to soar.

But the durability of Paul's product, coupled with a small turnover in the catalog houses' customer base, meant that eventually the catalog market became saturated. Sales began to fall.

Then a company called Comfortably Yours billed it in their catalog as "a must for petite women." This was a brilliant marketing idea, since many short women's backs hurt because their feet dangle a couple of inches above the floor when they sit. In fact, Paul recently conducted a survey that indicates that short women account for about forty percent of the BackRelax's sales.

But it's Paul's tall wife, Val, who has become Paul's best customer. Over the years, she has left quite a number of BackRelax footrests in restaurants, at theaters, and on planes. Every time this happens she reminds Paul that her forgetfulness is *his* fault rather than hers. Even her old wicker purse couldn't hold a candle to a footrest that makes her so comfortable she forgets it's even there.*

THE BOSARO: HOT OFF THE PRESS

Just as this book was going to press, an amazing new backrest — one that can be adjusted to accommodate lumbar spines with different dimensions and different needs — came my way. There wasn't time or space to include the story of its invention by a former accountant from Tanzania, Riyaz Adat. But I couldn't resist at least including a picture of the Bosaro (see Figure 11.4).

---

* For more information and an order form, contact BackRelax, Suite 607, 1 St. Clair Avenue East, Toronto, Ontario, M4T 2V7.

Bosaro is an East Indian word meaning "very nice" — quite the understatement when it comes to rating the world's only fully adjustable back support. I should admit that I was prejudiced toward Riaz Sadat more for his Tanzanian origins than for his talents as an inventor, which are awesome. When I met him, to learn about his Bosaro backrest, we spent a lot of time talking about his homeland, where I have spent the most interesting days of my life . . . and my back didn't hurt once.*

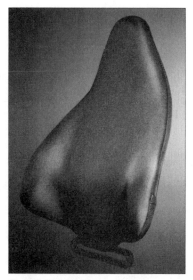

Figure 11.4 The Bosaro Backrest

STORES FOR BACKS

Thank God for these and all other ergonomic inventors. But I can tell you, most of them wouldn't stand a chance if it weren't for the entrepreneurs behind specialty stores for ergonomic products, of which I now present you with the promised list. My personal favorite is Backworks, where you'll find everything from the amazing Bosaro to novelty key chains that look like a human spine. I take my hat off to Auby, Alan, and Linda Bloomfield, who run it, and to all the small businesses out there making our lives a little easier.

In Canada

Back Stop	Back Comfort Shop
930 West Broadway	2535 Danforth Avenue
Vancouver, British Columbia	Toronto, Ontario
(604) 732-6546	(416) 694-7278
Owner: Brian McCoy	Owner: Ken Clarke
free catalog	*no catalog*

---

*   The Bosaro is available from Backworks and retails for $119.95.

Backworks
66 St. James Street
Winnipeg, Manitoba
R3G 3J6
(204) 774-6322 or
1-800-361-7788

Back Shop
78 Ottawa Street North
Hamilton, Ontario
L8H 3Z1
(905) 547-2225
Owner: Virginia Carmichael
free catalog

The Back World
110 Place d'Orléans
Suite 404
Box 242
Ottawa, Ontario
K1C 2L9
(613) 830-6166
Owner: Jason Pilon

In the United States

Better Back Store
7939 East Arapalo Road
Greenwood Village, Colorado
80112
(303) 773-2225
(which is 773-BACK)
free catalog —
fax to order (303) 773-2244

Relax the Back
3800 North Ramar Boulevard
Austin, Texas
78756
(512) 329-8980
Owner: Virginia Rogers
free catalog
51 stores across the United States

The Back Shoppe Inc.
8026 Germantown Avenue
Philadelphia, Pennsylvania
19118
(215) 247-0779
Owner: Larry Newman

12

Bed Rest Is for the Birds

I f you asked me to pick the person who has made the greatest positive difference to the treatment of back pain, I'd choose Dr. Gordon Waddell, an orthopedic surgeon and researcher from Scotland. Dr. Waddell became my human being of the century in 1987 at a conference in Rome. On a lovely June morning, in front of about 200 of the world's most eminent back surgeons, he presented a research paper that questioned the very basics of treatment for back pain.

Dr. Gordon Waddell's Bombshell

Gordon Waddell had concluded from his research that the standard method of treating back pain, long-term bed rest, the treatment of choice for decades, was for the birds. Back pain sufferers, explained Dr. Waddell, were routinely put to bed by their physicians for weeks and sometimes months, despite the fact that there was no hard research showing that this policy was effective. He felt that bed rest had become popular during the 1950s when researchers discovered that lying down put the least amount of strain on the discs of the lumbar spine. At the time, medical science was high on discs as the major cause of serious back pain — particularly back pain that radiated into the leg. Ergo, patients were instructed to remain supine.

Dr. Waddell pointed out that long-term bed rest was no longer being prescribed for any other ailment. In some cases — he mentioned knee injuries — it had fallen out of favor fifteen years earlier. Then he dropped his bombshell. His own research showed that long-term bed rest was doing more harm than good. Becoming active — gradually, but as soon as possible — worked far better.

For two days we had been listening to technical reports: how metal screws can be used to fuse the spine's vertebrae; how nerves can be surgically decompressed by entering the body from the front rather than from the back; etc. But it was Dr. Waddell's down-to-earth words that caused this roomful of physicians to literally stand up and cheer. In all the years I've been writing about back pain, I have never seen such enthusiasm among a group of surgeons; in my experience it usually takes a couple of tons of TNT to get a rise out them (see Chapter 17 for more on the humors of back surgeons!).

TOWARD A NEW TREATMENT MODEL

Today, Gordon Waddell's words have become gospel among expert clinicians, who can rattle off the conclusions of the best "active treatment" studies practically in their sleep. For example:

- Bed rest for two days almost always works better than bed rest for seven days. (A study from Norway suggests that, for many patients, reduced activity but no actual bed rest may be the best bet of all.)
- Staying in bed leaves patients **deconditioned**. In plain language, this means physically unfit — and therefore at increased risk of sustaining a second injury when they finally do get up.
- Long-term bed rest also increases the chances of becoming depressed, and depression often makes back pain feel a lot worse.

But the most amazing bit of information Dr. Waddell had to share with his colleagues was based on an anecdote rather than a formal study. The year before, at the Workers' Compensation Board (WCB) of British Columbia, Dr. Waddell had given a speech to 230 doctors. When he was finished, he decided — for interest's sake — to question his colleagues about their own backs. He asked how many of these 230 physicians had ever suffered from back pain; 138 hands shot up. When he asked how many had stayed in bed for as long as two weeks, 136 of those hands went down. It was a stunning story. And yet it's exactly what I would have expected from a couple of hundred busy doctors.

Dr. Waddell opened the minds of both researchers and clinicians — the majority of them physical therapists — to a *totally* new way of thinking about the treatment of a very common ailment. This does not happen all that frequently in medical science. Nor does the result: a 180-degree flip in treatment theory. Even more unusual was the way Dr. Waddell's ideas gained universal acceptance very quickly. In fact, even those who were skeptical to begin with have come to agree with his concept, which has been given the name **early active treatment**.

Early Active Treatment: A Physiotherapist's Perspective

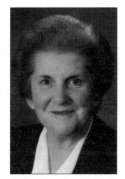

Mary Sauriol

Mary Sauriol has been a physiotherapist for forty-two years, which gives her a pretty interesting view of the changes we've seen. She teaches at the University of Toronto and runs her own community clinic, called Physiotherapy Associates. I thought it would be interesting for you to hear, in her own words, what early, active treatment can do, and how.

I've seen many changes over the years. But I think the greatest change is that we now know the importance of active treatment, started as early after an injury as possible. A decade ago, we didn't know that the clock starts ticking almost right away — that, if you don't get moving within a few weeks (or even sooner) the new tissue that forms at the site of your injury is less flexible than it ought to be.

We learned this from research on the body's cells. For instance, when you injure soft tissue, including a disc, a muscle, or a ligament, the body's repair system gets right to work. Within minutes, a clot forms. Within twenty-four to forty-eight hours, scar tissue begins to form.

To explain what scar tissue cells are like when they are first formed, I like to use an example that people can picture. If you throw pieces of straw on the ground one at a time, the pile that gathers is not orderly; it's higgledy-piggledy. That's how the cells in scar tissue form. They are not like normal cells, which are organized in neat rows. (If you look at a scar compared to normal skin, you can see that it is different.) Normal tissue is flexible — "elastic" is the word that professionals use. Flexible tissue is strong and resistant to injury. Tight, inflexible tissue works poorly and is much more easily strained.

But scar tissue can become flexible. Movement — gentle movement to begin with — actually stimulates those disorganized cells to get themselves organized into neat rows. However, you must begin this gentle movement soon after the injury, if possible within a few days, to initiate this process.

Imagine a man with a back injury who is told to stay in bed for several months and is then sent to physiotherapy. By this point, his injury has healed. But the new tissue is tight. Even the slightest movement causes terrible pain.

A decade ago, this frustrating scenario used to happen all the time. This man's recovery was likely to be limited. For one thing, he would be completely out of condition by the time I saw him. He would also have learned that the best way to help himself was to do nothing; that way his back hurt, but not dreadfully.

Now, take all this and ask yourself about this man's self-image. It's simple: "I am a person who can't do anything." So, in addition to all his other problems, he would feel depressed.

Sure, I could help him improve. But I had to do it by showing him how to get stronger. How to rely on other tissue to compensate for the rigid, injured area that could never be normal and flexible — again.

Now let's imagine that, instead, this man with the back injury comes to an active program after a week. Certainly he's in a lot of pain and can't move very well. And, of course, he's petrified out of his mind. But I can usually get him to do something — some little movement — that lessens the pain, at least a bit. At first, it may only be lying in a certain position. But it's something to send him home with; something he can do for himself.

The next day I might, for example, show him how to arch his back very gently — what we call passive extension. At the same time, I'll teach him a bit about what is happening inside. This is important because, if he can understand why a certain movement helps, then he can start to feel that he is in control.

As the days go on, he can increase the range of his movement and start to do some gentle exercises. But, as a physiotherapist, I know which movements and exercises he should do and which ones he should avoid. I can also show him how to do this without putting a lot of stress on the injured tissue until it has a chance to get stronger.

At the same time, this movement is stimulating the new cells to line up neatly. The result is that his new tissue works like normal tissue. He can recover and get back to work. What's even better is that he has less of a risk of injuring his back again. Plus he's never had a chance to get depressed.

HOW EARLY? HOW ACTIVE?

Dr. Waddell's findings offered some important answers, but they also raised a number of questions — a common occurrence in medical science. For example:

- Exactly what kinds of activities are better than bed rest? For instance, is *aerobic* exercise important in addition to remedial back exercises?
- How intensely, and how soon, after an acute bout of back pain should you start to become active?
- Should you persevere in the face of pain?

In order to come up with a precise definition for "early active treatment," it was necessary to answer these sorts of specific questions. In fact, researchers — for the most part physical therapists who specialize in exercise physiology — are still grappling with them today.

For example, clinicians still disagree about the answer to the first question. Some believe that specific back exercises (pelvic tilts, hamstring stretches, sit-ups, and so on) are the most important part of an early active treatment program. More and more, however, clinicians are coming to the conclusion that, while such exercises are important, aerobics are essential as well. These professionals believe that specific exercises should be done for *remedial* reasons — i.e., if your hamstring muscles are tight, you need to stretch them because tight hamstring muscles increase the strain on your lower back whenever you bend forward, which is frequently. But they also maintain that aerobic exercise is a crucial part of early active treatment. (Chapter 13 treats both aerobics and specific back exercises in more detail.)

Exercise specialist Linda Woodhouse (whom we met in Chapter 3) hails from the latter group. Her reasoning, she explains, has to do with cell behavior:

"As you become fitter from an aerobic standpoint, your body becomes better at delivering nutrients to tissue, including damaged tissue. The point is, in order for damaged discs, joints, muscles, ligaments, and tendons to heal and/or adapt over the long haul, good nutrition at the cellular level is essential."

The problem is, it usually takes a good three to six months for these benefits to pay off in terms of getting rid of pain.

"This is a tough bill to sell," Linda Woodhouse admits. "Patients come to rehab wanting to get rid of their terrible back pain. That's what the doctor promised would happen if they came to this clinic for intensive physiotherapy. It's hard to explain that, at least for the first few weeks — and probably for a whole lot longer — their pain won't decrease, although their ability to function will improve, often by leaps and bounds."

Linda Woodhouse and her colleagues tested this theory in a study of fifty patients who went through a six-week intensive rehabilitation program. Each patient's general aerobic fitness level was measured at the beginning of the problem, then after three weeks, and again after six weeks.

Their method was to measure — with the help of a special machine — how efficiently each patient's heart was able to pump oxygen to his or her muscles, and how efficiently the muscles could use this "fuel." Some years ago, studies showed that people with fairly sedentary lifestyles who followed a six-week aerobic exercise program were usually able to increase their fitness levels by 15 to 20 percent. Much to her surprise, Linda Woodhouse discovered that the fitness levels of the people in her study were increasing by 20 to 30 percent in a mere three weeks! After that the curve leveled off slightly, and the total increase by the end of six weeks averaged about 40 percent, which is downright dramatic.

Even more importantly, the study indicated that, when people worked out at a high level, their back pain was no worse than it had been when they worked out at low levels six weeks before. Better still, when they were doing low-level exercise — i.e., the levels you use when you do "ordinary things: walking, shopping, mowing the lawn" — the pain was a lot less.

"Part of the gain in function," Linda Woodhouse explains, "has to do with changes in the tissue, and part is learning how to cope with pain and do activities more efficiently, or in a slightly different posture that doesn't aggravate your particular problem quite as much." (How different postures affect different types of back pain is described in Chapter 13.)

The people in the study also learned to tell the difference between the signs of exertion and the signs of actual pain. Sometimes you can be so out of condition, so afraid, and so focused on your back problem that you interpret, for example, a rise in your heart rate or the need to breathe harder as pain. Says Linda Woodhouse: "For decades we've drummed the wrong message into people's heads: 'If it hurts, you shouldn't do it because it will make you worse.'"

Nevertheless, the bottom line is that, however much people appreciate the ability to function at a higher level, they want to be pain-free, and I can certainly get behind that. When you persevere for months on end, it's human nature to feel you deserve some light at the end of the tunnel.

However, a recent study from Denmark supports Linda Woodhouse's belief that it takes from three to six months before back pain sufferers can expect to exercise at a high level with no pain. I believe that knowing about such findings can help you keep the faith during periods of pain. (The theory as to *why* the process takes so long goes like this. During these critical months, the number of capillaries — tiny blood vessels that deliver oxygen and nutrients to cells — actually increase in number. This means that oxygen and nutrients are able to get into cells more easily and faster; as well, waste products are more efficient at getting out. Of course, you can't expect this kind of change to take place overnight; in my opinion it's incredible that it can happen at all!)

THE BIGGER QUESTION

Of course most back pain sufferers get better whether they undergo a regimen of early active treatment or not. The bigger problem is that so many people suffer a recurrence, and the second bout is often worse than the first. This fact begs a bigger question: Can early active treatment, especially if it includes an educational component, reduce the likelihood of repeat injuries — i.e., can it help prevent an acute episode of back pain from turning into a chronic problem?

The question is complex, in part because it's hard to separate the psychosocial factors that cause recurrences from the physical ones. But if the enormous cost of back pain to our society is going to be reduced, this question must be addressed. The small percentage of injured workers who suffer from an acute back problem and go on to become chronic sufferers account for the lion's share of the money we spend on compensation.

Let me hit you between the eyes. No matter what kind of treatment is provided (including none at all!), about 20 percent of people who experience an acute bout of back pain develop a chronic problem that ultimately renders them unemployable. But, over 80 percent of the compensation dollars spent worldwide goes toward this small group. Furthermore, once an injured person has been off work for six months, the chances of him or her *ever* going back to work are only 75 percent. After a year, those chances decline to 50 percent, and after two years, they are more or less zero.

A few studies on recurrences have been done. One indicated that, while something like 85 percent of injured people were getting back to work fairly quickly, not all of them were staying on the job. Not by a long shot. Between 40 and 60 percent were having recurrences. Each time, they would stay away from work longer, until eventually many of them became part of the small, chronically unemployed group that costs our society such a fortune.

Clearly, if we could only identify who was at risk of falling into this category early on, and find ways to help prevent that fall, a huge amount of money could be saved. But how to go about this? In the absence of further research, we have only logic: it makes sense that a person who goes back to work in excellent physical shape ought to have a wider safety margin than someone who goes back in the same — or worse — condition than he or she was in at the time of the original injury.

A SAD, SAD STORY

At the end of the 1980s, I and many of my colleagues who are passionate about the future of back pain research were heartened by the news of a major change that was being instituted by the Ontario WCB. It held out promise of answering, or at least providing some insight into, some of the important questions surrounding early active treatment, including the motherlode: could it help prevent recurrences? I was especially proud that such an important step was taking place in Canada.

Unfortunately, the story of this study has a sad ending — one so sad that it breaks my heart. I am including it here because it's an important reminder of how politics, infighting, and just plain bad judgment can screw up even the best-intentioned projects, and of how dangerous it can be to oversimplify complex data. If you suffer from back pain you owe it to yourself to understand the details of what took place.

The story began happily enough. For many years, the Ontario WCB has paid out over $750 million annually in compensation dollars for back pain. Around 1987, some WCB bureaucrats got to thinking about how they could reduce this amount. Because they were forward-thinking, they had been following the kinds of developments in back pain treatment research outlined above and had concluded two things:

1. It's important to get people with back injuries back on the job sooner rather than later because, as time goes by, the chances of someone becoming a chronic, unemployable human being increase.
2. It's no good getting people back to work in a condition that leaves them vulnerable to another back injury.

In other words, do whatever it takes to get people back ASAP: encourage — even *legislate* — employers to modify the jobs of returning workers for a time if it appears that this will help. But for God's sake, make sure that they are in decent physical shape when they return, and that they have the education needed to help them cope, without further loss of work time, when one of the inevitable minor bouts of back pain strikes again. In a nutshell, *prevent* recurrences.

Guided by these principles, the Ontario WCB introduced one of the most progressive changes in medical institution history when, in 1989, it paid (handsomely!) for 102 community clinics to open their doors to men and women who were off work due to low back pain. Some of these clinics were privately owned and freestanding; others were located in hospitals. One hundred were run by physical therapists (the other two were run by chiropractors). Their mandate was to provide injured workers with a six-week, intensive, active rehabilitation program.

The model was to be early active treatment, with emphasis on the "early" — the WCB stipulated that every clinic had to admit all referrals within five days. Education was also an obligatory component of the program; in 1990, this aspect became more formalized when the WCB began providing the clinics with educational material published by the Back Association of Canada (BAC). To put it mildly, I was in heaven; for a few weeks there my back scarcely hurt.

It wasn't a perfect scenario. Medical science was still defining early active treatment, and as I've explained already, different clinicians had differing ideas about what it meant. But within the constraints of what we knew at the time, it was the most exciting large-scale back pain experiment on this planet.

It goes without saying that a trial of this magnitude would have to be evaluated. About the time the program began, the WCB had given $5 million to the Ontario Workers' Compensation Institute (now called the Institute for Work and Health). Its mandate, among other things, was to conduct world-class research, and evaluating these clinics would provide exactly that. Specifically, the Institute was charged with evaluating both the quality of service provided by each of the community clinics and the overall efficacy of the early active treatment program.

A number of clinicians I knew, including Linda Woodhouse, were following this initiative with great interest. To them, it seemed pretty obvious what kind of questions the Institute needed to ask in order to come to a fair and useful conclusion. These included:

1. Were all the community clinics providing the same type of treatment program? (If so, its success could be evaluated; if not, it would be tough to judge.)
2. Were the injured people who were attending the community clinic

program getting back to work in a timely fashion? If not, why not? Were the delays due to physiological or bureaucratic problems? (In fact, in some cases, people whose recovery programs were right on schedule were delayed for weeks from returning to the job while waiting for the WCB to sign off!)

3. Did the program significantly increase people's level of fitness, as well as their coping skills and knowledge?

4. If there was an increase in people's level of fitness, was it resulting in a reduction of the number of recurrences of back pain?

As I have mentioned, this last question was the motherlode — a tough one to answer, to be sure, but even some reliable indications would have been incalculably useful.

Yet — and here the sad part of the story begins — the Institute chose to address only the first two of these four questions. Furthermore, many reputable researchers have questioned its approach even to answering these. For example, the Institute concluded that not all clinics were in fact offering early active treatment; some were offering mostly passive modalities. However, they did nothing to remedy this problem — they just plowed on ahead and asked all the clinics the next question: How long did it take participants to get back to work? Fat lot of good it does to compare apples to oranges.

Worse yet, the Institute failed to properly evaluate what the clinics that *did* offer active treatment actually meant by "active." Remember, increased fitness was supposed to be one of the goals — yet the Institute classified as "active treatment" anything that was not completely passive. No distinction was made between a clinic where patients lay down on the floor and did gentle stretching exercises while listening to a relaxation tape compared to a clinic where regular intense aerobic exercise was part of the regime.

All in all, the evaluation seemed to focus more on process than on programming. For instance, the Institute investigated whether patients were actually being treated by qualified clinicians for the right number of days and whether these clinicians had filled out certain forms correctly. These are not unimportant questions, don't get me wrong. But they are certainly not as important as whether the clinics were in fact meeting their obligation to deliver early active treatment programs!

Such investigation of programming as the Institute did do was pretty poor-quality research. About 8 percent of the community clinic patients were surveyed by telephone, and asked such questions as whether they *liked* the program and whether they personally *felt* that their ability to function had improved. Any researcher can tell you that such subjective judgments are of little use when you're trying to be scientific. Furthermore, a phone survey could not determine *how much* a person's ability to function had increased, if indeed it had.

The community clinic evaluation was no camptown racetrack in terms of money — the Institute for Work and Health spent about $600,000 on it. Frankly, for that price, I think they ought to have been able to provide the world with more accurate, more useful information.

A GOLDEN CHANCE LOST

In 1995, the Institute presented its findings — principally, that injured workers who had attended the community clinic program were going back to work no sooner (although no later) than those who had received rehabilitation somewhere else.

This information amounted essentially to a dubiously supported, incomplete answer to question number one in my list on page 217. Since the treatment was not even remotely standard at the community clinics, and not even always truly active, this finding actually said very little about the effectiveness of early active treatment at all. And the all-important issue of recurrent injuries was never addressed at all. Through the grapevine, I heard that the Institute felt that such an undertaking would have been too cumbersome and that tracking recurrences would have taken a couple of years.

A couple of years! You're darned straight it would have taken that length of time — but it doesn't seem a lot to ask for $600,000 never mind the millions that were being spent on the early active treatment program itself! My feeling is that the bureaucrats behind the evaluation, unlike the forward-thinking ones who introduced the program in the first place, were simply too arrogant to seek out the opinions of clinicians who might have pointed them in the right direction. At one point, I called the Institute's coordinator of health services half a dozen times to discuss it — but not one of my calls were returned. Okay, I'm a layperson. But I know a couple of things.

The final blow occurred on November 1, 1995. In the wake of the Institute's finding that community clinic patients were returning to work no earlier than those treated elsewhere, the WCB held a meeting of community clinic owners. Without so much as a word of consultation with the clinics (who had heretofore been billed as "partners" in the program), the WCB announced that, starting the next month, no one would be allowed to attend a community clinic program until he or she had been off work for at least twenty-nine days.

How can I explain my disappointment? For the majority of Ontario workers with back injuries it's no big deal to wait twenty-nine days for treatment — as I have said, most people get better no matter what you do. What matters is that a golden opportunity to study the benefits of early active treatment, including its effectiveness in reducing the number of chronic patients that cost us billions a year, was squashed because of bureaucratic ineptitude and sloppy research.

Worse was the coverage the news received in the lay press. I don't blame the media — how could a mainstream reporter be expected to understand the complexities of such a research project, or the importance of the early active treatment philosophy? But however unintentionally, harm was done. Shortly after the November meeting, for example, a story in the *Toronto Star* ran under the following subheadline: "Costly clinics make no impact, study says." To approximately one million readers, it sounded as if a trial of the latest treatment philosophy had been a failure — when the truth of the matter is simply that we still have no idea!

Why have I devoted so much space to this small, sad story about research? Because I think back pain sufferers, researchers, clinicians, journalists, politicians, and plain old voting, taxpaying, letter-writing citizens — in other words, all of us — have a responsibility to ensure that this kind of tragedy is prevented wherever possible in any field of medicine, or, for that matter, any human endeavor.

13

Fitness and Exercise

T his chapter is devoted to exercise for back pain. If you've read any
other books about back pain, you'll probably have already waded
through a similar chapter, since exercise is the one treatment everyone seems to agree is important. What I have to say, however, is a bit
different. Rather than leave it at "Do ten of each of the following exercises
once a day," I want to give you the information you need to play an *active*
role when it comes to taking responsibility for your own back. By the time
you have plowed through this chapter, you will have a good understanding of the meaning of fitness, the increased importance of fitness as we
age, and how exercise can help improve function as well as decreasing
pain (I touched on this last one in Chapter 12). I'll describe some specific
back exercises too, of course, but I'll also give you the general background
you need to design a program to meet your *particular* needs, including
altering your posture if necessary so that you can do daily activities without discomfort, and select aerobic activities that are appropriate for your
situation.

When your body is working well, you tend not to think about all the
tasks you ask it to do: walking, sitting, standing, reaching, lifting things,
carrying things, playing sports, etc. But each and every day, whether you

are aware of it or not, you make demands on your body, particularly on your back, that are very stressful. The fitter you are, the easier it is for you and your back to deal with these stresses.

WHAT DOES IT MEAN TO BE FIT?

Exercise experts identify five categories of fitness: body composition, flexibility, muscular strength, muscular endurance, and aerobic fitness.

Body composition refers to how your body is made up, specifically your height relative to your weight and the percentage of fat in your body relative to the percentage of muscle. Body composition is not something you can control completely because genetics plays a role. However, if you are willing to put in the effort, you can do quite a lot to make your body composition healthier. (For more on body composition and how to measure it, see "Value of Pound Plummets!" at the end of this section.)

Flexibility refers to your ability to move easily within your normal range of motion, including at times moving to the very end of this range without doing yourself harm.

Muscular strength refers to the *greatest amount of force* a particular muscle group (as opposed to your entire body) can produce, or withstand, for a very short period of time — for example, the greatest weight you are capable of lifting once.

Muscular endurance, on the other hand, refers to the ability of a particular muscle group to produce, or withstand, a *moderate force* over a longer period of time — for example, lifting 50 percent of your maximum four times per minute *for a few minutes.*

Aerobic fitness refers to how well your body can perform *low-intensity* tasks over a long period of time. An example is lifting 25 percent of your maximum ten or more times per minute for fifteen minutes or longer. You may not realize it, but you use your aerobic system when you sit at a desk typing, or on a couch just watching TV. Of course, in these cases, it is working at a *very* low level!

Your body uses different fuel systems for strength, endurance, and aerobic types of tasks. For instance, to create the energy that's required for a short but intense burst of activity (for example, lifting a ninety-pound box once) your muscles use fuel that is stored right in the part of the muscle that must contract in order to do the job. The bigger the muscle is, the more fuel it can store and the more force it can generate. If your lifestyle — your job and/or your leisure activities — demands a lot of muscular strength, that's what you should focus on when you set out to design your personal fitness program.

Muscular endurance comes into the act after you run low on this local fuel. Your muscles must ultimately change their fuel source to carbohydrates, some of which must be brought in by your circulation system. The fitter you are, the faster your muscles will be able to take in, and use, this form of energy. Pretty well everyone's lifestyle demands muscular endurance, but if you do a lot of housework that requires you to bend forward (washing dishes, making beds), endurance is extremely important. It's also important to find efficient ways of doing these sorts of tasks.

For tasks lasting more than a few minutes, your aerobic system comes into play. For this kind of long-haul activity, the fuel comes mostly from fats. In order to convert fat into energy, your body needs oxygen, which must travel to your muscles from your lungs. The fitter you are aerobically, the more efficiently your body will be able to use oxygen. You will also require less of it to perform a certain task. Aerobically fit people also heal faster from most injuries, including strained backs.

Whatever your lifestyle, flexibility plays an important role. If bending forward, or flexing, your back thirty degrees puts you at the very end of your normal range of motion, you will strain the muscles, ligaments, and tendons of your back every time you do this. This is true whether you are carrying a light load, a heavy load, or no load at all. In turn, every time you strain your muscles, the discs and joints of your back will be stressed as well.

If, on the other hand, you are flexible enough to bend forward forty-five degrees with ease, it is only logical that there will be far less strain on your back when you bend to only thirty degrees.

When you injure your back, it is usually because you are doing some-

BACK
MEDICATION

The following chart explains what back pain sufferers should know about the drugs that exist for their ailment.

At first glance it may seem a bit complicated. Back pain patients take more than 100 different kinds of medication and this chart contains information on just about all of them. That's a lot of material. But if you take a moment, you'll see that the information is well organized and easy to find.

- *Analgesics* are in the first row (Boxes 1-7).
- *NSAIDS* are in the next two rows (Boxes 8-21).
- *Muscle Relaxants* and *Anti-Inflammatory Drugs* are in the next row (Boxes 22-26).
- *Antidepressants* are in the final row (Boxes 27-30).

If you know the brand name of your medication, you can look it up in the alphabetical list on page C6, note the box number in the list, then locate the box on the chart. In it you'll find: the drug's chemical name, information on possible contraindications and side effects, and specific tips. (The symbols are explained in the Legend on page C5.)

You can also use the chart to compare drugs. For example, if you are taking a muscle relaxant and you are experiencing a side effect (such as sleepiness), you can read about other choices, then discuss them with your family physician or pharmacist.

It's your responsibility to know what drugs you are taking, how they work, and how they may affect you.

ASA – Non-narcotic. Also reduces inflammation.
(Anacin, Aspirin, Ecotrin, Entrophen, Supasa, Apo-Asa, Novasen)
C: BD ⬡ ⬡ ⬡ ⬡ ⬡ (M)
(anticoagulants, drugs for gout, oral medication for diabetes, corticosteroids, NSAIDS) ⬡ (with large doses).
S: GI D (when combined with ⬡).
• Don't make up a missed dose. Stay on regular schedule. Discuss use before surgery, and prolonged use. **EAT** or ⬡.   1.

ACETAMINOPHEN – Non-narcotic. Does not reduce inflammation.
(Actimol, Anacin-AF, Atasol, Panadol, Tylenol, 222-AF, Apo-Acetaminophen, etc.)
C: ⬡ ⬡ ⬡ ⬡ (M) (some anticoagulants, cholestyramine).
S: Very safe when taken correctly.
• Overdose can cause ⬡ ⬡ damage or be fatal, especially with ⬡. **EAT** or ⬡.   2.

IBUPROFEN
(Advil, Motrin, Actiprofen, Medipren, Apo-Ibuprofen, Novo-Profen)
C: ⬡ ♡ **HBP** ⬡ ⬡ (M) (other NSAIDS, diuretics, digoxin, lithium, anti-coagulants, antihypertensives) ⬡ (safety not known).
S: Fewer than most NSAIDS, **GI** (especially with ⬡).   8.

NAPROXEN
(Naprosyn, Naxen, Apo-Naproxen, Novo-Naprox, Nu-Naprox)
C: See notes on Ibuprofen.
S: GI (especially with ⬡) (H) **D S**.   9.

TIAPROFENIC ACID
(Albert Tiafen, Surgam)
C: See notes on Sulindac.
S: See notes on Sulindac + **D**.   16.

FLURBIPROFEN
(Ansaid, Froben, Ocufen, Apo-flurbiprofen)
C: See notes on Ibuprofen + (M) (oral medication for diabetes).
S: GI ⬡.   17.

METHOCARBAMOL (MR)
(Robaxin, Robaxacet [with Acetaminophen], Robaxisal [with ASA])
C: ⬡ ⬡ ⬡ **E** ⬡ ⬡.
S: S & **D** in a small number of patients (especially with ⬡, sedatives, narcotic analgesics, antidepressants, antihistamines).
• Avoid driving, hazardous work until you are aware of effects. Discuss use before surgery.   22.

ORPHENADRINE CITRATE (Norflex)
ORPHENADRINE [with ASA and Caffeine]
(Norgesic/Norgesic Forte)
C: ♡ ⬡ ⬡ ⬡ (M) (amantadine, haloperidol, or other phenothiazines, sulfite sensitivity).
S: S ⬡ **D** ⬡ **GI** (nausea, constipation), insomnia, possible sexual dysfunction.
• Avoid driving, hazardous work until you know effects. Don't stop abruptly. Discuss with doctor. Discuss use before any surgery.   23.

TRICYCLICS Clomipramine (Anafranil), **Trimipramine** (Rhotrimine, Surmontil, Apo-Trimip), **Doxepin HCI** (Triadapin, Sinequan), **Nortriptyline HCI** (Aventyl), **Amitriptyline HCI** (Elavil), **Imipramine** (Tofranil)
C: ♡ **E G** ⬡ **T BD** ⬡
⬡ **P** (M) (sedatives, anti-hypertensives, MAOIs).
S: S ⬡ **TS** ⬡ **D LB** (gain) ⬡ (increases sedative effects).
• Overdose can be serious, even fatal.   27.

ATYPICAL ANTIDEPRESSANT
Venlafaxine (Effexor)
C: ⬡ ⬡ ⬡ (M) (MAOIs, cimetidine, [Tagamet]).
S: S ⬡ **D** (H) **GI** (especially nausea, constipation), insomnia, possible sexual dysfunction.
• Discuss use before any surgery.   28.

CODEINE – Mild narcotic
+ ASA (222, 292, Fiorinal, which is also a barbiturate, etc.).
+ ACETAMINOPHEN (Empracet, Tylenol with codeine, Atasol with codeine, Parafon Forte [see Box 24], etc.).
C: ① ⊙ ⬤ Ⓜ (sedatives, antidepressants, antihistamines, especially with ⓨ).
S: GI (especially constipation) with Ⓜ (especially sedatives) effects are increased.
• Also see ASA & ACETAMINOPHEN notes. 3.

OXYCODONE – Strong narcotic
+ ASA (Percodan, Endodan)
+ ACETAMINOPHEN (Percocet, Endocet)
C: T ❔ ⬤ ♡ ✋ 🫁 ⊙ ⬤
Ⓜ (see codeine).
S: GI (nausea, vomiting, constipation) **D MC S**.

• See ASA & ACETAMINOPHEN notes.
• Lying down often relieves side-effects. 4.

KETOPROFEN
(Orudis, Oruvail, Rhodis, Apo-Keto)

C: See notes on Ibuprofen.

S: See notes on Naproxen.

• Some tabs must not be broken. Suppositories also available.
10.

DICLOFENAC
(Voltaren, Apo-Diclo, Novo-Difenac, Nu-Diclo)

C: See notes on Ibuprofen + Ⓜ (methotrexate, oral medication for diabetes) ⊙ .

S: See notes on Naproxen + **AB**.
11.

TOLMETIN
(Tolectin)

C: See notes on Sulindac + Ⓜ (lithium).

S: See notes on Sulindac.

• Adverse affects usually decrease during treatment. Higher risk factors than other NSAIDS.
18.

PIROXICAM
(Feldene, Apo-Piroxicam, Novo-Pirocam, Nu-Pirox)

C: See notes on Ibuprofen.

S: See notes on Sulindac.

• Large overdose may cause nausea/vomiting.
19.

CHLORZOXAZONE
(Parafon Forte C8)
C: ⬤ ✋ **AB** ⬤ ⊙ Ⓐ + other allergies, head injury.
S: S & **D** in a small number of patients (especially with ⓨ, sedatives, narcotic analgesics, antidepressants, antihistamines) ▦ (rare).

• Avoid driving, hazardous work until you know effects. Don't stop abruptly. Discuss with doctor. Discuss use before any surgery. 24.

CYCLOBENZAPRINE (MR)
(Flexeril)

C: Ⓐ use of MAOIs ♡ **T** ⬤ ⊙ .

S: S & **D** in a large number of patients (especially with ⓨ, sedatives, narcotic analgesics, antidepressants, antihistamines) ⬥ (rare).
• Avoid driving, hazardous work until you know effects. Don't stop abruptly. Discuss with doctor. Discuss use before any surgery. Not recommended for more than 3 weeks. 25.

MAOIs – MONOAMINE OXYDASE INHIBITORS
Phenelzine (Nardil)

C: E ❔ ⬤ ♡ ⬤ ⊙ Ⓜ (antihyperintensives, digoxin, phenytoin, sedatives, narcotics, antihistamines).

S: D ⓨ (increases sedative effects).

• Discuss use before any surgery. Reacts with some foods, such as cheese. (Ask for list.) With Nardil, avoid heavy red wine in particular. 29.

SSRIs — SELECTIVE SERATONIN REUPTAKE INHIBITORS
Fluoxetine (Prozac), **Sertraline** (Zoloft), **Paroxetine** (Paxil)
C: ❔ ⬤ ♡ **E** ⓨ Ⓜ (MAOIs, sedatives, tryptophan) ⬤ ⊙ .
S: Ⓗ 〰 **GI** (nausea, diarrhea) insomnia **LB** (loss) ⓨ (may increase sedative effects), possible sexual dysfunction.

• Discuss use before any surgery. 30.

PROPROXYPHENE – Medium strong narcotic – does not reduce inflammation except if boosted with ASA (642, Darvon, 692, etc.).

C: (particularly sedatives) .

S: **D GI** (particularly nausea, vomiting).

• Effects tend to weaken over time. Less addictive than similar drugs.

5.

MORPHINE – Strong narcotic – does not reduce inflammation unless boosted with ASA (Epimorph, Morphine HP, MS Contin, Roxinol).

C: (see codeine) .

S: **S & D** (particularly with), **GI** (constipation, vomiting, nausea).

• Slow release tabs (MS Contin) available.

6.

DIFLUNISAL
(Dolobid)

C: See notes on Ibuprofen.

S: See notes on Naproxen.

12.

FENOPROFEN
(Nalfon)

C: See notes on Ibuprofen + oral medication for diabetes.

S: **GI** **D S** (H).

13.

INDOMETHACIN
(Indocid, Apo-Indomethacin, Novo-Methacin, Nu-Indo)

C: See notes on Sulindac + (methotrexate, lithium).

S: See notes on Sulindac + **D** (H).

• Advise doctor if you have Parkinson's disease.

20.

PHENYLBUTAZONE
(Butazolidin, Apo-Phenylbutazone)

C: E BD

HBP (see notes on Ibuprofen + oral medication for diabetes).

S: **GI AB** H_2O.

• Side-effects can be severe. Not first choice. Take for 7 days only and blood tests should be taken during use.

21.

BENZODIAZAPINES (Anti-anxiety)

Alprazolam (Xanax, Apo-Alpraz, Novo-Alprazol, Nu-Alpraz), **Bromazepam** (Lectopam), **Chlordiazepoxide** (Librium, Solium, Apo-Chlordiazepoxide), **Diazepam** (Diazemuls, Valium Roche, Vivol, Apo-Diazepam), **Flurazepam** (Dalmane, Apo-Flurazepam, Novo-Flupam), **Lorazepam** (Ativan, Apo-Lorazepam, Novo-Lorazem, Nu-Loraz), **Oxazepam** (Serax, Apo-Oxazepam).

C: G alcohol/drug abuse, myasthenia gravis, (especially sedatives, antidepressants, narcotics, scopalamine, anti-psychotics, antihistamines, other drugs for anxiety).

S: **D S**.

• If stopped suddenly, withdrawal symptoms possible. Discuss with doctor.

26.

TIPS

• The three main Canadian generic 'brands' are called: Apo, Novo and Nu.

• Take with **full** glass of water.

• Take with food. **EAT**

• Please note that side-effects often increase for patients over the age of 60.

• Rare side-effects are too numerous to list. They are mostly the same as those already mentioned.

• Steroids are rarely indicated for back pain. They include: Cortisone, Prednisone, Dexamethasone.

• is usually contraindicated for people taking medication. Can increase **D** and **GI** problems (NSAIDS: **GI** problems especially).

MEPERIDINE – Strong narcotic – does not reduce inflammation.
(Demerol, Pamergan)

C: ♡ E ✋ T ❓ ⊙ ● U

▶ Ⓜ (MAOIs, sedatives particularly).

S: **GI** (particularly nausea, vomiting, constipation)
D S.

7.

NOTES on NSAIDS • EAT or 🅦. Wait 15 min. before lying down, so drug can reach stomach.
• Long-term use increases risk of **GI** problems. If taking NSAID for more than 3 weeks, don't stop suddenly. Consult doctor.
• Discuss allergy to ASA, other NSAIDS.
• Call doctor immediately in case of black or blood-stained stools/unexplained wheezing/ breathlessness.
• NSAIDS may increase/prolong bleeding. Discuss use before any surgery.

KETOROLAC TROMETHAMINE
(Toradol)

C: See notes on Ibuprofen plus ● ⊙
definitely not recommended.

S: See notes on Naproxen.

• New drug, minimal anti-inflammatory properties at normal dose for pain. Other **C** and **S** may be reported in future.

14.

SULINDAC
(Apo-Sulin, Clinoril, Novo-Sudac)

C: ▶ ❓ ✋ ❤ Ⓐ (ASA) ● ⊙
Ⓜ (other NSAIDS, anti-coagulants, antihypertensives, diuretics, corticosteroids) **HBP BD**.

S: **GI** (especially with Ⓨ) **AB** ❤.

• Notify doctor if extra dose taken by mistake and unusual symptoms noticed.

15.

LEGEND

C: Possible Contraindications – Discuss with Doctor

Kidney Problems	❓	Nasal Polyps	👃
Liver Problems	▶	Blood Disorder	**BD**
Heart Problems	♡	Use of Other Medications	Ⓜ
High Blood Pressure	**HBP**	Inflammatory Bowel disease	Ⓘ
Ulcers/ Stomach Problems	S	Epilepsy	**E**
Asthma	✋	Prostate Problems	**P**
Drug Allergies	Ⓐ	Glaucoma	**G**
Pregnancy	●	Thyroid Problems	**T**
Breast Feeding	⊙	Lung Problems (Bronchitis)	🫁
Alcohol	Ⓨ	Urinary Problems	**U**

S: Possible Side-effects – Discuss with Doctor

Gasto-intestinal Tract (nausea/ vomiting/diarrhea/ constipation/stomach irritation)	**GI**	Wheezing	🫁
		Abdominal Pain	**AB**
Dizziness	**D**	Dry Mouth	👄
Sleepiness/ Drowsiness	**S**	Rash	▦
Nervousness	∿	Blurred Vision	👁
Heartburn/ Indigestion	❤	Mood Change	**MC**
Headache	Ⓗ	Clammy Skin/ Sweating	
Swollen Feet/Ankles	👣	Weight Gain/Loss	**LB**
Ringing in Ears	〜	Trembling/ Shaking	**TS**
Water Retention	H_2O	Muscle Weakness	**MW**

Drugs Listed by Brand Name

222 – 2*
222 (+ codeine) – 3
222-AF – 2
292 – 3
642 – 5
692 – 5
Actimol – 2
Actiprofen – 8
Advil – 8
Albert Tiafen – 16
Anacin – 1
Anacin-AF – 2
Anafranil – 27
Ansaid – 17
Apo-Acetaminophen – 2
Apo-Alpraz – 26
Apo-Asa – 1
Apo-Chlordiazepoxide – 26
Apo-Diazepam – 26
Apo-Diclo – 12
Apo-Flurazepam – 26
Apo-Flurbiprofen – 17
Apo-Ibuprofen – 8
Apo-Indomethacin – 20
Apo-Keto – 11
Apo-Lorazepam – 26
Apo-Naproxen – 9
Apo-Oxazepam – 26
Apo-Phenylbutazone – 21
Apo-Piroxicam – 19
Apo-Sulin – 15
Apo-Trimip – 27
Aspirin – 1
Atasol – 2
Atasol (+ codeine) – 3
Ativan – 26
Aventyl – 27
Butazolidin – 21
Clinoril – 15

Dalmane – 26
Darvon – 5
Demerol – 7
Diazemuls – 26
Dolobid – 12
Ecotrin – 1
Effexor – 28
Elavil – 27
Empracet – 3
Endocet – 4
Endodan – 4
Entrophen – 1
Epimorph – 6
Feldene – 19
Fiorinal – 3
Flexeril – 25
Froben – 17
Indocid – 20
Lectopam – 26
Librium – 26
Medipren – 8
Morphine HP – 6
Motrin – 8
MS Contin – 6
Nalfon – 13
Naprosyn – 9
Nardil – 29
Naxen – 9
Norflex – 23
Norgesic – 23
Novasen – 1
Novo-Alprazol – 26
Novo-Difenac – 12
Novo-Flupam – 26
Novo-Lorazem – 26
Novo-Methacin – 20
Novo-Naprox – 9
Novo-Pirocam – 19
Novo-Profen – 8
Novo-Sudac – 15

Nu-Alpraz – 26
Nu-Indo – 20
Nu-Loraz – 26
Nu-Naprox – 9
Nu-Pirox – 19
Ocufen – 17
Orudis – 11
Oruvail – 11
Pamergan – 7
Panadol – 2
Parafon Forte – 3
Parafon Forte C8 – 24
Paxil – 30
Percocet – 4
Percodan – 4
Prozac – 30
Rhodis – 11
Rhotrimine – 27
Robaxacet – 22
Robaxin – 22
Robaxisal – 22
Roxinal – 6
Serax – 26
Sinequan – 27
Solium – 26
Supasa – 1
Surgam – 16
Surmontil – 27
Tofranil – 27
Tolectin – 18
Toradol – 14
Triadapin – 27
Tylenol – 2
Tylenol (+ codeine) – 3
Valium Roche – 26
Vivol – 26
Voltaren – 12
Wellbutrin – 28
Xanax – 26
Zoloft – 30

* Numbers refer to boxes on previous pages

thing that requires you to be fitter than you are in one, or more, of these various categories. Of course, nobody is *so* fit as to be able to perform any kind of task without risk of injury. Human backs were not built to toss around refrigerators, withstand serious falls, or remain in stressful postures for long periods of time.

You should, however, be able to become fit enough to be able to lift things within reason, play tennis, or tend your garden without great risk of injury, even if you have suffered from acute or chronic back pain in the past. This is part of the miracle of the human spine.

Value of Pound Plummets!

I'm a bit reluctant to admit this, but after years of procrastination, what finally got me walking on a regular basis was not my sore back but my desire to lose five pounds. I've always preached the gospel that there's little point in going on a diet unless aerobic exercise is part and parcel of the deal. But what moved me to actually do what I'd been urging others to do for years was understanding *why* this is true. It all has to do with body composition.

The penny dropped — that is, I grasped why exercise and weight loss must be a team — when I ran into a couple of guys who sell a computerized instrument called the *Body Composition Analyzer*, or BCA. As the name suggests, this type of analysis provides information about the composition of the pounds in your body in terms of lean tissue (muscle, organs, bone, etc.) and fatty tissue. But let's stop mincing words and call a spade a spade. What I mean when I say fatty tissue is FAT.

A BCA costs about $5,400. But that hasn't stopped hundreds of hospitals, health clubs, and universities from buying one. Over the past few years, the number of people who have become interested in analyzing their body composition before they start a fitness and/or weight loss program has grown by leaps and bounds.

BCA is pretty simple, really. You lie down. Two electrodes are attached with adhesive tape to one hand, and two to one foot. A high-frequency signal (a radio frequency of 50,000 hertz, actually) is created. Since human skin offers no resistance to such a signal, a weak field is set up inside your body when the machine is turned on.

What BCA measures is how easily your body is able to conduct this signal. The bottom line is that lean body mass conducts it with very little resistance. Fat, on the other hand, is a lousy conductor. BCA figures this out and computes a number. The higher the number, the greater the percentage of fat your body contains.

I tried it. Three painless, noninvasive minutes later, the computer spewed out all the gory details of my body's ability to conduct radio signals, and the software translated them into my own personal body composition report. I have no intention of sharing this information with any of you, but I will illustrate the concept and its implications with a couple of made-up examples.

Take two women, Joan and Jan. (See the illustration on the next page.) They are both age forty-six. They are both five feet, six inches tall and tip the scales at 130 pounds. They also eat the same number of calories each day. In fact, the only big difference between their lifestyles is that Joan exercises moderately, but consistently, several times a week, while Jan is a couch potato.

To people who are interested in body composition, however, the important difference between these two women has not yet been discussed. How many of those 130 pounds are composed of lean tissue and how many are composed of fat? Joan and Jan could stand on their bathroom scales every morning for the next decade and they wouldn't learn the answer to that important question.

BCA, however, can add this information to the picture:

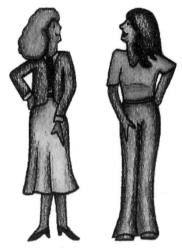

Joan and Jan

Joan's Analysis	Jan's Analysis
Total weight:	Total weight:
130 lbs	130 lbs
31.5 lbs of fat	43.8 lbs of fat
98.5 lbs of lean	86.2 lbs of lean
tissue	tissue
% of body fat: 24	% of body fat: 34

A normal, healthy female in her mid-forties should have a body with a fat content of about 22 to 28 percent. (At the same age, a male's fat content should be 14 to 20 percent.) That puts Joan right in the middle of the fit category. Jan, on the other hand, is a bit above; her body contains too much fat to be called fit in terms of composition.

But here's the punchline: If Jan goes on a calorie-restricted diet for a few months but retains her couch-potato lifestyle, she will lose some weight — let's say, eight pounds. The trouble is, most of what she will lose is precisely what she wants to keep: lean tissue. Even worse, she will keep almost all of what she wants to get rid of: fat.

At the end of her diet, Jan's body composition might look something like this:

Total weight: 122 pounds
37 lbs of fat
85 lbs of lean tissue
% of body fat: 30.3

For all her willpower, Jan's body composition has, in fact, become worse. Although she has lost eight pounds, her body fat percentage has actually increased. Worse, she has not become healthier at all!

This phenomenon has to do with the body's fuel systems. It so happens that human beings have three such systems. Two of them are called **anaerobic** systems because they do not use oxygen. The other is the **aerobic** system, which does use oxygen. It is also the only system that uses fat as its fuel.

The first fuel system uses glycogen, which is kept stored in our muscles for immediate use. If you walk over to the TV to turn the channel, for instance, the energy required will be provided by the fuel stored in the muscles of your legs. No fat will get used up.

The second fuel system kicks in if you do something that takes a couple of minutes — for example, stacking up half a dozen cartons of books. After the local fuel is used up, this system relies on carbohydrates as its fuel source. But you still don't burn up any fat.

In order to use fat as fuel, your body has to **metabolize** it. (That's health-care jargon for "breaking down.") The problem with fat is that it's difficult for your body to break it down. Doing it takes something like a hundred different steps, all of which take time and require oxygen as well. So the aerobic system only gets going after you've been exercising for at least three or four minutes or longer at a good, although not excessive, rate. That's when you start burning up fat.

Sprinting up one flight of stairs won't do it. This activity doesn't take long enough, plus it calls for a lot of energy very fast. Scrubbing a floor just might do it — a very big, very dirty floor. Taking the garbage out won't do it, although that kind of activity is good for building up strength. Walking will do it. There's no doubt in my mind about that because I've been doing it and I'm starting to see the results. By now there shouldn't be any doubt in your mind either! So get moving.

P.S. What do you think will happen to Joan if she eats normally but exercises regularly? She will build up lean tissue, which means she will actually gain some pounds. But she will also lose some pounds of fat. In the end, she may weigh about the same or even

a bit more since lean tissue weighs more than fat when you compare it volume for volume. But she'll look and feel better, and have
a lot more energy — and I bet you her back will hurt less!

For more information about BCA, contact Michael Donahue or Frank Mayne at Biotech Medical Inc., 1071 King Street West, Toronto, Ontario, M6K 3K2. Telephone: (416) 345-8392. Biotech Medical Inc. also does employee assessments for companies.

FITNESS AND AGING

As your back ages, its composition changes; for one thing, you end up
with less lean body mass and more fat. This translates into decreased ability in terms of muscular strength, muscular endurance, aerobic fitness,
and flexibility. This process is normal, but it can cause certain problems,
notably in your discs and joints. (These age-related back problems are
described in more detail in Chapter 2.) If your back is fit, you can avoid
(or at least be better able to cope with) many of these difficulties.

To become fit, you will have to work at it. If you have injured your back,
or strained it by forcing it to deal with poor posture every day for many
years, you will have to work a bit harder to get fit and stay fit.

On the other hand, your body — and that includes your back — is
much tougher and more resilient than you probably realize. If, due to an
injury or chronic strain, one part of your back cannot function properly,
nearby tissue — if it's strong — can usually compensate. For instance, if
some of your ligaments have become too lax to provide support, your
muscles can help take over the job. A fit back can *compensate* for an injury.

For these reasons, I urge those of you who are older especially not to be
afraid to start a back fitness program. Yes, getting fit will take some time
and may well cause you some discomfort along the way. But I promise
that it will be worth it in the end. Not only will increasing your fitness
reduce your risk of injury, it will also reduce the time it takes you to
recover if, like a lot of people, you have recurrent episodes of back pain.

IMPROVING FUNCTION THROUGH EXERCISE

As physical therapist Mary Sauriol explained in Chapter 12, the first focus of modern rehabilitation is to help you get back to normal in terms of function as soon as possible. This way of thinking has, in part, to do with our new understanding of how scar tissue develops. As your injury heals, *very* gentle stretching is usually all you can be expected to do. (As I explain in Chapter 18, massage is another way of stretching injured tissue, but the stretch is passive rather than active.)

In most cases, acute pain will begin to subside within two or three days. That's when the second phase of treatment — more strenuous flexibility exercises and aerobic exercise — can begin. After a few weeks, you can add strengthening exercises to your regime. If your lifestyle requires it, endurance exercises can be added after you have built up your strength.

When you begin to exercise, your pain may increase for a few weeks. However, this sort of pain usually feels different from the kind of acute pain of, for example, a bulging disc irritating a nerve. It is the pain of muscles getting used to new activity.

On the positive side, as I've explained in Chapter 12, your ability to function will also improve dramatically, and this should be your measure of success. At least that's the theory; in practice, trying to balance pain with increased function can be quite a challenge. To help pull it off, I urge you to listen to what your body tells you about the difference between *hurt* and *harm*. The toughest part is hanging in for the three to six months it so often takes for back pain sufferers to become almost or totally pain-free. By this time, you will probably have been in pretty good shape for quite a while. This seems so unfair!

Some people never get rid of all of their pain. In some cases, this is because they simply don't achieve a level of fitness high enough to cause their pain to disappear. Researchers do not fully understand why this happens. In other cases, the original injury may have been so extensive that, miraculous as the human body is, the tissue cannot heal 100 percent. Finally, I think that in some cases, some discomfort lingers simply because there are mysterious components to pain — especially back pain. This is true in my case: regardless of how much I exercise, my back pain has never totally gone away. Of course, I've never managed to really give up my sedentary existence. I have a great chair, but I sit in it for, I'd say, seventy or more hours a week when I'm writing to stressful deadlines, which is most of the time. But, what the hell! You wouldn't want me to stop even if it meant that my back would never hurt again — at least, not until I've finished writing this book.

Designing Your Own Exercise Program

Now that you know a little more about fitness in theory, you're ready to start on the nitty-gritty of creating an exercise scheme that works for *you*. I believe that this is far better than relying totally on a health-care professional to make the decisions for you. For one thing, running — okay, walking! — to clinicians takes up a lot of time; you'd probably be better off devoting that time to getting fit. For another, no one — not even the most brilliant exercise physiologist — can possibly get in touch with your back as well as you.

On the other hand, if you're not satisfied with your progress, or you're in doubt about which exercises are best for you, by all means consult a professional. Just be sure to choose someone who knows something about exercise and wants you to take an active role.

However, once you start your program, if at any time you are feeling frustrated by the pain, you shouldn't hesitate to consult a health-care professional — a physical or occupational therapist, or your family physician. At the very least, a professional should be able to see what you are doing and assure you that you're on the right track, even give you a little pep talk. In my book, you can't get too much encouragement when you're undertaking a task that demands such patience and perseverance!

Setting Goals

The first thing to decide is exactly what you want to accomplish. What area of fitness concerns you? Do you need to make forward strides in it, or just hold the line? Here are some guidelines.

To *improve* your flexibility, the best advice is to do stretching exercises daily. To *maintain* flexibility, four or five times weekly will do the trick.

To *improve* your muscular strength, three times a week (for at least fifteen minutes per session) is the minimum. Twice a week is usually enough for *maintenance*.

If you want to work on muscular *endurance*, you will need to add an additional fifteen minutes to your program: three times a week to *improve*; twice a week for *maintenance*. The easiest way to do this is to add an endurance component to the exercises you do for strength; this is explained in greater detail in the descriptions of specific exercises.

To *improve* your aerobic fitness, three times a week (for at least fifteen minutes each session) is the minimum. Again, twice a week is enough for *maintenance*.

The Basics of Aerobic Fitness

To improve your aerobic fitness, your heart — which is a muscle, remember — must work *continuously* at 75 to 80 percent of its maximum capability for a minimum of fifteen minutes. (Older, and very deconditioned, people should start at 60 percent of their heart's maximum. Athletes often work toward 85 to 90 percent.)

You can measure how hard your heart is working in beats per minute. To find out your maximum, subtract your age from 220. Seventy-five percent of that number is about the level at which you should be working.

For example, let's say you are forty-four years old.

220 − 44 = 176 (your maximum), and
75% of 176 = 132.

Therefore, to improve your aerobic fitness, your heart should beat around 132 times per minute, for at least fifteen minutes. Divide this number by six to see how often your heart should beat in ten seconds (in this case, 132 ÷ 6 = 22). Use your wrist or neck to take your pulse for ten seconds periodically while you exercise.

Aerobic exercise is any activity that uses more than half of your body's muscle mass: swimming, walking, jogging, cross-country skiing, skating, bicycling. Start off slowly for a few minutes, then begin to build up until you reach your target heart rate. (If you are swimming, there will be a slight variation; see page 246.)

Some people like to do strengthening and aerobic exercises each time they exercise — about fifteen minutes of each type. Others prefer to spend the entire half-hour doing strengthening exercises one day, then aerobic exercises the next.

Warming Up and Cooling Down

There are different theories about the best way to warm up before exercising. But you can't possibly go wrong if you ride an exercise bike, walk, or jog leisurely on the spot for about three minutes (an active warm-up) or take a hot shower (a passive warm-up). I always take a hot shower before I garden as well as afterwards. (*Mea culpa*: My environmentalist friends are going to kill me!)

After your workout, to ensure that you don't get dizzy, it is important to do an active warm-down — sometimes called cooling down — for three minutes before you take a hot shower.

General Tips

- Always do flexibility exercises first. Start at one end of the body — the feet, for example — and work toward the head. Hold your stretch for at least six seconds and don't bounce.
- Breathing is important. Breathe out to a count of two as you lift up, as in a sit-up. Breathe in to a count of four as you go back to your resting position.
- When you work on a muscle that has a right and left side, it's best to switch sides each time, rather than doing all the repetitions on one side before switching to the other side.
- Muscle strengthening exercises can be adapted if you want to work on local muscular endurance. Generally, you lower the load and increase the number of repetitions. It is important to build up muscle strength before working on endurance.

- Most of us spend too much time bending forward. Get a little extension into your life. Arch your back for a few seconds before you lift. (A
  good example is to arch before you put groceries into your truck or take
  them out. Arch while you are vacuuming and while you are sitting for
  long periods of time, in your car or at your desk — in fact, whenever
  you think of it. If you can't lie down to do this, do it standing up: put
  your hands on your hips, thumbs on your back, and extend.)
- Always wear proper shoes when you exercise. These can be comfortable walking shoes, or running shoes, with a cushioned sole.
- If you miss exercising for a few days, it's not the end of the world.
  But you can't make it up. Exercising once a week for three hours is
  simply not the same as exercising three times a week, for an hour
  each time.

Now you're ready to start building your program. The sections that
follow should help you find flexibility and/or aerobic exercises that will
suit your goals, ability, and category of back pain.

A sample program may look something like this:

- three minutes to warm up;
- ten minutes for flexibility exercises;
- thirty minutes for strengthening and/or aerobic exercises;
- fifteen minutes for endurance exercises, if you are doing them;
- three minutes to warm down.

Note: When I suggest a number of repetitions for the exercises below, if it's
a muscle group you have two of, I mean per side!

EXERCISES FOR FLEXIBILITY

1. Gastrocs/Soleus Stretch

The **gastrocnemius muscles** run up the back of the leg, from the heel to just
above the knee. The **soleus muscles** start at the ankle and run to mid-calf.

To stretch your right gastrocs muscle (Figure 13.1), stand facing a wall, about an arm's length away. Place your feet in a walking position, with your left foot ahead of your right foot, your toes pointing forward and your feet about shoulder width apart. Your right knee should be straight and your left knee, slightly bent. With your elbows straight, place your palms against the wall. (A tree is fine if you are outside.)

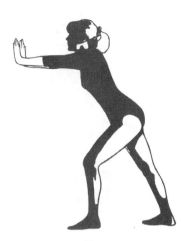

Figure 13.1 The Gastrocs Stretch

To stretch the left gastrocs muscle, lunge forward, allowing your left knee to bend farther. Make sure that your right knee remains straight and your right heel stays flat on the floor. As you push forward, your hips will move forward and down. You will feel the stretch high up in your right calf. Hold this stretch for six seconds, then relax. Do a minimum of three repetitions.

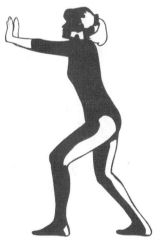

Figure 13.2 The Soleus Stretch

To stretch the right soleus muscle, the position is the same except that both knees are bent (Figure 13.2). As you lunge forward, your right knee should bend even more, but your right heel should remain on the floor. You will feel the stretch slightly lower — at about mid-calf. Hold for six seconds. Then relax. Do a minimum of three repetitions.

To stretch the gastroc and soleus muscles of the left leg, switch your position and repeat.

Tip: If you want to strengthen your **abdominal (stomach) muscles** as well, do a pelvic tilt before you start and hold it through this exercise. (See exercise 3 and Figure 13.4.)

2. Quad Stretch

The **quadraceps** are the large, strong muscles that run from just above the hip down
the front of the thigh to just below the
knee. You use them when you kick a foot-
ball, climb stairs, or move from a sitting
to a standing position. If your quads are
tight, you will have a tendency to overextend your lower back. This will put
additional strain on your facet joints.

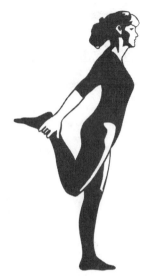

Stand sideways to a wall, placing the
palm of your left hand against the wall for
balance. Keep your back straight. With
your right hand, grasp your right ankle,
then pull it back and up (see Figure 13.3).

Figure 13.3 The Quad Stretch

You will feel the stretch along the front of your thigh. Hold for six
seconds, then relax. Do a minimum of three repetitions. (If your quads are
very tight, you may find it easier to sling a towel around your right ankle.
Grasp both ends in your right hand and gently stretch your leg back and
up.) Switch legs to stretch the left quads and repeat.

3. Knee-to-Chest/Hamstring Stretch

This version combines these two stretches very nicely. As well, it puts
less strain on the hip joints and on the back, which helps if you have a
disc problem.

The hamstrings start at the hip and run down the back of the leg to just
below the knee. The knee-to-chest part of the exercise stretches out some
of the muscles of the low back, buttocks, and hips, as well as the upper
portion of the hamstrings.

The first step to this stretch is to get into the **pelvic tilt** position (Figure
13.4). Lie on your back with your knees comfortably bent and your feet
flat on the floor. Relax your leg muscles and breathe normally. Press your
lower back into the floor by tightening your abdominal muscles; you will
feel your hip joints move toward your face.

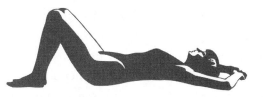

Figure 13.4 The Pelvic Tilt

Tip: You can strengthen your abdominals with pelvic tilt exercises alone. They can be done during an acute phase of back pain, while you are standing or sitting. If you do them while sitting, the change in position will be good for your back as well.

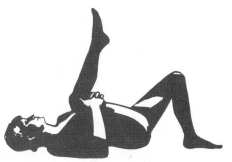

Figure 13.5 The Hamstring Stretch

Now for the knee-to-chest / hamstring stretch: Lie on your back with your left knee comfortably bent. Using both hands, grasp the back of your right thigh, just behind the knee. Pull the leg tightly against your chest and hold it there. Straighten your right leg as much as possible (Figure 13.5). (It is not essential to straighten your right leg completely but it is important to keep the knee pressed *tightly* against your chest.) You will feel the stretch down the back of your leg and, if your hamstrings are very tight, into your buttocks as well. Hold for six seconds. Then relax. Do a minimum of three repetitions.

To stretch the hamstring muscles of the left leg, switch your position and repeat.

4. Low Back Extension Stretch

This exercise stretches the abdominal muscles and some of the muscles that run across the front of the hip. It also helps the deep muscles of the back to relax.

Lie on your stomach. Place your hands next to your shoulders

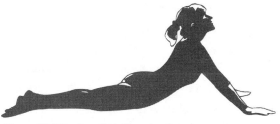

Figure 13.6 The Low Back Extension Stretch

with your elbows bent and your palms flat on the floor. Using your arms only, push up to arch your lower back (Figure 13.6). Do not allow your pelvis to come off the floor. Your arms should be as straight as possible and your elbows should be close to the body rather than pointing out to the side. The first time, hold for six seconds, then relax. Then work your way up to ten seconds. Start with three repetitions and work your way up to six.

Modified Version: If the above exercise causes acute back pain — or leg pain — try this modified version. (It often helps reduce the pain associated with an acute disc problem; do it every couple of hours.)

Instead of pushing yourself up onto your hands, push up onto your forearms only. Hold this position for five seconds. If this still causes pain, consult a health-care professional; extension exercises may not be good for you.

5. Mid-Back, Shoulder, and Neck Stretch

Very few exercises stretch the muscles of the mid-back (the thoracic

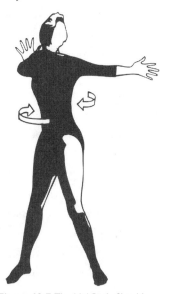

region). This exercise will do that, as well as stretch the muscles of your shoulders and neck. If these muscles are flexible, you will find it easier to do lifting tasks, especially those which require you to lift and twist at the same time.

Stand with your back to the wall, about a foot away from the wall. Your feet should be about shoulder width apart. Keeping your knees straight, stretch and twist to the right (clockwise) until your upper body is facing the wall (Figure 13.7). Your palms should be against the wall. Your right elbow should be straight; your left elbow should be bent. Push gently through the right arm

Figure 13.7 The Mid-Back, Shoulder, and Neck Stretch

to increase the stretch, which you will feel in your mid-back. Hold for six seconds, then relax. Do a minimum of three repetitions. If you want to stretch your neck as well, look over your right shoulder while you are holding the stretch. (See Chapter 19 for more detail on neck pain.)

To stretch these muscles the other way, twist to the left (counter-clockwise.)

EXERCISES FOR STRENGTH AND ENDURANCE

6. Half Sit-up (with rotation)

Easy Version (Figure 13.8): Place your arms at your sides with your palms flat against the floor. Do a half sit-up by sliding your hands forward about one hand's length. Only your head and shoulders should come off

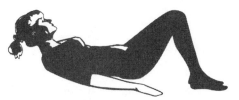

the floor. (Don't arch your neck.) Hold for six seconds. Then relax. Do three to five repetitions. Over the course of about two weeks, work up to fifteen or twenty repeti-

Figure 13.8 The Half Sit-up

tions. (To strengthen the two other sets of abdominal muscles — the transverse and obliques — add rotation. After your head and shoulders come off the floor, stretch your right shoulder toward your left knee and hold the sit-up in *that* position. The next time, stretch your left shoulder toward your right knee.)

Moderate Version: To work your abdominal muscles a bit harder, place your hands over your ears instead of by your sides. The rest is the same.

Difficult Version (Figure 13.9): To work your abdominal muscles even harder, stretch your arms straight back over your head, with your palms up. Your hands should not touch the floor. The rest is the same.

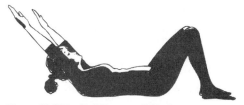

Further Progressions: Now add weights! Start again with the easy version but, instead of putting your arms by your sides, clutch a soup can in each hand and bend your

Figure 13.9 The Half Sit-up — Difficult

elbows to ninety degrees. Work your way through the moderate and difficult versions until you can do fifteen half sit-ups. Then increase the
weights — use your imagination! — until you can do fifteen repetitions of
the moderate version holding ten pounds. (Two to four pounds is enough
weight for the difficult version.) Be patient. It takes most people several
months to build up this much strength.

Endurance Version: To improve your endurance, focus on increasing the
number of repetitions rather than adding weights. Start with the easy version and work your way up to fifty half sit-ups. Then progress to the
moderate and difficult versions. You can also add rotation to about twenty
of the fifty sit-ups.

7. Back Extension Exercise (with rotation)

There are many different **back extensor muscles**. The longer ones are
close to the surface; the shorter ones, which are important for rotation as
well as extension, are deeper. When your back extensors are strong, bending forward and lifting will cause less strain. The rotational component is
important if you must lift and twist at the same time. Add it last.

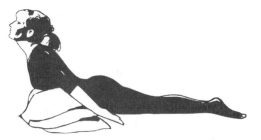

Easy Version: Lie on your
stomach with two or three
pillows under your pelvis.
Hook your feet under a sofa
to keep your legs from coming up off the floor. (You
can also do this exercise by
hanging over the end of a

Figure 13.10 The Back Extensor — Easy

bed, but someone will have to hold your legs down.) Let your arms rest
comfortably at your sides. Arch up into extension (Figure 13.10). It is not
enough to arch into a neutral position. Hold for six seconds, breathing
normally. Return slowly to the resting position. Do a minimum of three
repetitions, then work your way up to six.

Moderate Version: This is the same as the easy version except that your
hands should rest on your shoulders, or behind your head, whichever you
find more comfortable.

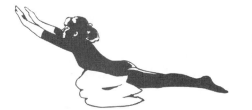

Figure 13.11 The Back Extensor — Difficult

Difficult Version: Same as above except that your arms, which should be straight, are extended over your head.

Endurance Version: For endurance, increase your holding time. Start again with the easy version. Work up to being able to hold this position for one minute. (Your head should be in a neutral position with your face looking at the floor.) Then progress to the moderate and difficult versions, working your way up to one minute.

Adding Rotation: Add this last, after you have built up both your strength and your endurance. Work on the easy version first. When you are in extension, roll your right shoulder up and back toward your left side. Go back to the neutral position and then roll the left shoulder, then relax. Now progress to the moderate and difficult versions. Finally, if you wish, you can do this exercise, with the rotational component, for endurance.

The Perfect Workout

One morning several years ago, I was watching David Goulding, who cleaned my house. I had a brain wave: David has the perfect job for a healthy back: constant motion, little heavy lifting, and a variety of postures. Here's how he sees it.

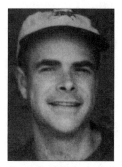

David Goulding,
Freelance Housekeeper

I got into the cleaning business because it offered me a way to earn money while keeping a flexible lifestyle. But, over the past few years, I've come to realize that my work is also great for me in a physical sense.

I didn't appreciate this to begin with. For instance, there were things I resented doing, such as cleaning bathroom tiles. I'm not sure how I came to change my attitude and make this particular task work *for* me rather than *against* me. But now, when I wipe a tile wall from ceiling to floor, I stretch my back, and I really feel the stretch, and I take the time to enjoy the way it feels. In a sense, it's like getting a mini-workout without having to go to the gym.

Another example? Take dusting the top of door frames. Door frames are a bit high if you just stretch your arm up. But if you stand on your tip toes and stretch out the muscles in the back of your legs, you can reach the top of a door and it feels great. You've made a chore into a fun little flexibility exercise. I guess what it comes down to is attitude, which is true of everything.

As far as I'm concerned, the more positions I can get my body into — and the more often — the better. Which means, for instance, that I don't spend two hours mopping, then dust for three hours. At some point, I learned to change tasks as often as possible. Now it's just something I do naturally.

The thing is, when you're cleaning a house *you're* in control. It's too bad that a lot of people who have cleaning jobs in, say, hospitals can't be so flexible. First they mop the floors. Then they have to clean the counters, because someone else has created the routine. Somehow, someone has gotten the crazy idea that doing one task for hours at a time is more efficient!

The workout I get from cleaning is great for toning and flexibility. But it doesn't give me an aerobic workout. I get that through biking, which is how I get around downtown Toronto. I arrive at my job warmed up and ready to go.

The truth is, for many people exercising is boring. Just say the word "exercise" and think of a routine on a schedule. It's separate, rather than a part of, their lives. But if you exercise by cleaning your house, you can kill two birds with one stone! We could do this with a lot of things if we were just a little more creative.

And, by the way, it's true my back never hurts!

AEROBICS, POSTURE, AND THE FIVE CATEGORIES OF BACK PAIN

I have discussed already how the three different mobile postures — flexion, rotation, and extension — affect the different categories of back pain. In Chapter 3 I explained how checking out which postures increase your pain can help you figure out which category you fall into. Posture is also an important factor in choosing an aerobic activity that is good for you.

Before embarking on an aerobic exercise program, spend some time figuring out which postures tend to make your pain worse.

You may recall from Chapter 2 that the five basic categories of back pain are: strains and sprains of the muscles, ligaments, and tendons; disc problems; spinal stenosis; facet joint syndrome; and osteoarthritis.

Strains and Sprains of the Muscles, Ligaments, and Tendons

Positions that put you into extreme ranges of motion, and particularly rotation, will increase your pain. So will any kind of jarring move, or a move that you must do without warning. The key is to stay in control of how you move. Therefore, sports that allow you to decide when and how to move — not, for instance, squash! — are best for you.

Disc Problems

Flexion, as well as rotation toward the side on which the disc is bulging, usually causes the most discomfort. Flexion is probably toughest to avoid since so many of our daily activities involve forward bending, so it's not a wise idea to pick an aerobic activity that requires you to spend even more time in flexion. For example, biking may or may not bother you depending on the setup of your bike (for tips on cycling with back pain, see the next section.) Hockey, on the other hand, probably will bother you no matter what precautions you take; you simply can't alter the design of your hockey stick in a way that allows you to avoid flexion.

Spinal Stenosis

If you suffer from spinal stenosis, you'll likely find that being in an extended posture over a period of time aggravates your condition. If you like to walk — a wonderful, low-risk activity that does, however, put your body into a slightly extended posture — you can learn to adjust your posture so that you flex just a bit. Often, this will solve the problem.

Another tip recommended by exercise specialists is to lower the intensity of your exercise sessions. In other words, it's probably better for you to exercise at a lower rate for a longer period of time rather than intensely for a shorter period. One advantage of lowering intensity is that your legs will not have to work quite so hard.

Facet Joint Syndrome

Extension also tends to increase the pain of a facet joint problem, especially prolonged extension. As I mentioned in Chapter 3, if you suffer from a facet joint problem, it's also likely that you will suffer from chronic rather than acute back pain, though if you experience the occasional acute flare-up you will want to avoid rotation as well.

Osteoarthritis

As with strains and sprains, extreme ranges of motion generally increase pain caused by osteoarthritis. So will vibration and compression — so avoid sports that involve jumping up and down. Remember that the pain caused by osteoarthritis often develops a few hours later, or the next day, rather than while you are doing an activity.

SOME LOW-RISK AEROBIC ACTIVITIES FOR BACKS

Here are a few suggestions for ways to get aerobic exercise that are not likely to stress most backs unduly. You'll have no trouble guessing my favorite. . . .

Walking

Why, in recent years, has walking become the most popular aerobic exercise among Canadians? Because it's cheap, virtually risk-free, and perfect for people who want to lose weight. It's also easily accessible; you can easily build a walking program into your regular daily activities by, for instance, walking home from work. (A cautionary note for extremely overweight people: to begin with, you may do better riding a stationary bike, which will put less strain on your joints than walking.) Recent studies show that walking at a pace of only four miles per hour for thirty minutes is enough for most people to improve their aerobic fitness. Buy shoes that are designed for aerobic walking, as opposed to jogging.

Tip: The normal walking posture is slightly extended. If you suffer from stenosis, or worn facet joints, you may have to work on changing your posture while walking. If this doesn't work, consider changing to biking.

Tip: It's also important for walkers to have flexible hamstring muscles.

Bicycling
Adjust the height and angle of your handlebars to minimize discomfort. Some mountain bikes are built so that you can sit in a normal, erect posture, rather than in flexion, which puts strain on the discs and ligaments of your lower spine. You can also buy extenders for the handlebars of a regular bike. Adjust your seat height so that when your foot rests on the lower pedal your knee is just slightly bent.

Horseback Riding
The main pitfall is poor technique; if you don't know what you are doing, you can hurt yourself by falling, or by bouncing, which can aggravate a vulnerable back. But if you are good at it, riding will put your spine in the best possible posture (half standing, half sitting). On top of that, riding gives your lower back what amounts to a gentle stretching session, almost like a massage. (Riding is used as a therapeutic activity for people who suffer from cerebral palsy because the rhythmic motion has been found to have a relaxing effect on muscles.)

Aquabics (Aqua Aerobics)
This is an excellent, low-risk aerobic activity for back pain sufferers. The only thing to watch out for — and it may not be a problem for you — is

loading the upper body with weights held in the hands. This can increase the stress on your spine and is of particular concern when you rotate. A better alternative is to wear sweatpants, which load the body from the waist down.

Swimming

This activity has been touted as a great aerobic activity for back pain sufferers for years. It is, but there are some things to keep in mind. The first is picking the right stroke. If you suffer from facet joint syndrome or spinal stenosis, the breast stroke will be stressful because it puts your body into extension (also, probably, the front crawl). The backstroke is a great alternative except for the fact that many people — including me! — seem unable to do it in a straight line! Probably the side stroke is your best bet, but do remember to change sides every few lengths.

Also bear in mind that your maximum heart rate decreases by fifteen when you are in a horizontal rather than a vertical position. Adjust your calculations accordingly. For example, if your target heart rate is 132 beats per minute while walking, this changes to 117 beats per minute (or approximately 16 beats every ten seconds) when you swim.

Gardening

I gave up tennis to garden, and since it's the fastest-growing hobby among Canadians, I have to assume that many back pain sufferers tend plants as well. If you choose to join us, here are a few pointers that I've picked up along the way.

First of all, for Canadians — and most Americans — this passion is a seasonal activity. Remember that different types of activities use different muscle groups; just because you ski or walk during the winter months does not mean that you are physically fit to garden the moment spring arrives. (Although washing floors on your hands and knees will help you gear up!) So, you should warm up and stretch your muscles before you dig up your beds, using the same motions as you use when you garden. Go slowly and hold each stretch for about ten seconds. It's also important to do some gentle stretching after gardening.

Once you start work, pace yourself, alternate activities, and take breaks in between: shovel, dump, rake, weed, rest. Then repeat.

Remember all the standard posture-related tips when you garden. You shouldn't spend more than fifteen minutes in any one position before you change to something else. Don't bend forward with your knees straight; if you can't bend your knees, lean on the handle of a long tool and bend with your back straight, one leg extended back slightly. Try not to lift and twist at the same time. Hold objects close to your body.

Reorganize your tool shed to store heavy supplies at waist level. And invest in some tools that will help: a kneeling bench with push-up handles; long-handled grass shears, shovels, and weeders; and a swan-necked watering can.

V

THE HEALTH-CARE PROS AND THEIR WARES

14

Getting the Best
from the Pros

After seventeen years and what seems like a zillion encounters with health-care professionals from every discipline under the sun, an important truth has finally permeated my gray matter: I know as much about my back problem as they do; we just know different things. For instance, a particular health-care professional may know the latest method of coping with stress, but I can best figure out when it's stress that has caused the dull roar in my lumbar spine to go through the roof. He or she may be able to show me how to alter the way I do a certain exercise, but I'm in charge of determining that the exercise is hurting my back in the first place. *I* know when my back pain has heated up because I've done something stupid like hauling eight cubic yards of Triple Mix into my garden single-handedly (see Chapter 8). And I know when the court of last resort — taking painkillers and, perhaps, muscle relaxants for a few days — is the only way to make it through a week from hell; when this is the case I make it clear to my family physician that medication is what I want and need.

Basically, I no longer consider the role of the patient to be compliant, *carte blanche*. I regard health-care professionals as consultants. The aim is to combine my knowledge with their knowledge in the hope that, together, we can arrive at a conclusion that's greater than the sum of its parts. In the end, however, the decision taken must be *mine* — which means I must also take responsibility for what results. That, I admit, is the tough part!

These days, a great many back pain sufferers and health-care professionals concur with this philosophy. In fact, the professionals whom I respect and enjoy the most welcome it with open arms. At least they do in principle. In reality, decades of baggage can sometimes get in the way of equitable relationships between patients and their health-care professionals.

WAY BACK WHEN

At the beginning of this century, patients and health-care professionals (for the most part, I mean doctors) were content with a model of health-care management that put the doc in charge. In many ways, this suited the times. The vast majority of patients were less educated than their doctors, and so, early-twentieth-century doctors had no choice but to direct and prescribe. They knew stuff that their patients would never have an opportunity to learn.

This model actually worked pretty well. Had I lived back then, I probably would have gone along with it without making much of a fuss. In return, my turn-of-the-century physician would have been a man of infinite kindness who devoted his life to his vocation. He would have known everything about me both medically and emotionally. He would have known my entire family as well, and as often as not, he would have made house calls without blinking an eye. If necessary, he would have accepted produce — or one of my famous lemon chiffon pies — in lieu of cash. Within the limits of his science he would have treated my illnesses and sewed up the gashes I got mending the garden fence. But even more important, he would always have been there to counsel and console. He would have been the quintessential holistic practitioner; and if his job was not always lucrative, it was interesting, and came with the built-in bonus of status and respect.

THE DAWN OF SPECIALIZATION

The technological revolution brought a lot of science to medicine but, in some ways, it also bunged up the works. By the 1930s, medical students were spending so much of their time packing facts into their heads that the philosophy of holism began to slip. When it became clear that no human brain could possibly take in everything there was to know about the mechanisms of the human body, the concept of specialization was born. Those who opted to become specialists — and their numbers increased exponentially — learned more about a particular body part or illness than was previously imaginable. At the same time, I think many of them lost the ability (perhaps because they lost the opportunity) to see their patients as human beings. Little by little we started to look like livers, stomachs, or hearts.

Technology also came with a rhetoric: medicine was going to cure everything that ailed mankind. It soon became apparent, however, that such a promise was pure fantasy; no matter how much doctors learned, there would always be ailments that could not be cured. (Chronic illnesses with psychogenic components — back pain is the perfect example — were at the top of the list.) Meanwhile, patients were becoming more educated and more demanding, which made them less satisfied with a system that, in some ways, was beginning to resemble a machine.

THE HOLISTIC REACTION

For every action there is a reaction. I believe that mainstream medicine's loss of holism, coupled with its inability to cure every illness, was the impetus for the surge in "alternative" therapies of more recent years. (By 1990, Americans were spending almost $14 billion (U.S.) on alternative therapists. A more recent Ontario survey indicates that approximately 12 percent of people have tried alternative therapies.) While these therapies were often short on scientific proof of their validity, their practitioners, almost without exception, were compassionate and took the time to listen to people's woes. It should come as no surprise that this went a long way in the eyes of patients.

Just a few decades ago, alternative therapies such as hypnosis and chiropractic were different from mainstream medicine in another sense as well: patients who were starting to enjoy the luxury of socialized medicine — at least in Canada — had to pay for them. Pretty soon, alternative practitioners and their devoted patients lobbied both public and private health insurers. Eventually, their demands for financial subsidies were addressed, to a degree. In 1970, for example, the Ontario Health Insurance Plan (OHIP) began to pay a five dollar stipend to chiropractors; patients topped up that amount. (Today, OHIP pays about nine dollars toward most visits. Chiropractors, unlike physicians, have the right to "extra bill.") More recently, alternative therapies such as massage, hypnosis, and biofeedback have started to be covered, in part, by the private insurance plans of many large companies.

What happened next was inevitable in many ways. Realizing that its revered position was less secure than it once had been, the medical establishment began to pay attention, and to make some demands — principally, that if public money was going to be spent on alternative therapies, those who practiced them must demonstrate their efficacy. Clinical and anecdotal evidence might be interesting, but it was not good enough. Scientific studies had to be conducted and their results, if positive, had to be replicable.

Doctors had a point, of course. Some of the more vociferous alternative therapists acted like faith healers with business degrees from Harvard. Who knew what they were doling out and whether, in fact, their treatments were doing more good than harm? (Personally, I believe that, in the vast majority of cases, the only harm alternative therapists ever did was to play their patients for financial suckers.)

On the other hand, as alternative therapists were quick to point out, a number of the therapies that were being used by physicians had never been scientifically proven either. In some cases — long-term bed rest for back pain is a perfect example — it was ultimately revealed that some mainstream treatments were based more on theory than on evidence.

In any case, slowly but surely, practitioners who had spent their lives doing clinical work started to get involved in research projects, mostly in their spare time. For alternative therapists in particular (most of whom had no access to well-endowed universities), lack of finances as well as inexperience in scientific methodology had to be overcome.

But somehow these obstacles were addressed and data began to trickle in. Like the growth of specialists, the growth of research was exponential. Today, there are so many studies about back pain (with so many conflicting conclusions) that I can't begin to keep track of them all, let alone digest and weigh them. I can say, quite unequivocally, a respectable number of excellent studies have been conducted by alternative therapists over the last decade. When they have shown their treatments to be efficacious from a scientific standpoint, even the most skeptical mainstream practitioners have had to open their eyes.

My own impression is that, as a result of this surge in research, three additional things occurred.

The first was a merging of minds and money from various disciplines. These researchers should be lauded for their efforts. Today, physical therapists, physicians, chiropractors, massage therapists, and others are pooling their knowledge in the name of research. The results of their studies, a large number of which are top-notch, can scarcely be dismissed by anyone. I'd like to see a lot more of this type of interdisciplinary effort.

My second observation is that there has been a resurgence of holism among physicians. (I don't think nurses and physical therapists ever let the concept of holism lapse in the first place.) The importance of the bedside manner is now emphasized in every medical school. Courses on patient communication skills that used to be elective are now mandatory. In some medical schools, students are videotaped during their consultations with patients and their performances are critiqued. It also seems to me that the majority of young men and women who are going into medicine today are committed to the type of practice that's come to be known as "patient-centered." While they expect to make a decent living, they don't expect to get rich.

My third impression is less positive. While many mainstream

practitioners are honing their communication skills and becoming more respectful toward their patients, some alternative clinicians, in their desire to gain respectability and acceptance, have become more aloof. Many chiropractors, for example, now insist on being called "Doctor," while more and more physicians introduce themselves by their first names. I've also heard a few chiropractors spew out technical jargon with impunity. Perhaps they think that highfalutin language impresses patients; or maybe they hope a patient who doesn't understand the diagnosis is less likely to pick it apart.

It has been said that money is the root of all evil. Sometimes I worry that our society's current lack of money is causing much of the discombobulation and rivalry among health-care professionals who must vie for their share of a shrinking pie. I also worry that it's going to get a lot worse before it gets better. As dollars are chopped from our virtually bankrupt health-care system, clinicians, like the rest of us, are focusing on their own economic needs. When they chose their careers, the vast majority of health-care professionals did so because they were inclined to care for people who were sick and/or in pain. At the same time, they expected to be able to pay their bills. Each time I see a hospital closing, or a merging of departments, I try to remember that more health-care professionals are going to have to work their guts out to stay alive. While none of this is your fault, or mine, I think it behooves us all to keep in mind that the health-care professional from whom we are seeking treatment and sympathy may be having a day that's even worse than ours!

RESEARCH ON RELATIONSHIPS

But enough of history and philosophy. It's time to get down to the practical aspects of dealing with the health-care practitioners of today. To begin with, I'd like to pass on the conclusions of a few studies on professional/patient relationships.

The research clearly shows that, as a patient, you're more likely to improve from a physical standpoint if you and your health-care professional are able to communicate well. (Some researchers connect this fact to the patient's sense of being in control.) While it's your job to be an active partner, it's your health-care professional's job to make this easy for you to do. This involves many things, of course, but two of the most important are giving you the time you need to explain how you feel, and asking you for your opinions — then treating them as valuable.

Most of the research on how health-care professionals measure up has been conducted by physicians on their colleagues. But I think the lessons of the following example — an analysis of seventy-four doctor-patient interviews — can be extended to other disciplines. I also think that the physicians who took the time and trouble to do this work should be congratulated.

This study was done in 1984, and much has improved since then. Nevertheless, the results were extremely disturbing. On average, these doctors waited a mere eighteen seconds before interrupting patients who were trying to describe what was wrong. At this point, the doctors took charge. They tended to ask questions that demanded one-word answers, effectively putting the kibosh on the patient's narrative voice.

A second study applies mostly to doctors because it concerns the use of prescription drugs. (You could, I suppose, apply it to therapists who recommend vitamins and homeopathic remedies, although for the most part, such potions are far less likely to cause harm.) In any case, the study showed that patients who didn't understand what their doctors were telling them had a fifty percent chance of taking the prescribed medicine incorrectly.

THE SMART PATIENT'S HALF-DOZEN BASICS

So how can you get the most out of your relationship with a health-care professional? Here are six basic rules I've picked up over the years for savvy patients.

1. *Take notes.* Bring a small notepad, a tape recorder, or even a friend with a good memory with you, especially for a first visit, or

whenever you expect that your diagnosis or treatment will need to be clarified. Dr. Ahmed Sakoor, the family physician I interviewed for Chapter 3, puts it this way: "At the time you might be certain that the six-syllable word I used to describe your condition — spondylolisthesis is a wonderful example — will remain imprinted in your brain for the rest of your life. But it's a better idea to write it down." Many terms sound similar: was that spondylitis, spondylolisis, or spondylosis . . .?

2. *If you don't understand what's being explained to you, say so.* Don't be afraid to say so again if your health-care professional does no better the second time around. If you feel that you do understand the explanation of a diagnosis or a procedure, confirm this by repeating, in your own words, what you think you heard. For example: "Are you saying that you think I have a bulging disc but you're almost positive it will get better without surgery and you think we should wait for a month and see?" This may sound silly, but it works.

3. *Think carefully ahead of time about what you need to know.* If you're going in for a diagnostic test or procedure, even a minor one, you may find it helpful to write down any concerns you can think of at home, where you're bound to be more relaxed and clear-headed. Here's what happened to a woman I know who missed one important point: Hilary was going to law school at the time and had a summer job as a waitress. During the last week of May, she went into hospital for some "minor surgery" on her foot. Well, the operation was minor. But the recovery required her to wear a walking cast for two weeks. The trouble was that her waitressing job started on June 1! Not realizing she had a summer job that required her to be light on her feet, Hilary's doctor had said she could go back to work in a week. As a secretary, she could have!

4. *Agree on the number of treatments before you start.* This is true of any series of treatments — massage, acupuncture, manipulation. . . . When that number is up, you and your health-care professional should review your progress together. *Your* opinion is as important as his or hers. By now you know my philosophy: all back pain sufferers need to do a variety of things for their backs. But you must

tell your health-care professional what else you are doing. For example, if you're going to try manipulation for a few weeks, swimming might be a good adjunct as far as aerobic exercise is concerned. However, the sidestroke might be better for your back than the breaststroke, which can aggravate certain types of problems. The point is, if you are no better at the end of the agreed upon time, you don't want the blame to be attributed to your swimming. That won't happen if you both agree on what you're doing at the start.

5. *Have a look at your medical chart.* It's your right. Quite frequently, patients discover a few details they didn't know about, and this knowledge often results in a more productive discussion. If you've been in hospital, you will be sent home with a discharge paper, which can be pretty vague. Ask your doctor to write or call the hospital for a copy of your record. It will contain the names and results of all the tests and procedures you had, a list of current prescriptions, and so on.

6. *Ask a lot of questions.* Ask about your health-care professional's interest in other disciplines, and what continuing education courses he or she intends to take. In the case of a family physician, ask about hospital privileges and access to specialists. Ask everyone about their philosophy of returning phone calls. (Some health-care professionals return all their calls at the end of the day; others can take several days to get back to you. Personally, I like same-day service!)

JUDYLAINE'S PERSONAL RULES OF THUMB

The basic tips given above should be of use to almost everyone. But I'll also share with you some more personal habits I've developed over the years when dealing with health-care professionals. Some of them may work for you; others may strike you as off the wall. In any case, I think they'll give you a chuckle, and that's always good for back pain.

About a decade ago, it hit me with the force of a hardball that I could count on the fingers of one hand the number of doctors and chiropractors who had ever addressed me as Ms. Fine. On the other hand, almost without exception, these same people had introduced themselves as "Dr. Smith." (There are exceptions. My experience is that nurses, physical therapists, yoga, Feldenkrais and Alexander technique teachers, massage therapists, and stress-management professionals tend to use their first names right off the bat.) On that day I made a resolution in the name of equity: any health-care professional who calls me Judylaine gets his/her Christian name in response. In other words, "How's your back, Judylaine?" gets, "I think I'm making some progress, Bob!" I try to do this in as charming a way as possible no matter how vulnerable I'm feeling, or how much pain I'm in. But I never make an exception, because I believe it establishes the right balance.

If on a first visit to a health-care professional I'm ushered into a consulting room by the receptionist and told to wait, I always make it a point to sit in the chair rather than hopping up onto the examining table. When the health-care professional comes in, I gesture toward the table in a way that says I'm inviting him or her to take that seat. (No one, by the way, has ever refused!) I want to make it clear that I expect a conversation before getting down to business. (I may be a child of the sixties, but I have my principles, one of which is that I never take off my clothes for someone with whom I've exchanged less than ten sentences!)

To get off to a good start, I smile. If my back is *killing* me, I smile! I believe that a first meeting with a health-care professional is not completely different from a first meeting with some other business associate — for example, a bank manager from whom you want a loan. In that case, the *worst* way to begin is with a grimace or a groan, especially if you're on the verge of bankruptcy! By the same token, if you want a health-care professional to take an interest in your case, it's best to present an image of a competent human being. Yes, you are in need of information and sympathy. But no one likes to start a relationship with someone who opens with a kvetch. (In an emergency, all rules are off; I'm not *that* cruel.)

A survey done by *Consumer Reports** indicates that back pain sufferers

---

*   This excellent article is worth the time it will take you to look it up in your public library. It was published in February 1995.

are more likely to be dissatisfied with their doctors than any other patients except those who have chronic headaches. I would like to suggest that, by the same token, many health-care professionals shudder when a new back pain patient walks through the door; who in their right mind would be thrilled by the spectre of failure? This is their problem, of course. Notwithstanding, I find it helpful to remember that, when they come across as distant or cool, some health-care professionals are merely feeling uncomfortable. Experience may have told them that whether they listen for three minutes or three hours I am likely to walk out dissatisfied. I often try to begin by explaining that I realize how complicated back problems are to diagnose and treat. Then I tell my story.

Finally, I've developed some tricks for dealing with health-care professionals who think nothing of making me wait for half an hour: I book the first appointment after lunch. (The first appointment in the morning can be dicey; many doctors start their day by seeing patients in hospital, and who knows how long that can take?) If this doesn't work, I try booking the last appointment of the day, then phone ahead to see how far the doc has fallen behind. That way I can judge when to set out.

INFORMED CHOICE

A final note on dealing with the health-care pros. As general respect for patients has risen in the health-care system and patriarchal attitudes have declined, the notion of informed choice has gained increasing attention. This principle involves "the exchange and understanding of relevant information so that an informed, reasoned, and unpressured decision can be made by someone who has the competence and legal capacity to make such choices."*

It used to be argued that patients should not have a major say in treatment decisions, especially when the treatment is risky — that patients

---

* This quotation is from the New Zealand Medical Association's "Principles and Guidelines for Informed Choice and Consent," reprinted in *The Journal of Manual and Manipulative Therapy* 2 (1994), p. 3. The importance of this issue is gaining recognition not only across all the health-care professions but across the globe.

couldn't comprehend the information presented, and that they might be unnecessarily frightened and refuse procedures that were in fact only minimally risky.

Today, however, the health-care professions recognize that patients have the right to control over their own lives. Informed choice allows them that control; it also promotes trust between the health-care user and provider, and encourages people to take responsibility for their own health.

It is the responsibility of the health-care provider to present information about treatment, and any associated risks, clearly and completely so that the patient can make a truly informed choice. If the decision is made to go ahead with a procedure, the patient is then able to give informed consent.

Steer clear of any health-care provider, from any discipline, who shows the slightest signs of not respecting the principles of informed choice and informed consent. If a professional attempts to coerce you, or seems unforthcoming with information, run for the hills. It's your body, your back — your choice.

15

Physical Therapy:
A Profession in Evolution

I'm not cut out for the life of a health-care professional. Part and parcel of the deal is to park your own troubles at home, and my style is to wear my heart on my sleeve. But if the heavens were to open with a thunderous voice that declared health care to be my lot — "Madame, choose your discipline!" — I'm pretty sure I'd become a cutting-edge physical therapist.

For one thing, I feel comfortable with the philosophy of physical therapy (also called physiotherapy), which is to help patients (whom they respectfully call "clients") get back to normal functioning, or as close to it as possible. Physical therapists consider it essential to educate clients so they can do this on their own. In other words, people are discouraged from becoming dependent on a health-care professional; the goal of treatment should be to put an end to treatment. By now you know that independence is my number one credo and that, when it comes to chronic back pain, I'm zealous about my belief. Other than such treatments as massage, yoga, or tai chi, it's simply too tempting — and, in the end, counter-productive — to get into the habit of relying on a sympathetic pro. Besides, our health-care system can't afford it.

My second reason for choosing physical therapy as my hypothetical profession is that I dislike repetition. Dispensing the same treatment to every back pain patient who came through the door would drive me up the wall. I mean, can you imagine being a back surgeon who does lumbar disc surgery year after year, or a dentist who only fills teeth? My practice, of course, would be a state-of-the-art, hands-off, active approach, which — in addition to education — emphasized exercise and postural modification. Plus I'd damn well expect every client to play an active role, for instance, setting goals and sticking to them. I think this part would be the most fun.

To me, the fact that physical therapy isn't married to one modality would be an additional plus. By definition, it would mean that I could evolve whenever research demonstrated the efficacy of a new treatment, or a better way of doing an old one.

Of course, I'd have a postgraduate degree — probably in the area of sports medicine, which interests me more than orthopedics, cardio-respiratory care, neurology, pediatrics (children's rehabilitation), exercise physiology, administration, or ergonomics in the workplace, although ergonomics would be a close second choice.

In any case, I wouldn't be a full-time clinician. I'd devote two or three days a week to helping athletes with back pain, which would leave me enough time to conduct research as part of a multidisciplinary team. On our team would be chiropractors, physicians, occupational therapists, psychologists — all of whom were open-minded and turned on by the concept of collaboration. We'd conduct small studies — say on fifty to seventy-five patients — and we'd design them to demonstrate the efficacy, or inefficacy, of specific aspects of treatment. One of *my* jobs would be to write up the results of our studies for publication — and I'd bloody well do it in a way that laypeople could understand.

Plus I'd teach one course to undergraduates at the University of Toronto and do my best to fire my students up!

If I was good at what I did — and I would be — I'd never worry about being unemployed. At the end of 1995, 13,500 physical therapists were practicing across Canada but they couldn't — they still can't — keep up with the demand.

In fact, about the only aspect that would niggle at me is the salary I'd be likely to earn, although it would be more than I make as a fairly successful writer! If, for instance, I was a senior physical therapist working in Toronto with some management responsibilities and ten to fifteen years of experience, I'd make around $50,000 — and Toronto's pay scale is as high as it gets. That's after a bachelor of science degree and three more years of university training. (That two-year postgraduate degree wouldn't make much difference.)

However, I would have known the financial score since the day I signed on. With the exception of a handful of the already small number of physical therapists with private clinics, the profession has never been well paid. The fact that the vast majority of physical therapists have traditionally been women probably has a lot to do with that fact. The percentage of men, however, is increasing. Today, about a quarter of Canada's full-time physical therapists are men, and only half of the 1,100 physical therapists who graduated in 1996 were women. I wouldn't be surprised if the financial status of the profession changes somewhat over the next decade, although in terms of economics it's a damn tough era during which to make a great leap.

Actually, I've already said a great deal in this book about physiotherapy, because the early active treatment philosophy I advocate in Chapters 12 and 13 is embraced by physical therapists more than by any other class of clinician.

A BIT OF HISTORY

Physical therapy became a profession because of the need to rehabilitate soldiers who had been wounded during World War I. Before 1914, there were professionals in Europe who practiced massage and what was then called "remedial gymnastics," but virtually no one in North America had training in either of these techniques, which meant that Canadian and American soldiers had to be admitted to French or English military hospitals thousands of miles from their families.

Toward the end of the war, twenty-eight men and women were trained in rehabilitation medicine at the Ontario Hospital in Whitby. Soon afterward, the Military School of Orthopaedic Surgery and Physiotherapy became part of the University of Toronto. By 1929, U of T was offering a degree course in physiotherapy.

Today in Canada, all physiotherapists must complete a three- or four-year university program, and the best universities require an undergraduate science degree before they let you through the door. All thirteen of Canada's physical therapy programs are located at universities that have medical schools, which means that students train in a milieu with links to teaching hospitals as well as the tradition of research. (This is not true in the United States, where many physical therapists receive their training at a college rather than at a university.) It has also become fairly common for physical therapists to do postgraduate work — specialty programs, masters' or doctorate degrees.

For decades, virtually all physical therapists were employed by hospital rehabilitation departments. Other than people recovering from surgery, most of their back pain patients were referred by their physicians on an outpatient basis. The doctors would send these men and women along with both a diagnosis and a prescription. While physicians felt comfortable delegating the responsibility for treatment to physical therapists, there was no question as to who was in charge.

In the early days, exercise and massage were the two main forms of treatment for back pain. To increase circulation, heat was often applied first. By the 1940s, **short-wave diathermy**, which can deliver heat to deep tissue, had been invented. Within a decade it became popular. In the late 1950s, **ultrasound** took diathermy's place. Today, some physical therapists still use such passive treatments to decrease muscle spasm, relieve pain, and speed up the healing process. But cutting-edge physical therapists consider these modalities to be adjuncts to treatment rather than treatments in their own right.

Passive Modalities for Physical Therapy

With these descriptions comes the following caveat: if all you're getting is passive treatment, you're not getting state-of-the-art physical therapy, and my advice is to look for another physical therapist. As I have explained, today's top-notch physical therapists consider these passive modalities to be supplements to treatment rather than treatments in their own right. Nevertheless, people are always asking me about them, so here they are. If nothing else, this section will save you the expense of purchasing another book!

Ultrasound

How **ultrasound** works is to deliver high frequency sound waves to tissue, which results in a sort of micro massage — that is, each cell, as opposed to a mass of tissue, is affected. Those who use ultrasound feel that, when used after an injury, it reduces swelling and increases the elasticity of the new tissue that the body must produce. It also stimulates cells to be more efficient at taking in nutrients and getting rid of waste products.

Transcutaneous Electrical Nerve Stimulation (TENS)

TENS (also called TNS) is used to relieve pain. The machine delivers a painless electric current to nerves via electrodes that are placed on the skin. Those who use it believe that it works either by stimulating the production of endorphins, or by lessening a patient's perception of pain when large sensory fibers are stimulated (see Chapter 6). Proponents of TENS say that it is successful — to varying degrees — for about a third of chronic patients who try it, which is no higher than the success rate of a placebo. A recent review of TENS studies questions our ability to judge its efficacy for acute back pain.

Cold and Hot Packs

Cold packs are used to reduce swelling and increase circulation, most often during the first forty-eight hours after an injury. **Hot packs** are used after the first forty-eight hours with the objective of increasing circulation to an injured area as well as decreasing muscle spasm. Both are used as a prelude to treatment. You can easily use cold packs and hot packs at home.

Short-Wave Diathermy

Similar to ultrasound, **short-wave diathermy** sends out sound waves whose deep heating effect is meant to increase circulation and relax muscle tension. These days, few physical therapists use it. In fact, Toronto's Orthopaedic and Arthritic Hospital sent its machine to the dumpster last July!

Interferential Current

Similar to TENS, **interferential current** uses two different frequencies of electric current to alleviate pain and reduce swelling. You can often identify a person who has had this treatment by the tell-tale suction cup marks on his or her back.

Traction

Used to reduce pain, **traction** involves the application of either intermittent or continuous force in a way that elongates the spine. Studies on its efficacy are, at best, inconclusive.

Mobilization and Manipulation

In a joint that is stiff, **mobilization** is used to increase movement. The joint is moved by the therapist, but not beyond its physiological range of motion. Manipulation, which moves the joint slightly beyond its physical range of motion, is described in Chapter 16.

During the 1960s and 1970s, high technology entered many areas of medical science; physical therapy was no exception. In those days, it seemed as though money grew on trees and, as more of it was spent on sophisticated weight-training machines, hands-on modalities such as massage were used less. By the beginning of the 1980s, computerized equipment for both assessment and treatment (i.e., strength and endurance building) was the talk of the town. I remember how exciting it was to write about an American machine called the Lido Lift. It weighed 800 pounds and looked like a Nautilus that had undergone a face-lift in California's Silicon Valley. It also had a price tag of $100,000 (U.S.). But high tech has had its heyday. When the Lido Lift company went into receivership in 1996, none of the physical therapists I knew were shocked or particularly upset — at least not on behalf of their patients. These days, such equipment is used mostly for research and testing, and the main impact of the company's demise on the profession is the lack of service when the machines that are still in existence break down.

What's more interesting is what stimulated so much interest in high tech in the first place. During the early 1980s, the numbers of people with musculoskeletal injuries who were being referred for treatment literally exploded, and the majority of them were back problems. By the middle of that decade, back ailments were costing industry a fortune in workers' compensation board (WCB) claims. If high-tech machines could ultimately save money, employers said to themselves, then the hell with the initial cost.

During this decade, physical therapists were literally reeling from the number of patients who were being referred to them in a steady stream. In many clinics, this translated into less individual time for each patient. In too many cases, clinics began to crank out assessments and dole out exercise regimens. Some patients were even sent home to cope on their own, which only works if the therapist has had time to instruct them properly before they go. In response to the increasing numbers, workers' compensation boards across the country set up work-hardening programs (occupational therapy designed to "toughen up" workers before their return to the job), but these too were bogged down by the never-ending stream of injured workers.

At this point, the number of private physical therapy clinics increased by leaps and bounds. The services they provided were paid for by employers who didn't want their injured employees at the back of an ever-lengthening line. (Since 1966, no freestanding physical therapy clinics in Ontario have been given the right to bill OHIP. When the demand for services has increased, private clinics opened; today there are about 700 of them in operation. They bill patients directly or bill third parties — for example, supplementary insurance plans — or the WCB.) The point is, the profession was stretched beyond its limits — and back pain patients got short shrift. In Ontario, the WCB tried to deal with the problem by instituting their community clinic program, but it, too, was fraught with kinks (see Chapter 12).

Two Shining Stars: Robin McKenzie and James Cyriax

But the 1980s came with some positive aspects. Particularly worth describing are the stories of two innovative individuals who had the courage to promulgate their beliefs on their own steam.

It's difficult to pin down the exact chronology of this tale, and to assess the impact it had with any amount of accuracy. But it seems to me that, because of two men — and isn't that ironic! — the profession of physical therapy rose to a new level.

One of them was Robin McKenzie, a physical therapist who still practices in New Zealand. Among other things, Robin is an advocate of extension — both as an exercise and as an important aspect of posture — and because of him, medical science dramatically changed its definition of good posture as well as its attitude toward exercise.

The second person was the late James Cyriax, a British orthopedic surgeon, who always regarded the physical therapists he worked with as equals. As a proponent of manipulation (as well as many other methods of treating back pain), he brought this modality into the physical therapist's realm. It has always been legal for physical therapists — and, for that matter, physicians — to use manipulation as a therapeutic technique, but before James Cyriax took North America by storm, it was pretty well used exclusively by chiropractors and Canada's handful of osteopaths. While physical therapists use manipulation far less frequently than chiropractors, the fact that they use it at all has caused a considerable amount of friction between the two professions.

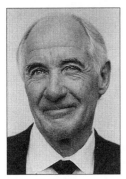

Robin McKenzie

The first time I met Robin McKenzie was at a 1988 conference on back pain in Chicago. Robin was in great demand but, as always, he made time for everyone. During the two hours he found for me, he related the story that changed his own life, the lives of many back pain sufferers, and the lives of many of his colleagues.

In the mid-1970s, Robin McKenzie ran his own clinic in Wellington, New Zealand, an off-the-beaten-track location if ever there was one. This was during the reign of flexion, when back pain sufferers were advised to flatten their lumbar spines and avoid extension exercises like the plague. Like the rest of his colleagues, Robin McKenzie had graduated from this school of thought and believed in its efficacy. He certainly helped many back pain patients, but he was by no means successful all of the time.

Then the most ridiculous thing happened. A patient with acute back pain (which was radiating down one leg) hobbled in. Robin told the guy to go into the examining room and lie down on the table on his stomach — he'd be right there. What Robin didn't know is that someone had left the front end of the table tilted upward, which meant that, when the patient lay down in a prone position, his back would go into extension with a capital E!

Meanwhile the phone rang. Robin took the call, which delayed him for twenty minutes. When he finally walked into the examining room, he was horrified. The guy's lower back was arched like a gymnast doing a back bend, and Robin was certain that he was going to get sued.

Gingerly, Robin asked his patient how he felt. The response made him wonder which one of them had taken leave of his senses: the guy insisted that he felt terrific. His back still ached but, for the first time in weeks, his nagging leg pain was gone.

Robin breathed a sigh of relief, but he couldn't stop thinking about it. Eventually, he cautiously tried extension on a few other patients with similar problems and got similar results. To make a long story short, Robin spent the next several years developing the **McKenzie method**. Then, using his own resources, he flew off to tell the world. The McKenzie method approaches disc problems in a totally new way that focuses on soft tissue (mostly muscles and ligaments). Part of the method is that treatment should be as short as possible and that the client should be taught independence. But its most revolutionary aspect is the use of extension exercises and the maintenance of the lumbar lordotic curve. (Recent research has confirmed that, from a mechanical standpoint, Mother Nature is no dummy. Your lumbar spine is at its strongest when you maintain its natural lordotic curve.)

Not everyone agrees with all aspects of Robin McKenzie's theory as to *why* extension works — I don't! — but almost everyone agrees that, for disc problems in particular, extension exercises should be part of the treatment regimen. The fact that our current definition of good posture is dramatically different from what it was just a decade ago has a lot to do with Robin McKenzie.

In 1983, Robin McKenzie became the first physical therapist to be elected to the membership of the prestigious Society for the Study of the Lumbar Spine. To many people, myself included, it felt as if the entire profession was being knighted, not just the man himself. I also believe that Robin McKenzie's contribution to both back pain and his profession has been a lot greater than the sum of its parts. Physical therapists would never use the term, but I can say it: Robin McKenzie was the profession's first star.

During the same decade, James Cyriax (who had a long-standing and somewhat controversial reputation in Britain going as far back as the 1950s) started to lecture and give workshops in North America. Some physicians, but physical therapists in particular, eagerly signed up to learn the methods he advocated and taught. (Physicians who practice according to the philosophy promulgated by James Cyriax call themselves **orthopedic physicians**.)

During the 1980s, James Cyriax became an octogenarian, and was still going strong by anyone's standards until his death in 1985. During the last years of his life, his physical therapist associates did most of the teaching, and all of them always called him "James." I frankly doubt that he ever gave the issue of titles more than a passing thought. It was just the way he was, and it looked good on him.

James Cyriax also brought some new modalities into the physical therapist's armamentarium, the most important of which was manipulation. Physical therapists certainly use manipulation far less these days than they did back then. The active treatment approach has largely taken manipulation's place, at least where physical therapists with up-to-date training are concerned. But physical therapists have always used manipulation far more sparingly than their chiropractor colleagues because they believe that, if it's going to work, it generally works right off the bat. If the first few treatments show no improvement, they will usually discontinue manipulation more quickly than chiropractors.

But the point I want to make is this: when chiropractors could no longer claim a monopoly on manipulation, a number of questions arose, and the first ones to ask them were physical therapists. One of these questions was: What can chiropractors offer that the physical therapist/physician "team" can't? Chiropractors countered by insisting that they have more training in the technique and therefore do it much better. In any case, the issue put physical therapists on a new footing and raised their sense of self-esteem. When, more recently, chiropractors trying to prove the efficacy of manipulation cited quite a number of studies that had been conducted by physical therapists, more than a few eyebrows went up. (For more on the issue of who can and should perform manipulation, see Chapter 16.)

RECENT TRIUMPHS

It could be that I'm off the mark when I theorize that the increased confidence in the profession following the debate about manipulation was at least in part responsible for the flourishing of physiotherapy in recent years. In any case, it's just a theory and I'm certainly prepared to admit that it emerged from my gut rather than my brain. But it's a fact that, during the mid-1980s, physical therapists began to pursue greater status and authority; just as chiropractors, of course, had been lobbying for this for many years. More times than not, physical therapists have been successful in their quests and many people are of the opinion that the status quo has changed. Only a few years ago, the most talked-about power struggle in health care was the one between physicians and chiropractors. Today, when it comes to treatment, you're just as likely to find research that compares chiropractic to physical therapy.

The physical therapy profession has accomplished a great deal over the past decade or so. Physical therapy clinics often have a similar mandate to chiropractic ones. In 1993, Ontario's physical therapists and chiropractors became self-governing, a status that physicians have always enjoyed. Physical therapists also won the right to provide primary health care, although in reality the vast majority of patients are still physician-referred. In 1994 the regulations of the Ontario Insurance Commission were amended to authorize physical therapists to certify disability claims made by people injured in motor vehicle accidents. Other jurisdictions usually follow Ontario's lead in these areas.

Furthermore, a large number of physical therapists have become involved in research; quite a number of the studies are being conducted by multidisciplinary teams. The areas physical therapists have been studying are so numerous that it would be impossible to list them all here, but basically the push has been to produce scientific evidence that determines which modalities are, in fact, efficacious — as well as when they are efficacious, and for whom. Clinicians who endorse this philosophy are committed to what's called an **evidence-based practice**, which means basically that if a modality does not stand up to scientific scrutiny, they toss it out.

But more often than not, years pass between the time research studies begin and are published. Furthermore, in order to make sound conclusions, a number of studies must produce similar results. To complicate the matter further, health-care professionals are always disputing the findings of even the most lauded studies: everything from the study's design to the skill of the clinician involved is commonly dragged through the mud.

Clinicians need to be able to measure the effectiveness of the treatments they are using, and they need to do this *today*, not five years from now. In order to do this, they rely on tests called **outcome measures**, which objectively measure the degree to which a client has improved. (Outcome measures are also important to researchers, who must ensure that each person in a study is being judged objectively.) Until recently, however, the validity and reliability of even the best known and most often used outcome measures tests had not been evaluated in a scientific way.

In 1994, four Canadian physical therapists published a 200-page manual that describes and rates both the reliability and validity of sixty outcome measures — everything from ways of measuring how much a person's pain has decreased to ways of measuring how much more efficiently a patient is able to use oxygen when exercising. The manual, which was funded by the Canadian Physiotherapy Association as well as Health and Welfare Canada, was a milestone. Within a short time it began to be used worldwide.

And yet, these accomplishments, laudable as they are, don't touch me as much as the simple fact that it has become common for physicians to sign their referral letters to physical therapists, "Thanks from Bob!" This is evidence that many physicians now see the difference between and value of the two jobs. Theirs is to make a differential diagnosis (discussed in Chapter 3); the physical therapist's job is to rehabilitate. In this case, referral letters are short and to the point: "Please assess this patient and treat."

Of course, the road has had its bumps and potholes. Not all North American physical therapists have renounced the antiquated passive modalities for the up-to-date philosophy of active therapy and an evidence-based practice.

Physical therapists themselves have studied this issue. In 1994, U.S. physical therapist Alan Jette and his colleagues published the results of a nation-wide survey. They found that the care given to back pain patients varied substantially from therapist to therapist in terms of the number of visits per episode, the length of time care went on, and the kind of rehabilitation program that was offered. (The study had no access to outcome data so it could not evaluate the efficacy of care.)*

Most therapists said that they used a combination of therapeutic exercise and other modalities; only a small number said that they incorporated manipulation and/or mobilization into the mix. But the combination varied from clinic to clinic and there was little consensus about what intensive exercise meant.

This, of course, is one of the most important issues of the community clinic program described in Chapter 12, from which physical therapists learned a lesson from the school of hard knocks. From the start, physical therapists should have been collecting and analyzing their own data. And they should have been screaming blue murder at any of their colleagues who failed to measure up.

The importance of self-reliance was underscored when, during 1996, a few community clinics were the subject of an embarrassing investigation by the WCB. One issue was the overtreatment of a number of back pain patients. The other, which was far worse, was a conflict of interests; it appeared that a small number of physicians were referring patients to clinics in which they themselves had a financial share. (In my opinion, the affair might have been nipped in the bud if a considerable amount of the Ontario Physical Therapy Association's energy had not been tied up in a dispute with a small group of members over the OPA's representing them in negotiations with OHIP.) At the time of this writing, the investigation had yet to be concluded.

A FEW NEW STARS

Several dozen names spring to my mind in the same instant, but it would take up pages to tell you about them all. Those who should be here will forgive me because that's the way they are. In fact, you've already come across most of these names; their accomplishments are noted throughout this book. The truth is, I couldn't have written *The Ultimate Back Book*

---

*   This study was published in 1994 in *Physical Therapy* 74(2): 101–10.

without the hundreds of hours physical therapists have donated to the Back Association of Canada over the past sixteen years.

But if the heavens ever *do* open and in a thunderous voice assign me to the vocation of physical therapy, my wish would be to accomplish at least half as much as the people I describe below.

Linda Woodhouse

A researcher, senior physical therapist, and exercise physiologist at Toronto's Orthopaedic and Arthritic Hospital, Linda Woodhouse could be dubbed Linda Powerhouse. She has a mind like a steel trap in which she methodically stores facts by the thousands. They are mostly about research, but she also remembers who said what about any subject you can think of, as well as when. Even better, she has the ability to spit out all these facts in plain English, allowing me, in turn, to explain them to you. Linda is soon to receive her Ph.D. in Community Health from the University of Toronto — a feat by anyone's standards. But I predict that Linda Woodhouse will go down in history as the gutsy professional who, on the basis of research, stuck like glue to her belief in early active treatment, even when it meant flying in the face of adversaries whose power was far greater than her own.

Molly Verrier

As the director of physical therapy at the University of Toronto, as well as a professor and researcher, Molly has made enormous changes in the university's physical therapy program, the most important of which has been to augment the profession's commitment to practices that are evidence-based. Perhaps more than anyone, she has encouraged her colleagues to conduct research and aspire to postgraduate degrees. To that end, she was the force that got the university's graduate program off the ground and to a level that's respected worldwide. My spies tell me that Molly goes at ninety miles per hour, eighteen hours a day. Nevertheless, they can't figure out how she manages to accomplish so much.

Elspeth Finch

Elspeth is an associate professor of physical therapy at McMaster

University and a research associate at the Center for Studies in Physical Function, which is a clinical teaching and research unit at Toronto's Orthopaedic and Arthritic Hospital. As well, she does her own research, and it has earned her an international reputation in the design and validation of functional questionnaires, a skill that's tougher than most of us think. Elspeth also figures out ways to measure the efficacy of treatments, so it shouldn't come as a surprise to hear that she is one of the authors of the *Physical Rehabilitation Outcome Measures Manual* I discussed earlier.

Lina Santaguida

A physical therapist at Toronto's Sunnybrook Medical Centre and a Ph.D. candidate at the University of Toronto, Lina's specific area of expertise is the biomechanics of lifting, a subtopic of dynamic posture (see Chapter 10). For instance, when Jane Smith is on the go, what is the precise impact on a particular joint in her lumbar spine if her psoas muscles happen to be tight? This kind of question may sound pretty esoteric but answering it could in fact produce some very practical results. For example, it could be that excellent posture means very little if your body lacks flexibility in certain ways. Back pain sufferers also need to know which muscles figure most in this equation as well as to what degree. Spending years on such a narrow topic takes tenacity and dedication. I couldn't do it, and I bet you couldn't either; we should all take our hats off to someone who can.

Sharon Thornton

Have you noticed how Toronto's Orthopaedic and Arthritic Hospital keeps popping up throughout the pages of this book? The reason is simple: the director of its department of rehabilitation, Sharon Thornton, is light years ahead of her time. Back in 1987 — before the WCB of Ontario's community clinic program was launched — Sharon put a bug in the ears of the hospital's executives. She wanted her department to get into the business of assessing active treatment for people on WCB claims. Sharon believed that her prestigious hospital had an obligation to rehabilitate injured workers. For one thing, it was one of the few hospitals devoted to the philosophy of early active treatment for musculoskeletal injuries, and it was important to find out if active treatment worked. In addition, her gut told her that the time was right.

Just about everyone — the hospital's top brass, directors of other hospital rehabilitation departments — said she was nuts. Who needed the headache of a population known to be poorly motivated, not to mention the WCB paperwork, which drives everyone up a wall? But Sharon pressed her point and got her way, and a few years later her phone was ringing off the hook. "How can *we* get into this high-profile, lucrative business?" everyone was asking her. Each time she chuckled, then told them everything she knew.

But that's not Sharon Thornton's only claim to fame. Her department is the envy of every rehabilitation director in town. She is rarely short-staffed, and her physical and occupational therapists have years of experience, as well as more graduate degrees than you can shake a stick at. That's because she encourages and makes it possible for her employees to pursue graduate studies and work at the same time, which is the way life ought to be.

OCCUPATIONAL THERAPY: PHYSICAL THERAPY'S QUIET RELATION

I would be remiss if my chapter on physiotherapy didn't include some discussion of this important, if less glamorous, related discipline.

The profession of occupational therapy was born around the same time as physical therapy, based on the same need: to rehabilitate disabled war veterans. The professions merged in the 1970s, then separated again. Throughout their development, they have followed similar, often over-lapping paths.

The most important distinction is this: physical therapists are con-cerned with an individual's physical capabilities; **occupational therapists (OTs)** are concerned with **activities of daily living (ADLs)**, which include self care (feeding, bathing, dressing, toileting, and mobility), productivity (paid and unpaid work), and leisure (hobbies and recreation).

Historically, OTs used purposeful activity, or "occupation," to improve function in the needed areas. They carefully selected and modified activities in order to engage participation by the client. Carpentry or basketweaving, for example, were used to improve hand function, increase self-confidence, or improve attention, concentration, and problem solving.

Some OTs specialize in vocational rehabilitation, which concerns the client's ability to perform the demands of work. Ideally, individuals who are ready to return to work after an injury or disability leave will be assessed by a skilled OT working in cooperation with the physical thera- pist, the treating practitioner, the employer, the insurance carrier, and of course the client. More and more OTs are developing their skills in the area of workplace ergonomic intervention (see Chapter 20), which is a natural developmental step for the profession.

OTs can be a lifesaver to those with acute or chronic back pain. Often an individual's ability to perform ADLs is affected by back pain. Tasks such as dressing, bathing, housework, child care, and work can all be difficult if not impossible to perform with a sore back. OTs can help identify how to improve function by doing any or all of the following:

- modifying the method in which the activity is performed (e.g., squatting instead of bending to retrieve laundry from the dryer);
- modifying the activity, often by breaking it up into smaller, achiev- able components to reduce the weight or time spent (e.g., washing smaller loads of laundry at a time); or
- using adaptive equipment (e.g., lightweight tools, lifting devices, etc.).

Like physical therapists, OTs in Canada graduate from a university affil- iated with a medical school and must be registered with the appropriate provincial college of occupational therapists in order to practice. OTs may also continue the formal education process to achieve a masters' or doctorate degree in rehabilitation or a related field.

Occupational therapy is less well known than physical therapy mostly because it is smaller and has less lobbying power. Another factor may be that the majority of OTs are women, so a higher rate of practitioners leave the profession to raise families than in physical therapy or medicine.

Like other health disciplines, occupational therapy today is focusing its attention more on outcome measures and research. As a profession, it is responding to government and public pressures to demonstrate the effectiveness of intervention. Its continued growth is proof of its success, despite continuing reductions in health-care funding and the fact that occupational therapy tends to be the quiet member of the therapeutic family.

16

Chiropractic: A Few Questions, a Few Answers

Twenty-two years ago, on a blustery February day, fifty-eight chiropractors, osteopaths, scientists, and physicians met at a conference center in Bethesda, Maryland — just down the road from the infamous Watergate Hotel. They had been invited by the National Institute of Neurological and Communicative Disorders and Stroke (NINCDS) to discuss the research status of spinal manipulation. As far as American organizations went, this was about as prestigious as you could get. Furthermore, it was the first time in North America that a world-class medical and biological organization was treating chiropractors and medical experts as equals.

When the NINCDS conference was over, however, it was evident that the cloudy waters that had surrounded the profession of chiropractic for almost a century had yet to clear. American osteopath Dr. Murray Goldstein summed it up this way: ". . . analysis of available data clearly indicates that specific conclusions cannot be [drawn] either for or against the efficacy of spinal manipulation therapy or the foundations from which it is derived. . . .

"Chiropractors, osteopathic physicians, medical manipulative specialists [physical therapists] and their patients all claim that manipulation provides relief from pain, particularly back pain, and sometimes cure; some medical physicians, particularly those not trained in manipulative techniques, claim it does not provide relief, does not cure, and may be dangerous, particularly if used by non physicians. The available data, however, do not clarify either view. . . ."

The Bethesda meeting had been organized for one important reason: chiropractors were making so many inroads into territories traditionally sacrosanct to the medical profession that physicians could no longer turn a deaf ear. As well, some of the physical therapists to whom physicians were referring their patients were, on occasion, performing manipulation. So were a few physicians. Clearly, this was not a treatment that was going to disappear.

In both Canada and the United States, chiropractors had already lobbied and won (in the early 1990s in Canada) the right to call themselves "Doctor of Chiropractic," although most were shortening this to plain "Doctor." They were also well on their way to having both governments and private insurers pay for a portion of their services. (In Ontario, OHIP pays $8.40 toward a regular chiropractic visit; unlike physicians, however, chiropractors can extra bill; most chiropractors ask patients to pay an additional $16 to $20 per visit.)

As well — and this was especially important to the profession — they gained the right to provide primary care, meaning that patients could consult them directly rather than having to be referred by their family physicians. (Physical therapists became primary care providers in 1993 but few of them exercise this right. For the most part, they can't even begin to keep up with the referrals!)

But, in return for these sorts of privileges, the public, governments, and private insurance companies were starting to demand answers to some basic questions, to wit:

1. Is manipulation, the mainstay treatment of chiropractic, truly efficacious? If it is helpful, *when* is it helpful and for *whom*?
2. Should chiropractors have a monopoly on performing manipulation?

3. What should be a chiropractor's scope of practice? For example, should back pain sufferers getting treatment from a chiropractor consult their family physician as well? Should chiropractors manipulate people in the name of prevention? Should chiropractors be allowed to imply that manipulation may also affect diseases of the internal organs?

Manipulation for Acute Back Pain

Over the past two decades, millions of dollars have been spent on research about manipulation. However, when you get down to the nitty-gritty, not all that much has been learned.

The most prestigious work in the area of manipulation for acute back pain was done by a well-respected California group called the RAND Corp. For $1 million — part of which came from the American Chiropractic Association (ACA) — RAND analyzed twenty-two studies on manipulation that had been done over the years. The studies used in this meta-analysis were chosen because they were **controlled studies**. This means that manipulation's efficacy was compared to the efficacy of something else — for example, passive physical therapy treatments such as TENS.

Some studies have certainly shown that manipulation is effective, but in a limited way. In a nutshell, RAND research indicates that manipulation is helpful for some people who are suffering from *acute* back pain that has not gone on for more than three weeks, and where there is no evidence of nerve damage. Twelve years ago, when I wrote *Your Guide to Coping with Back Pain*, I said more or less the same thing. The difference between now and then is that now there is scientific evidence to support what clinical experience had already suggested was true.

It's important to realize that the RAND study was talking about manipulation as opposed to chiropractic. In fact, more of the studies were performed by physical therapists, osteopaths, and medical doctors than by chiropractors. Perhaps not surprisingly, however, chiropractors often cite the RAND research as supporting the efficacy of chiropractic!

MANIPULATION FOR CHRONIC BACK PAIN

As for chronic back pain, the research indicates that manipulation *may* be useful in some cases. The problem is (and I admit that I've said this ad nauseam), chronic back pain is often a complicated affair. When you're talking about an ailment that's fraught with psychological overtones, whatever works does so because it addresses these overtones along with the physical aspects. That's why I keep insisting that most chronic back pain sufferers need a combination of treatments. Manipulation may be beneficial as part of the roster, but personally I doubt that it will ever become a substitute for exercise, postural and ergonomic improvements, and stress management.

Right now, one study is generally cited by people who want to make a case for the efficacy of manipulation for chronic back pain. A controlled study published in 1990 in Britain by Dr. Tom Meade showed that chiropractic treatment was more successful than physical therapy at the end of three years. This, however, is only one study, and even the person who conducted it acknowledged that it was flawed. For one thing, the back pain patients who were treated by physical therapists were all hospital outpatients; the chiropractic patients were all private. (In Britain, which has a two-tiered medical system, private patients tend to receive more time and attention than patients who are treated within the public system.) As well, in two hospital clinics the physical therapists happened to specialize in manipulation, and their results were as good as or better than the chiropractic clinic results.

For another thing, manipulation has not yet been compared to state-of-the-art active treatment as I define it in Chapter 12. As Dr. Meade himself has said, "Until further trials have been carried out, the superiority or equivalence of any particular technique . . . remains an open question." (God, I wish these researchers would learn to write in plain English!)

WHAT IS MANIPULATION? HOW DOES IT WORK?

There are many different ways of manipulating the human spine, but they can all be defined in the same way. **Manipulation** is an assisted passive motion applied to the spinal facet joints or the sacroiliac (SI) joints. ("Assisted passive motion" means that the patient is passive and the manipulator assists.) Dr. David Cassidy, a Saskatoon chiropractor and researcher, once gave me the best plain-English explanation I've heard: "You have a stiff joint and you manipulate it and that makes it move. You're increasing the range of its motion — and we know that a mobile joint is less likely to be painful than a stiff joint. That's true for the elbow, for the ankle, and for the spine."

If you're scientifically inclined, you'll be interested in joint range of motion (ROM). If not, you can skip the next few paragraphs.

Toward the end of a joint's normal physiological range of motion is a buffer zone. At the end of that, there is an elastic barrier of resistance. This barrier has what chiropractors describe as a "springlike end-feel," which is the result of negative pressure within the joint capsule. (This negative pressure is one of the mechanisms that helps to stabilize the joint. Muscles, ligaments, and the capsule itself are the others.)

If the joint surfaces are forced beyond this elastic barrier by someone who is performing manipulation, they move apart with a cracking sound and enter what is called the paraphysiological ROM. This constitutes manipulation. (Mobilization, for example, is different because the joint stays on the buffer zone side of the elastic barrier within its normal physiological range of motion. See Chapter 15.)

The cracking sound of a manipulated joint is the result of the sudden liberation of gases contained in the synovial fluid of that joint's capsule. Physicists call this phenomenon **cavitation,** and have demonstrated that, if an X-ray is taken right after a joint is manipulated, bubbles of gas can be detected for several minutes; for approximately thirty minutes the elastic barrier of resistance between the buffer zone and the paraphysiological ROM is absent. During this time, further manipulation is unsafe.

In some cases, the manipulative thrust is thought to stretch a contracted muscle, thereby relieving spasm. This makes a lot of sense to me. In fact, when I was a kid, my father used to see a chiropractor once every couple of years when, as he explained it, he put his back out by lifting and twisting at the same time. For him, it worked with one visit.

There is also some evidence that manipulation may decrease pain itself in the same way as acupuncture. One theory is that, like acupuncture, manipulation stimulates the body to produce endorphins.

HOW MUCH SKILL DOES MANIPULATION TAKE?

Chiropractors feel that considerable training and experience are necessary to perform a manipulation competently, and I'm the first one to agree. Toronto chiropractor Dr. David Drum, who has a long-standing reputation for keeping National Ballet of Canada dancers on the stage, puts it this way: "Manipulation is not particularly demanding to learn, but it takes about five years of constant practice to get really good, and you have to do it all the time to stay good. Otherwise you lose it." Personally, I think that manipulation is as much of an art as a skill, and that this accounts for the fact that some clinicians get better results than others.

Whether or not other types of health-care professionals can become really good at manipulation is a controversial question. Physical therapists who take postgraduate courses in manipulation believe that they can. Chiropractors often maintain that they can't — that you must be a licenced doctor of chiropractic to manipulate safely and well. If this is so, then it seems to me that chiropractors can't have it both ways. In my book, it's not cricket to argue that physical therapists are amateurs, then trot out the results of their studies when they show that manipulation works. Yet I've heard a number of chiropractors do just that, sometimes labeling manipulation done by physical therapists as the "chiropractic method." Pardon the pun, but that really cracks me up.

THE ISSUE OF DIAGNOSIS

I could devote pages to this issue; in fact I could write an entire book. But to help sustain your interest, I will limit myself to a few comments.

First of all, I've changed my position over the past twelve years in a couple of ways.

When I wrote *Your Guide to Coping with Back Pain*, I said that back pain patients who choose to be treated by a chiropractor should be in contact with their family physician as well during the treatment. Today I would simply say that you should consult your family physician *first*, but perhaps only once.

The first time your back packs up on you, it's important to consult a professional whom you know. This is nothing if not pure logic. A health-care professional who knows your personal and medical history, as well as how you tend to react to stress, is in a much better position to reassure you. If — as is true in most cases — muscle strain is at the root of your back problem, this is extremely important. (See Chapter 6 for more about the contribution of stress.)

Some chiropractors will argue that this is precisely why you should see a member of their profession *before* your back hurts. They're entitled to that opinion, but I'm afraid I don't agree — not, in any case, unless you are prepared to cover the entire cost, since I'm not interested in contributing my tax dollars to such treatment. But as you know, I think people should learn to cope independently. That costs even less.

The second way I have changed my mind is this: I used to believe that chiropractors were less able than medical doctors to make a **differential diagnosis**. This includes being able to rule out anything serious that may contraindicate manipulation as a treatment, as well as determining the cause of the pain. Now I think that, in the very unlikely case that your back pain is due to an infection or a tumor, virtually any intelligent, modern-day chiropractor has enough training to figure this out and send you right back to your family physician where you belong. I'm sure mistakes have been made, but over the past decade I've never heard of any other scenario taking place — at least in Canada. Anyway, physicians and physical therapists are certainly not perfect, either.

For the record, my bottom line is this: any caring, intelligent practitioner of state-of-the-art chiropractic is as capable as any caring, intelligent practitioner of state-of-the-art medicine or physical therapy of determining when a patient with back pain needs medical care, as well as when manipulation is contraindicated because of, say, an unstable joint. But I still like the idea of staying in contact with your intelligent, caring family physician.

I would also like to point out that the education chiropractors receive is very different from the education that medical schools provide. (The training of physical therapists is discussed in Chapter 15.) Over the past few decades, chiropractic education has certainly come a long way. But, as Dr. Craig Nelson, a world-respected chiropractor/researcher who teaches at the Northwestern College of Chiropractic in Bloomington, Minnesota, writes, classroom lectures are simply not the same as clinical experience, and, whether it is fair or unfair, chiropractors have no access to teaching hospitals, which is where physicians learn to translate theory into practice. Chiropractors get their clinical experience in a chiropractic clinic, where hardly anyone comes in with a serious disease.

"How could one argue," writes Dr. Nelson, "that a thirty-hour lecture class (no lab) in pediatrics, or a thirty-hour lecture class (no lab) in infectious disease, is in any way the equivalent of spending six weeks in a patient-care facility in each area?" Need I say more?

THE DIAGNOSTIC WORKUP

But let's say that you feel you are a candidate for manipulation and that you have chosen an excellent chiropractor as your clinician. I asked Marcel Reux, a chiropractor who practices in Toronto, and who has also been trained as a physical therapist, to take me through the steps of a chiropractic diagnosis. As is true of an excellent family physician or physical therapist, a good chiropractor will first listen to the history of your back problem. "The history is the most important part of the diagnostic workup that I do during a first visit," says Dr. Reux. For someone with a history of back pain, this can easily take half an hour.

"During this time, the chiropractor will ask you (among many other things) to describe the pattern of your back pain, as well as its chronology and quality. For instance, is your pain a "burning" pain or does it tend to nag at you? What causes it to improve? What causes it to get worse?" It takes patience and good listening skills to sort out many people's stories, whether you are a chiropractor, a physician, or a physical therapist.

Although it happens very rarely, Dr. Reux will on occasion hear a story that doesn't jibe. Let's say, for example, that someone lifted a flowerpot three months ago and is still experiencing acute pain that keeps him up all night but is not affected by movement. In this case, Dr. Reux would consider the possibility of a tumor, and his response would be to refer the patient back to his family physician. "Having the privilege of making a diagnosis," he says, "involves a tremendous amount of responsibility."

Of course, the original diagnosis may also change. If, after two or three visits, the patient is not getting better or is, in fact, getting worse, a good chiropractor will always think his or her diagnosis through a second time, perhaps calling the patient's family physician to talk it through.

Like many chiropractors, Dr. Reux rarely uses X-rays, especially to begin with. (One exception would be ordering an X-ray for a suspected fracture if, for instance, a patient has recently taken a bad fall and the family physician did not order an X-ray.) In almost all instances, he prefers to rely on the "hands-on" part of his clinical examination. This involves a neurological examination, which is not dissimilar to the one a good family physician will perform (see Chapter 3). After that, Dr. Reux conducts a **motion palpation exam**. In plain English, this means he examines your back — how it feels, as well as how *you* say it feels — while he gently moves you into and out of various postures. Some parts of the motion palpation exam are conducted while you are standing; other parts while you are lying down. But basically, he is trying to discover what reproduces your pain.

SPECIFICITY IN MANIPULATION

Manipulation is the mainstay treatment of chiropractic. What distinguishes a chiropractor from most other health-care professionals, as well as an excellent chiropractor from a mediocre one, is the ability — when necessary — to be specific about which joint he or she is manipulating. This too is both a science and an art; however, if manipulation (rather than, say, exercise) is going to be your treatment, I think it's fair for you to expect that the joint that gets manipulated is the one that's "fixated," or stiff.

Chiropractors say that there are ten to twenty different ways of manipulating every moveable joint in the body. Some maintain that when they have mastered the technique, they can be very specific about which joint is being manipulated. Others are not so sure. In any case, there is no scientific evidence. Twelve years ago I put the question to Dr. Cassidy, and he replied, "I've practiced for ten years and I used to think that I could manipulate L4-L5 on the right side if I wanted to. I tend to think now that when I try to do that I might also move the facet joint below or above, but I still think I can be fairly specific." Now he has practised for more than twenty years but his opinion has not changed.

Specificity becomes particularly important in several cases. One is when a patient has an unstable joint, or joints. Joints, you will remember, are unstable during the thirty minutes after a manipulation, but they can also be unstable due to degenerative changes, most commonly disc degeneration. I do not mean to imply that disc degeneration and joint instability necessarily go hand in hand. But it does sometimes happen that, when a disc becomes narrow, the facet joint at the back of that disc becomes **hypermobile**, which means that it moves extremely easily and, possibly, beyond a safe range. Lax ligaments, due to years of poor posture, can also contribute to joint instability and, in extreme cases, a joint will actually wobble slightly when you move. The point is, if you repeatedly manipulate a hypermobile joint, you'll just increase this instability.

I'd also like to point out that when manipulation is used to reduce muscle spasm, specificity probably doesn't matter quite as much. Muscles more frequently go into spasm in a general area rather than one tiny muscle in one tiny spot. (Perhaps this is one reason why the technique works well for simple, acute back pain, which usually involves simple muscle strain.)

SCOPE OF PRACTICE

The answer to my question about the profession's scope of practice depends upon whom you ask. The point is that chiropractors themselves cannot reach a consensus about whom they ought to treat and when. In the words of Craig Nelson, the image they present to the public is both "muddled and confused."

Some chiropractors restrict their scope of practice to the treatment of acute back pain, although most are prepared to try manipulation for a short time on patients with chronic back problems. The ones I respect the most don't make any promises; they also advise chronic back pain patients to exercise and correct their posture.

Another group believes in treating acute back pain and chronic back pain but, in addition, they believe in the use of manipulation on an ongoing basis. In this group, some chiropractors believe in "supportive care," which means that they treat people whenever they happen to have a bad bout. Others believe in "preventive care," which means that they will treat back pain sufferers even when they are pain-free. To my way of thinking, stiff joints cause pain, and if a joint's not stiff it doesn't make much sense to manipulate it. That's my opinion and I'm entitled to it.

At the far end of the spectrum are those chiropractors who believe that manipulation actually plays a role in the cure of various diseases. Within this group, some also believe in manipulating children and, when they promulgate this point of view, health-care professionals from other disciplines often go wild. But even within this group of chiropractors there are subgroups. There are those who believe that the children they treat will grow up with better backs, while others treat children for specific ailments such as bed-wetting and asthma. Fortunately, the number of chiropractors who fall into this last, almost fanatical, group is far lower here in Canada than in the United States.

To be honest, I am sometimes amazed that a profession so lacking in consensus has managed to progress so far. People like Dr. Nelson agree with this sentiment. They do not believe, however, that this state of affairs can continue. Our health-care system, they point out, is in such financial straits that *all* health-care professionals are now being held accountable for the treatments they offer. The argument that chiropractors have used for decades — that the medical profession has never been expected to prove the efficacy of *its* methods — is wearing very thin.

This puts chiropractors in a difficult position. Unlike medical doctors and physical therapists, chiropractors are married to one main method of treatment. They may advise patients about posture and/or exercise and even stress management, but these areas are not their forte. Chiropractors *need* to prove the efficacy of manipulation because it's what sets them apart from others . . . or it does if manipulation is restricted to licenced chiropractors.

My point is this. When, as I described in Chapter 12, Dr. Gordon Waddell stands up in Rome and says bed rest is for the birds, doctors can prescribe activity instead. While I agree that it may take some of them quite a while to change, they will eventually come around. The same thing can be said about physical therapists. When passive methods of treatment are shown to be inefficacious, with-it practitioners change like the wind. Eventually, the rest follow suit. But what would chiropractors do if, in the end, research shows that manipulation is no more effective for acute back pain than early active treatment? I ask this because, as I've said, manipulation has not yet been compared to state-of-the-art active treatment. I urge you to keep this in mind over the next few years.

THE HISTORY OF CHIROPRACTIC

Manipulation came long before chiropractic. In fact, people have been adjusting joints for thousands of years. Chinese artifacts from as early as 2700 B.C. describe the technique, and a Greek papyrus from 1500 B.C. gives instructions on how to manipulate the lumbar spine for back pain.

During the Renaissance, manipulators were known as "bone-setters," and by the middle of the 1850s, apothecaries had added the therapy to their mixed bag of potions. It was around this time that British physicians and surgeons began a joint campaign to have the profession legislated.

Being hospital-trained rather than apprenticed, these two groups united against the inclusion of the apothecary as a legitimate doctor. At the time, however, apothecaries were regarded favorably by the rural gentry who, of course, had a sizable membership in parliament. As a result, when physicians and surgeons became a legal entity, they were forced to include apothecaries, who have become today's family physicians.

Had medicine decided to incorporate manipulation into its roster, chiropractic as a separate entity would in all likelihood have never developed. What happened instead is that the apothecaries were forced to relinquish their apprenticeship training and move into the hospital setting.

There they studied such courses as anatomy, physiology, pathology (the science of disease), and the treatment of fractures. But they had no opportunity to acquire the knowledge to manipulate bones, joints, and ligaments.

Because they realized that manipulation worked, even if they didn't know exactly when, a number of physicians began to advocate its study. The eminent British surgeon James Paget was one. "By their practice of [manipulation]," he wrote, "bone-setters . . . are held in repute. Their repute is, for the most part, founded on their occasionally curing a case which some good surgeon has failed to cure. . . . Learn then," he told his students, "to imitate what is good and avoid what is bad in the practice of bone setting."

Paget's sensible advice was not followed by his colleagues and his worst fears came true. In 1874, in Missouri, Andrew Taylor Still founded osteopathy, proclaiming that all diseases were caused by improper nourishment of the nervous system by the blood and could be corrected by manipulation. Twenty-one years later, Canadian-born Daniel David Palmer "discovered" chiropractic.

Oddly enough, Palmer, who operated a "magnetic healing studio" in Davenport, Iowa, claimed that when he discovered chiropractic he was totally unaware of the existence of osteopathy. In any case, he was trying to restore the hearing of his deaf janitor by manipulating one of the vertebrae in the man's thoracic spine.

The janitor regained his hearing. Palmer's theory was that he had relieved pressure on a spinal nerve that had been affecting the man's hearing for seventeen years. The manipulation, he maintained, is what had removed the blockage. What Palmer didn't realize was that the nerves associated with hearing do not emerge from between two mobile vertebrae in the thoracic spine. They don't, in fact, emerge from between any of the mobile vertebrae, and, therefore, they cannot be affected by manipulation. These nerves are inside the head.

Nevertheless, Palmer and his followers established the basis of chiropractic: that misaligned, or **subluxated**, vertebrae were the cause of most disease. He also said that a subluxated vertebra exerts pressure on a spinal nerve, which interferes with the body's "innate intelligence," thereby causing disease.

Most modern chiropractors think of the word "subluxation" as outdated. In fact, most of the ones I know don't even bother to use it. Toronto chiropractor Sandra O'Connor, an assistant professor of radiology at the Canadian Memorial Chiropractic College, says that you can't see a subluxated vertebra on an X-ray, which further explains why modern chiropractors don't use the term.

In fairness, Palmer's beliefs and doctrine were not as outrageous at the turn of the century as they sound today. At the time, some medical doctors were still using leeches, which they applied alongside the spine as a therapeutic treatment. Louis Pasteur had only recently demonstrated the existence of germs as a cause of disease, and many physicians still regarded the spine as the "heart" of most human ailments.

By the beginning of the twentieth century, however, medicine had abandoned such practices and begun its scientific revolution.

Modern-day chiropractors recognize the role of bacteria, viruses, and other factors in illness. They simply focus on the musculoskeletal system. Some, however, still retain a philosophical bent toward seeing the spine as the focal point of disease.

However, even when it comes to the musculoskeletal system, I think it's fair to say that, over the past few years, some chiropractors — and some of them are Canadian — have been distorting the facts. Some have made sweeping generalizations and, unfortunately, some American journalists have reported them at face value. After the RAND study, all sorts of articles that read like PR pieces for the profession started to appear in national newspapers and magazines. One of them, entitled "Back Manipulation Gains Respectability," was published on the front page of the lifestyle section of the *New York Times*.

To put it mildly, the profession was in seventh heaven.

In June of 1994, however, *Consumer Reports* published a major cover story on chiropractic. Its title was "Chiropractors . . . Can They Help? Do They Harm?" As is true of all *Consumer Reports* articles, it was extremely well researched. In addition, because its readership is so enormous, it had a huge impact on the profession.

A great portion of the article was devoted to topics that drive people crazy, for instance, advertising and manipulation for kids. But even its opinion of the RAND report was lukewarm. One of the people they quoted was Dr. Paul Shekelle, the physician who headed up the RAND team. His comments were balanced. For example, he said, "We now have more evidence for the use of spinal manipulation as a treatment in low back pain than for many other medical therapies currently used."

But just a few months later, there was an article in *The Back Letter* (a for-profit U.S. newsletter that reports on the current back pain literature, which it translates — quite well, I think — into layperson's language.) Its title was: "Has a Leading Researcher Changed His View of Manipulation?" Again, Dr. Paul Shekelle was quoted. But this time, he was angry.

"I wanted to put the brakes on those who would overextend our results into sweeping generalizations," he said. "I've had to write dozens of letters to newspaper and magazines that had tremendously overgeneralized our study. . . ."

But I'd like to end this section on a positive note. To put it mildly, manipulation can be brilliant when it works. (If anyone takes *this* comment out of context I will start throwing well-aged fruit!) What's more, as Craig Nelson points out, millions of people suffer from the kind of back pain that is most responsive to manipulation — simple acute pain that does not radiate into the leg. Therefore, it is conceivable that a huge number of people could benefit from manipulation.

But first, as Dr. Nelson puts it, the profession of chiropractic is going to have to get real.

THE FUTURE OF CHIROPRACTIC

I'm the first one to admit it. It's tough to be a chiropractor out there on your own. To begin with, the Canadian Memorial College of Chiropractic gets no public funding. While government subsidizes the amazing education we give to our physicians and physical therapists at universities, chiropractors must pay their own way. When they graduate, most are in debt. And that's before they've gone to the bank to borrow money to set up a practice.

Nevertheless, that's not my problem, nor should it be yours. Nor should the fact that by and large chiropractors cannot rely on referrals from family physicians, at least not when they start out. Furthermore, only 10 percent of the population considers "alternative" therapies, and, however far it has come, chiropractic still bears that label in the general population's mind. Making a living — especially when you believe that you should earn as much as a family physician earns rather than, say, a physical therapist — is tough for a chiropractor, particularly one who is just starting out. It's even tougher if you are going to confine yourself to treating people who suffer from acute pain.

What do I hope will happen? I'm ready to throw my lot in with those who want the profession to set up a faculty at York University; negotiations are already in the works. If and when that happens, subsidized education is inevitable, although it may take a number of years. That, I think, will give the profession the boost it needs to read the riot act to those who overtreat or overstep the boundaries of science. I also believe it will encourage chiropractors to become members of multidisciplinary clinics, as well as encouraging multidisciplinary clinics to invite them. I only wish that York University had a faculty of medicine. (As I said in Chapter 15, the fact that, in Canada, all faculties of physical therapy are located at universities that also train physicians is a very good thing.)

Until all that happens, however, I cannot keep myself from asking the profession to please cease and desist from doing one thing that drives me up a wall. I am talking about advertising. Chiropractors (both as a profession and individually) advertise their services, although, again, this happens a lot less in Canada than in the United States. My position is that we live in a society which has a convention for better or for worse. The convention is that health-care professionals are supposed to act like genteel individuals who neither promote themselves nor their wares. Chiropractors not only flout this convention but they sometimes do it in ways that are more fitting for selling real estate than health care — even in Canada.

In the spring of 1995, for instance, a chiropractor who practices in my neighborhood delivered packages of forget-me-not seeds with a flyer to every house on my street! In 1996, the Chiropractic Association took out several multi-page ads to promote the profession in both *Maclean's* magazine and *Toronto Life*. One of them featured a bungee jumper under which appeared the following message: "Some people will go to great lengths to straighten out their backs . . . You just have to turn the page."

I mean, really!

In the meantime, I think the best advice has already been written in *Consumer Reports*. In that 1994 article, they advised people to be suspicious of any chiropractor who — and these are only some of their suggestions — does the following:

- takes full-spine or repeated X-rays;
- fails to take a comprehensive history and do a clinical exam to determine the cause of your problem;
- claims that the treatment will improve the immune function, or benefit or cure disease;
- solicits children or your family members; or
- wants you to sign a contract for long-term care.

I couldn't have put it better, so I didn't try.

17

Surgery: Less Is More

Quick, what's the difference between God and a back surgeon?
God doesn't think he's a back surgeon!

CHANGING A PRICKLY IMAGE

If there's a group of health-care professionals whose image could do with a facelift, it's back surgeons. Too often I've heard patients describe them as prickly, humorless, uncommunicative, and impatient, especially when it comes to answering questions. I was thinking about this a couple of years ago while setting out for a walk in the desert near Phoenix, Arizona, with four world-class orthopedic surgeons. What occurred to me was that these sorts of stereotypes often fall apart when people are taken out of their regular settings.

I'll need to give you three important pieces of background information before I get to the story. First of all, the five of us were playing hookey from a conference on chymopapain — an enzyme that can be injected into a herniated disc as an alternative to major back surgery, which I'll discuss in detail later in the chapter. The second thing is that I happen to know all the juicy gossip that has surrounded chymopapain like a shroud for three decades. So whenever the subject is front and center, health-care professionals love to pick my brain. That accounts for why these guys invited me to join their little desert trek. Third of all, I have a brother who lives near Phoenix. Therefore, I can be relied upon to rattle off the names and characteristics of the region's numerous cacti.

Now, try to picture the scene.

We are walking along, chatting about Dr. Lyman Smith, the genius orthopedic surgeon from Chicago who developed chymopapain treatment. I spy a lovely jumping cholla. Now, a jumping cholla is a type of cactus. It has a main body, which some people refer to as the "mother" because it produces little jumping chollas. When these babies grow to the size of a squash ball, the mother tosses them about her to form a sort of spiny moat. The babies protect Mom (a rather odd quirk of nature) even when they must lay down their lives to do it. There is some controversy about whether baby jumping chollas actually *jump* at passers-by or just appear to jump. I say THEY JUMP!

I am explaining these unusual characteristics while warning the docs to stay clear. Stupidly, I wag my finger at a baby jumping cholla to illustrate my point, and — *Vromp!* — it jumps on. I can assure you, this hurts like bloody hell.

Now, *don't panic*, I say to myself. Don't dwell on the possibility of a thirty-minute ride to the nearest emergency in the back of a bouncing Jeep with a cactus sticking out of your swollen-to-the-size-of-a-mango finger. And don't even let it cross your mind that emerg will probably refuse to treat you in any case once it discovers you are covered by a foreign public health plan.

Try instead, I tell myself, to keep your mind on the fact that you are in the company of four world-class orthopedic surgeons.

I sit down on a rock.

One of the surgeons points at my hand. "Shake it," he suggests.

I shake vigorously, which turns out to be an extremely bad idea. It causes about ten additional cactus spines to join the two dozen or so already embedded in the lowest layer of my epidermis.

"Yipes," I shout. "You guys are supposed to know about spines." I am still capable of making a play on words, but the truth is I'm on the verge of tears.

The other three surgeons form a circle around me. "Grand rounds," one quips. It strikes me that one set of keys, which the designated driver is twirling, are the only stainless steel instruments within a twenty-mile radius. I know I look pathetic but I put on a smile. I think, these guys must know that a journalist can poke an awful lot of fun at four surgeons who can't manage to make history out of one baby cactus stuck to one baby finger! Surely they will put on their thinking caps and think of something.

"This would make a great story," I say carefully.

"One paragraph and I'll sue," says the third surgeon. Then he strikes a caveman pose, wraps the hem of his sweater around his fingers for protection, and tries to yank the cactus out.

"Shit!" he screams as cactus spines penetrate virgin wool. Now about twenty needles are sticking out of *his* hand and my predicament is status quo.

I try to stay cool but it's clear that panic is the theme of my inner life. It's also clear that I would swear on the life of my child that I'd never tell a soul, never mention the incident, so help me, where do I sign? Just get the damn thing OUT.

But luckily, it doesn't come down to secret oath-signing.

The fourth surgeon, a shaggy-haired Englishman from Leicester, whips his camera out of its leather case, zips the case up around the baby jumping cholla (thus saving the world-class surgeon hands), and applies negative force with the enthusiasm of Hercules. A moment later, with a gracious bow, he presents me with the deceased baby cholla.

"Take it home as a souvenir," he says. "And feel free to tell the world if you think it'll give them a laugh."

I promise to do exactly that and now I'm keeping my promise. My hope is that it might help to change the image of the orthopedic surgeon just a little, which ultimately can only do all of us a lot of good!

THE TROUBLE WITH BACK SURGERY

If you suffer from chronic back pain you probably live with a fantasy that surfaces from time to time: if the pain becomes too terrible, you can always resort to surgery. Unfortunately, nothing could be farther from the truth. Back surgery is not — and never will be — a viable option for the vast majority of sufferers. One British researcher estimated that, for every 10,000 people who experience a bout of back pain, only four could possibly benefit from an operation. The other 9,996 people may be suffering from excruciating pain, but they do not have a problem that a surgical procedure can ameliorate.

Furthermore, back surgery is no panacea even when it is indicated. Most of us have heard of someone whose life has taken on new meaning after a back operation; I personally know six such individuals and I intend to remain jealous of them for eternity. On the other hand, I know a lot more people who insist that they are no better, as well as quite a few who say they feel a lot worse, for having had back surgery. This is particularly true in the case of three people I know who have undergone two surgeries, the second operation having been performed to correct the first. (Rhoda Reisman describes all this far better than I can because this happened to her. She tells her story at the end of the chapter.)

The trouble with back surgery is that it can usually fix the problem but it can also create problems. Cutting through tissue — a *lot* of tissue, about three inches' worth, in the case of the lumbar spine — is a fact of life when it comes to surgery, and the bottom line is that tissue that has been sliced through by scalpels and other surgical instruments cannot be expected to function perfectly even after everything has healed.

As well, some people heal better than others. That's simply a fact of life. Therefore, even if you choose the best surgeon in town (and who doesn't!), the outcome has partly to do with your body's ability to produce new tissue that functions nearly as well as the old. (How scar tissue is formed and why it doesn't always function well is described in Chapter 12.)

Surgery is further complicated by the fact that a number of judgment calls must be made. For instance, if you have a herniated disc, your surgeon must decide whether to simply remove the herniated portion of the disc, or to fuse the joints above and below as well to increase stability.

If the disc is going to be removed and no fusion performed, is the standard procedure the best tack, or would it be better to perform micro-surgery, which involves less cutting? Or one of the newer techniques that require no cutting at all? Of course there are pluses and minuses to every procedure.

There is one additional issue, which many surgeons fail to discuss with their patients for reasons that escape me. Maybe it's because, to them, this fact is so obvious that they assume everyone else on the planet knows about it as well. The purpose of back surgery is to correct a technical problem, most often one that is interfering with the ability of a certain nerve to perform its job. Surgery is *not* performed to eliminate pain. I suspect that a good number of back pain sufferers would think again about surgery if they understood this fact.

Of course, every surgeon hopes that correcting the technical problem will also relieve, or at least ameliorate, the patient's pain, and in many cases it does. However, back pain is a complicated affair (I think I've mentioned this before!), so the outcome of surgery is far more complex than simply fixing pathology. For instance, some studies show that how much a back pain sufferer likes his or her job is as important an indicator of a successful outcome as whether or not the technical problem has been rectified. This does not apply to patients with a broken leg, even when the break is so severe that surgery is required to repair the problem.

A LOOK BACK

Back surgery was born in the 1930s in response to the novel theory that herniated discs were the cause of most back pain. In 1934, two American surgeons teamed up to perform the first discotomy/fusion operation. One of them was a neurosurgeon whose job was to remove the herniated portion of the patient's disc. The other was an orthopedic surgeon whose task was to fuse the joints above and below that disc. Many surgeons hailed the procedure as a major breakthrough that would turn out to be a panacea. Within a short time, they found out they were wrong.

Nevertheless, for a couple of decades, back surgery became more and more popular, particularly in the United States. However, by the 1960s there were so many failed back surgery patients hobbling about that surgeons were forced to face the truth: in many cases, they were doing more harm than good. When *Time* did a cover story on back pain in 1981, they put the dilemma wisely: operating on a back, they pointed out, is a bit like using a hammer to kill a fly that has landed on a piece of glass. It's fairly easy to render the fly dead as a doornail — but look at the mess you must make.

By the 1970s, many back surgeons were removing herniated discs without performing a fusion. They believed that their patients were happier with the results. (This meant, by the way, that either a neurosurgeon or an orthopedic surgeon was needed, not both.) Others remained skeptical about whether the results were significantly better, but within a decade it did appear that the number of horrible failures was starting to decline. Since few outcome studies were being done back then, it was hard to say for sure.

In any case, a new philosophy emerged: where back surgery is concerned, "less is more."

With high technology at the forefront, this philosophy was able to be translated into reality. During the 1970s, the operating room microscope was developed and microsurgery became possible. In many instances this worked better, but, as is true of everything in life, when you gain something you give something else up. In this case, it was the ability to inspect the area near the herniated disc, and in some cases, surgeons missed a **sequestrated fragment** that had broken off and migrated beyond the area of vision.

During this time, X-ray equipment also became more sophisticated. For instance, a radiologist could insert a needle into the center of a disc using a sophisticated machine called a **fluroscope** to help guide the way. (For such blind procedures, where the person doing one can't actually see the way, an enormous amount of skill and experience is required.) To begin with, a test called a discogram was performed. A discogram is horribly painful for the patient but, during the early 1970s, it was all that was available. Later, myelograms, which hurt less, were developed, and today a CT scan or magnetic resonance imaging (MRI) (neither of which hurts at all) will do the job in the vast majority of cases (see Chapter 4 for details on these diagnostic tests).

Pretty soon, this sophisticated diagnostic technology was used to treat patients as well. As I mentioned in the opening, Dr. Lyman Smith developed chymopapain (which, procedurally, is similar to a discogram) and, eventually, other less invasive, high-tech surgical procedures were born, such as laser surgery.

Then the oddest thing happened — at least, I find it odd. During the 1990s, back surgeons started to do more fusions once again, only this time they started to use metal screws rather than chips of bone. Once again, the concept of "less is more" was under scrutiny.

Today, I believe we are at a crossroads where back surgery is concerned. We have come full circle, but the lessons of the 1930s still apply: back surgery is no panacea.

It's interesting — and slightly comforting — to see what world-class back surgeons have to say about the future of back surgery. Dr. John Kostuik, a Canadian orthopedic surgeon who left Canada to practice in the United States, believes that primary prevention could reduce the need for spinal surgery and ultimately be cost effective. "There is no doubt in my mind," he says, "that if students in Grade 1 are taught proper . . . ergonomics and [the importance of] physical fitness, costs could be considerably curtailed. . . ." I couldn't agree more. Alas, few institutions are interested in funding education.

The observations of Dr. Robert Keller, an American surgeon and researcher, are less comforting. For one thing, he believes that, in the United States, there are far more orthopedic surgeons than necessary and that this may account for the fact that, despite everything we know, the rate of back surgery in that country is going up rather than down. Even more alarming is the fact that disc surgery is performed twice as often on the American West Coast as on the East Coast, where there are far fewer back surgeons. I have yet to piece together what's happening in Canada, where few statistics have been collected and analyzed. Ask me next year!

Right now my conclusion is the one I seem to arrive at so often that I worry about sounding like a bore: *caveat emptor*. It's your back, and the harsh reality is that, if you choose to undergo back surgery, you, not your surgeon, will have to live with the consequences.

Of course, which type of operation you choose is as important as making the decision to have surgery at all. "Less is more" is the best philosophy overall. But there are times when a radical procedure does make sense. In other words, on occasion "more is less."

PRE-OP: BE PREPARED!

If it has been determined that you are a suitable candidate for back surgery, consider this: research shows that patients who are well prepared psychologically and are in good physical condition have better outcomes than those who are not well prepared. It's also true that chronic back pain patients who are not addicted to medication such as painkillers or alcohol generally do better as well.

However, it's difficult to define exactly what constitutes being well prepared psychologically because it means different things for different people. As I pointed out in Chapter 5, people from different cultures tend to react in certain ways to both stress and pain. The same, I think, can be said about back surgery. And of course, everyone has his or her own concerns. Some people want to know precisely how the procedure that's been chosen will be done; others are less interested in the technical details than the risk factors and how long it may take to recuperate.

I think my best bet is to tell you what *I* would want to know going into surgery — which, as you can imagine, is everything! In the sections that follow, I outline the most common back surgeries in as much detail as I can. (I am discussing mainly low back surgery here — neck surgery has its own problems, which are discussed in Chapter 19.) Take from it what interests you and what is relevant. But please take it seriously.

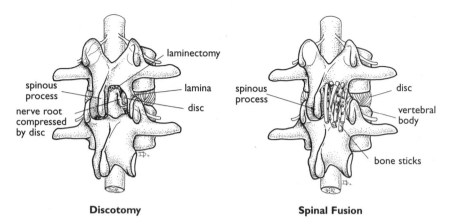

Figure 17.1 A Discotomy and Fusion

THE ANATOMY OF A DISCOTOMY AND FUSION

Discotomy

The most common type of back surgery is the removal of a herniated disc that is compressing, or pinching, a nerve. Technically, the procedure is called **decompression surgery**, although **discotomy** is a more commonly used term.

In 1992, 319,000 discotomies were performed in the United States. In 1986, the only year for which I could acquire data, about 11,000 were performed in Canada, which has a population about a tenth the size of the U.S. population. As is true in many aspects of medicine, we are far more conservative north of the 49th parallel.

Before surgery, the surgeon must decide which disc is causing the problem. Sometimes there is more than one. Either a CT scan or an MRI (see Chapter 4) will be performed to confirm what was learned from the clinical examination. Hopefully, these tests will pin down the precise location of the problem.

Once the patient has been anesthetized, the surgeon makes an incision. If one disc is involved, the cut is generally about two inches long. Next, various layers of muscle and ligament must be cut through or, if possible, gone around. Eventually, the lamina, or back portion, of the vertebra in question is exposed (see Figure 17.1). On a man of medium build and normal weight, the lamina of a lumbar disc is about three inches from the surface of the skin.

As I explained in Chapter 2, the majority of disc herniations occur in the back section of the disc's annulus, or outer casing. (The annulus tends to be weaker at the back, but lifestyle is usually a factor as well. Most of us spend far too much time in flexion, which strains the posterior part of the lumbar discs.)

In order to gain access to the disc, the surgeon must first remove a portion of the lamina, which I sometimes think of as the vertebra's roof. This is technically called a **laminectomy**.

These days, most surgeons use a microscope or special magnifying glasses. Either way, the next step is to peer through the hole in the lamina and, for the first time, actually view the problem.

The surgeon gently pushes the nerve root aside, then enlarges the rupture in the disc. Finally, he or she uses a tiny scoop to remove what is left of the nucleus, thus decompressing the nerve. The nerve root muscles and ligaments are put back into place, and the patient is sewn up. Over the course of several weeks, scar tissue forms where the nucleus used to be.

Fusion

In some cases — perhaps 10 to 15 percent — the surgeon will decide that it is also necessary to do a fusion to make the spine more stable. There are several possible reasons. Perhaps the joints in the area have suffered a lot of wear and tear. Or maybe a large amount of bone had to be removed in order to get at the disc. In any case, the decision to fuse is a judgment call made by the surgeon. (Often, the dual procedure, technically called a "discotomy/ fusion," is referred to simply as "fusion." What's confusing is that a fusion is sometimes performed without a discotomy, as with surgery performed to sta-bilize one or more levels of the spine in cases where the discs are just fine!)

Performing a fusion is more complex than simply removing a disc. It requires bone chips, which until recently were almost always taken from the patient's pelvis. These days, however, artificial bone from a bone bank is sometimes substituted. (On rare occasions the surgeon will decide to use some of each.)

There are advantages and disadvantages to both options. When the patient's own bone is being used, there is usually a lot of postoperative pain from the chip removal. In fact, several people I've spoken to say that they suffered more hip pain than back pain, and one or two people I've talked to say that their hip pain never completely subsided. On the other hand, human bodies sometimes reject artificial bone, in which case the procedure will fail.

If the patient's bone is being used, the surgeon makes an incision in the patient's pelvis, then carefully carves off about a dozen tiny strips of bone. (This is done before the disc is removed.) Each piece is about an inch long and not much thicker than a matchstick.

With a special surgical instrument, the surfaces of the vertebrae that are to be fused are roughed up. This is essential because it activates the healing process; the body is "tricked" into thinking there has been a fracture and sets about repairing the break.

Next, the bone strips are packed against the vertebrae. They are positioned somewhat like tiny splints, then tucked snugly against the vertebrae's damaged surfaces. Over the course of a couple of months, the bones become fused and movement is no longer possible. Health-care professionals call this **spine stabilization**.

If artificial bone is being used there is, of course, no need to make an incision in the patient's hip, but otherwise the procedure is similar.

In the vast majority of cases, fusions are performed posteriorly — that is, the patient is positioned on his or her stomach and the surgeon enters from the back. On very rare occasions, the procedure will be performed anteriorally — that is, the patient will be positioned on his or her back and the surgeon will enter from the front. Anterior back surgery is so new that there is very little data on its success rate, let alone the advantages and disadvantages. In Canada, only a few surgeons have even attempted the procedure.

Surgery for Spinal Stenosis

On rare occasions, surgery is performed on people suffering from spinal stenosis. As I explained in Chapter 2, most of these patients are elderly.

The success rate is not impressive; one meta-analysis has indicated a success rate of only 64 percent.

In fact, some recent studies suggest that conservative therapies offer more hope than was previously thought, and that the symptoms of spinal stenosis are not all that likely to worsen over time, so a "wait and see" attitude to surgery is indicated.

When decompression surgery is indicated for spinal stenosis, the procedure is a laminectomy to remove a piece of bone. Spinal stenosis, you will recall, is a narrowing of the spinal column. If surgery is indicated, chances are it is a case of lateral spinal stenosis, where the intervertebral foramen at the back of the vertebra has narrowed, usually because of a bone spur developing there. The laminectomy removes this bit of bone so it no longer compresses the nerves that pass through the foramen.

Only very rarely is surgery used to correct central spinal stenosis, where the actual spinal column has narrowed; the laminectomy has to be quite extensive and it is very difficult to correct this condition.

CHYMONUCLEOLYSIS: THE FRUIT OF CONTROVERSY

Chymopapain — an enzyme made from the flesh of the papaya fruit — is sometimes used as an alternative to traditional disc surgery in a procedure called **chymonucleolysis**.

Here's how it works: The physician inserts a stout needle into the nucleus, or center, of the disc. Then chymopapain is injected and the nucleus dissolves. Like a discogram, chymonucleolysis is a blind procedure requiring great skill and experience. The surgeon must use a fluroscope to see the way, but even a fluoroscope cannot provide a three-dimensional view.

Chymonucleolysis has some advantages over surgery, at least in theory. It can be done under a local anesthetic. It takes only about thirty minutes. There is no scarring, and the recovery time is short. The success rate — when the procedure is used by a skilled doctor who knows how to pick the right patients — is about 75 percent. If it doesn't work, open surgery is still an option.

In 1987, I spent months doing research on chymopapain because I wanted to find out why it had been plagued with so many complications, but only in the United States. In Canada, Europe, and Australia, a few well-trained surgeons and radiologists used the procedure on well-selected patients and got excellent results.

In the United States, however, about 3,500 doctors injected chymopapain into about 80,000 patients during 1983 and 1984. By the summer of 1983, complications started to be reported, and by mid-1984, the use of the procedure ground almost to a halt. Thousands of back pain patients who had undergone chymonucleolysis were no better than they had been before; worse yet, a few dozen had become paraplegics and a few had actually died. Over the years, the use of chymopapain picked up again, but cautiously. In 1995, 1,400 procedures were performed in the United States; less than a hundred were performed in Canada.

What was the problem, and why the disparity? This is what I found out: In Canada, Australia, and Europe, the use of chymopapain had developed slowly and steadily, which is exactly what's supposed to happen with new medical procedures. Every year, a few more surgeons learned how to use chymopapain by spending several days apprenticing with an experienced colleague, then going home to try it themselves. Very few serious complications have arisen amongst the patients whose physicians learned the procedure this way. Today, in all three regions, they are still using chymopapain on small numbers of well-picked patients with a success rate of about 75 percent. And of course, as I have mentioned, the patients for whom chymonucleolysis is unsuccessful can still go on to have traditional surgery.

In the United States things happened differently.

When chymopapain was approved by the U.S. Federal Drug Administration, there was so much demand for it that doctors rushed to "acquire" the procedure. Many learned it at a one-day course sponsored by two medical associations — a course which was designed by the drug company that manufactured and sold chymopapain. As a result, some of the doctors who used chymopapain in 1983 had never performed a blind procedure on a human subject in their lives. They had practiced sticking needles into plastic mannequins for about fifteen minutes, and spent another hour watching colleagues do the same thing at the practical portion of the seminar. This could only happen in America!

U.S. papaya fruit futures hit rock bottom, but the search for a less invasive procedure lived on.

PERCUTANEOUS DISCOTOMY

Metaphorically speaking, **percutaneous discotomy** is the child of chymopapain. Here's how it works: A hollow tube, called a **nucleotome**, is inserted into the nucleus of a disc. Bits of nucleus are sucked into the tube, chopped up — then flushed out.

In America, percutaneous discotomy, like chymonucleolysis, was introduced with great fanfare. Some predicted that it would put an end to regular surgery, which was what others had promised about chymopapain less than a decade before. But this time, many physicians refused to try it; lots of others tried it only a few times. The problem was not serious complications but the lack of scientific data to show that it worked. I also have a hunch that some doctors became disillusioned because they had picked their patients poorly.

Why do I think this? Because again, in other countries, the story was quite different. In Canada, for instance, a handful of surgeons use the percutaneous technique on carefully chosen patients, with generally good results. One reason so few physicians ever do it is that it takes much longer to perform than chymonucleolysis, but our provincial health-care plans will only pay the same amount.

LASER SURGERY

Laser surgery, technically called **percutaneous laser discectomy**, is the next step in the progression of noninvasive treatments for a herniated disc. Here's how it works: A thin, hollow needle — much thinner than the one used for percutaneous discotomy— is inserted into the nucleus of the disc. A strand of optical fiber is inserted through the needle. Then a few bursts of laser energy are sent through the fiber and a tiny bit of disc material — which is mostly water — is vaporized. This causes the pressure within the nucleus to drop, and a vacuum is created. As the old saying goes, nature abhors a vacuum. In an attempt to get the pressure back to normal, the nucleus sucks the herniated portion back in.

Well, sort of. What actually happens is far less dramatic. The herniated portion of the disc *is* sucked away from the nerve it is pinching, but only by a fraction of a millimeter. According to Dr. Daniel Choy, a surgeon at St. Luke's–Roosevelt Hospital in New York, who believes in the procedure and has used it on a fair number of patients, that's enough to do the trick.

The pluses? Laser surgery can be done with a local anesthetic. It takes about thirty minutes, and, except for heavy lifting, patients can return to their normal activities within a few days.

The minuses? Well, for starters, as one Canadian surgeon says, "if you're not careful about needle placement, you could vaporize something other than the disc." For another thing, the effectiveness of laser surgery, especially in the long term, is still unproven. Some recent studies show high rates of complication and reoperation; others suggest that the results often deteriorate over time. Surgeon Rick Delamarter of the UCLA Spine Center has compared the success rate of laser surgery to "a flip of a coin."

Other surgeons, however, argue that that the key is careful patient selection — that the procedure is valuable for single-level, contained herniations.

The future of laser surgery is up in the air, but in my opinion, it won't fly. Of course, I may be proven wrong. It depends upon who does it . . . and on whom. Once again, stay tuned.

ARTIFICIAL IMPLANTS

The latest trend in spinal surgery seems to involve the use of artificial devices implanted in the spine. These aren't completely new — rods and wires have had occasional use in spinal surgery for decades — but the 1990s seems to have brought on an increase in these procedures, most of which remain controversial.

Pedicle Screws

Rather than using either bone chips from the patient's hips or artificial bone pieces to achieve spinal fusion, surgeons can fix metal pedicle screws to the vertebrae at either end of the area to be fused, and fix to them plates or rods to hold the area rigid while fusion takes place.

For years, pedicle screw devices held only experimental status with the U.S. Federal Drug Administration (FDA), and controversy about their effectiveness and level of complication raged. Proponents argued that they provided excellent, rigid fixation, required reduced operating time, and, according to at least one study, allowed patients to recover much more quickly and feel pain relief right away.

Detractors pointed out the drastic consequences of misplacement (this is another blind procedure — the surgeon can't see the tip of the screw when implanting it), the high complication rates found in some studies, the difficulty the screws cause in subsequent diagnosis with high-tech imaging (a pedicle screw gets in the way of a CT scan), and the lack of conclusive evidence of their superiority.

Add to this allegations that the FDA seems to have been remarkably lax in policing their use in this period — many surgeons continued to use them in a wide variety of spinal fusion situations despite their experimental status — and you get a juicy controversy indeed. (It was even the subject of an ABC 20-20 segment in 1994.)

In 1995, however, the FDA approved the use of pedicle screws in certain applications — not because of more evidence in their favor, but because a manufacturer succeeded in showing them to be substantially similar to an item that was available before 1976, when the current standards for medical devices were implemented. They were "grandfathered" — but only for the treatment of severe spondylolisthesis, which is one condition for which there are few other surgical options.

Other conditions for which pedicle screws are proposed as indispensable include fractures, severe deformity, ankylosing spondylitis, and spines damaged by previous surgery. The 1995 FDA ruling probably has opened the door for wider approvals.

Artificial Discs

I almost didn't include these as they are so rare, but they are in the very early stages of human trials and may become more common if results are good. As with pedicle screws (as with every new treatment!), artificial discs have their defenders and detractors. The potential advantages have primarily to do with a speedier recovery than traditional fusion: patients don't need to wear a brace, can sit up immediately, and are immediately mobile. These advantages have yet to be proven in controlled human trials, however.

POST-OP: THE RECOVERY PROCESS

Patients who go into hospital to have a disc removed but no fusion generally stay in for about a week, or less. But anyone who is counting on having a nice rest will be disappointed. The rehabilitation process after back surgery should begin right in the recovery room; postoperative patients are put to work almost as soon as they open their eyes!

The first goal is to deal with the effects of the anesthetic. To help clear the airways, patients are encouraged to breathe deeply and to cough.

Foot and Ankle Exercise

The next item on the agenda is getting the circulation back to normal. When you remain still, blood tends to pool in your veins. So a simple movement called the foot and ankle exercise is recommended.

Lie on your back and pull the toes of your right foot toward your nose. Alternate between this movement and pointing your toes down. Then repeat, this time with the left foot. Patients are usually encouraged to do this exercise four or five times each hour.

Log Roll

The next important thing to learn is a safe and comfortable way of turning in bed. This is called the log roll; it's also the first part of the routine patients go through when they learn how to sit up.

Lie on your back with your knees bent. Bring your knees up toward your chest and place a pillow between them. Then, keeping your body rigid as if you really were a log, roll to one side. Most people find it comfortable to let their hands rest on their stomachs.

Sitting Up

Years ago, back surgery patients were confined to their beds for days on end. Not any more. Within twenty-four hours of surgery, just about everyone is encouraged to sit up. If possible, standing up and taking a short walk is also recommended for most patients. (If someone can't stand

Figure 17.2 Sitting Up

up, it's usually because of the effects of the anesthetic rather than the back surgery itself.)

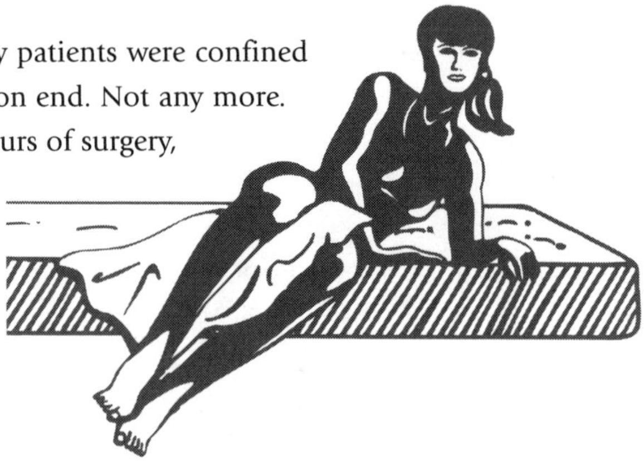

Sitting up and getting out of bed after surgery can be an effort. A physiotherapist will teach you how to do it and be on hand to help the first couple of times.

Start off lying on your back (see Figure 17.2). If you want to get out of the right side of the bed, the first step is to log-roll toward the right. Your body should be positioned so that you are near the right edge of the bed, but not so near that you can fall off! The next step is to let your feet drop over the edge of the bed. Then, using your right forearm and the palm of your left hand, push your body up into a sitting position. As your body moves into a sitting position, your legs, aided by gravity, will drop toward the floor.

Once you are sitting up, remove the pillow. Then, using your hands for support, slide your body forward until your feet are touching the ground.

For their first walk — which is usually no more than ten feet — most patients use a high-wheeled walker for support. Over the next few days, increasing distance is the goal. The next step is to get rid of the walker and walk with crutches, then unaided.

Knee-to-Chest Stretches

Gentle stretching exercises done right in bed are also important during the first days after surgery. A bit of extension (as much as the patient can tolerate) and some knee-to-chest stretches will do the trick. In fact, the single most important exercise for a discotomy patient is the knee-to-chest stretch, which keeps the spinal cord and surrounding tissue mobile.

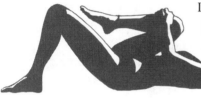

Lie on your back with your knees bent (see Figure 17.3). Using both hands, pull the right knee up to the chest, stretching the muscles of the lower back only to the point

Figure 17.3 The Knee-to-Chest Stretch

at which you feel pain. Hold for five seconds and relax. Then switch legs. Repeat ten times with each leg. To stretch the upper back, tuck your chin in and raise your head off the ground while you are holding the stretch. Over the course of a few days, gently increase the range of your stretch.

In the best of circumstances, a patient will continue to have access to both physical therapy and occupational therapy for as long as is necessary. In the worst of circumstances, patients are sent home with only a few tips. As always, if that happens, it's the patient's responsibility to get what's needed and sometimes that requires a degree of tenacity.

A TALE OF TWO SURGERIES

I first met Rhoda Reisman at an American Back Society conference in 1991. She looked great — slim and very pretty — and she never once complained about her back. But when she moved, it was in that delicate manner that said, to anyone who cared to see it, that she was in pain. Rhoda had had a one-level fusion in December of 1988 and, while she could move better, the pain did not go away.

Rhoda was doing something wonderful. In the spring of 1990, she had flown down to the Dallas Spinal Rehabilitation Center in Dallas, Texas, where she battled her way through a five-week program for chronic back pain sufferers. When she returned home to Montreal, she decided to set up a chronic spinal pain support group there so that others with back pain could also learn how to cope. She developed a program and received funding from the Jewish General Hospital Auxiliary. The first group met in the fall of 1990.

Three years after her first surgery, her mobility began to decrease once again. In February of 1992 she had a second, more complex, surgery. This time, her spine was fused at three levels and several nerve roots were decompressed. Not surprisingly, this forced her to slow down for a while.

As well as running support groups, Rhoda is one of the few laypeople who have been asked to put on workshops for health-care professionals at American Back Society conferences. There is a gap, she tells them, between what health-care professionals can provide and what chronic pain patients need. She explains how her support groups can fill that gap.

Rhoda is still recuperating and still pacing herself. But, as she says, she can at least depend on being pain-free most mornings, which is a big step in the right direction. She hopes the number of pain-free hours will continue to increase.

Rhoda Reisman's story is atypical in some ways. For one thing, her two surgeries were both spinal fusions; these days, far more discotomies — which are less complex — are performed. But, in many other ways, Rhoda's story is completely typical. Along with her pain, she has experienced fear, anger, depression, and the scary kind of hopeful acceptance that goes along with the decision to have surgery. I am dazzled by her ability to describe all of these things.

In the years since she wrote this story, she has become even more determined in her belief that people need to take control of their lives — and that spinal surgery should be only a last-resort option. "If I had known then what I know now," she says, "I never would have had my first surgery." I am also overjoyed to report that in 1996 she married a very lucky man.

A Surgery Patient's Perspective
RHODA REISMAN

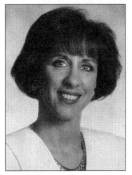

Rhoda Reisman

In my case, the original problem, which started in 1987, was in my facet joints; my lumbar spine was unstable. It may have originated from the high-impact aerobic exercise classes I went to in the 1970s.

Then I started to have trouble sitting, which affected my life socially. I had trouble in restaurants. While driving. At movies. But I went to physiotherapy, and, for a while, I felt better.

But eight months later, the pain returned. For a time, it came and went, but each bout lasted longer than the one before. Finally, it did not get better at all and back pain became part of my life.

I had to give up school — which I'd gone back to — because I couldn't sit. I had to give up community work, which I loved. I couldn't do many activities with my sons, who were ten and twelve at the time. It was hard on them, especially the younger one. My husband had a hard time dealing with it too.

I tried everything I could to avoid surgery: exercise, physiotherapy, corsets, anti-inflammatories, chiropractic, acupuncture. When every conservative option did not work, I started with the invasive procedures: discograms, CT scans, facet joint blocks, nerve blocks, a myelogram, a nuclear magnetic resonance, and finally, a rhizotomy during which some of the nerve roots in my spine were cauterized to try and stop the pain.

When you first have limitations like this, you're scared. I didn't know anything about chronic pain. All I knew was that I was an incredibly active person who could no longer do the things I used to do.

Psychotherapy was helpful to a point. But the pain was increasing and my mobility was decreasing. And, not surprisingly, I was getting more and more discouraged.

At the end of 1988 I decided to have surgery. If I had known then what I know now, I would have decided against it. But I didn't have the knowledge. I only knew that, apart from being in pain, I couldn't walk around the block. I couldn't walk *halfway* around the block.

I knew what procedure I was going to have: a one-level fusion to stabilize my lumbar spine. In fact, when it came to asking questions, I was my surgeon's star patient. The night before my operation, he came into my room with his staff and said, "Okay, Rhoda, tell them what we're going to do to you tomorrow morning." So I told them, step by step. The next morning, I joked around before they put me under. "Listen," I told my surgeon, "if you need me — if there's something you don't understand — don't hesitate to wake me up!"

What I didn't understand was how traumatic surgery can be, or how long it can sometimes take to recover. My surgery was successful in terms of restoring my mobility for a while. I could walk! I could drive! But I never got rid of my pain. I began to feel that I was out of the mainstream of life. I felt isolated and very depressed.

It soon got to the point where I couldn't ignore it. Sometimes, I'd go into my room and close the door and cry. If you haven't been through it, you can't really understand what it's like to feel pain all the time. You have to pace yourself because the number of hours you can be up during the day are limited.

But I was determined to give it the year my surgeon said it would take. At the end of the year I consulted another surgeon, and he told me to give it two years. But after about eighteen months, I went into a severe depression. I saw myself as a failure to my children, to my husband . . . even to my surgeon, as if it were my fault that what he did hadn't worked. I couldn't see myself living such an inactive life. And I didn't understand why I couldn't just learn to cope with the pain.

The fact that I was on different forms of medication made it more complicated. At the time, low levels of antidepressants were being prescribed for chronic pain. So I was on that. I was taking Valium as well as anti-inflammatories and painkillers.

As I describe it all now, I sound so rational. But back then, while it was happening, it wasn't rational at all. I didn't want to get out of bed but I couldn't sleep. I had no appetite. Nor energy to call people up. Life was a black tunnel with no light.

However, I was lucky. My orthopedic surgeon, Dr. Alexander Hadjipavlou (who has since moved to the United States) referred me to a pain clinic in Dallas, Texas, so I could learn to cope with chronic pain. There was no similar program here in Canada.

When I arrived in Dallas, I was completely debilitated emotionally and physically. They had to help me get off certain drugs as well as build me up physically and psychologically. Every day, I had an hour of psychotherapy, as well as two group sessions. I did occupational therapy — learning new ways of doing daily activities, even something as simple as how to get into and out of a car. I did physiotherapy, which included aerobics, as well as strengthening and stretching exercises.

There was also an educational component: anatomy, nutrition, sleeping and back pain, sex and back pain, relaxation techniques. It was the hardest, most challenging thing I had ever done in my life. I had to fight the physical pain and deal with the emotions that go along with it all at the same time.

One of the most important things I learned was to start thinking about the pain as being external rather than internal. Then it's easier to realize that you are not to blame. And in turn, you can get angry at the pain rather than feel depressed.

I also learned how to juggle. (Not literally!) Activity is very important when you have to deal with pain. So is rest. But if you get too much rest you end up stiff and deconditioned. So you have to find a balance. It's important to get it right and to be positive about having to adapt.

I believe that the greatest problem about chronic pain is that it is invisible and inconsistent. This issue has come up many times in the support groups. For reasons that medical science cannot explain very well, chronic pain changes. It is different from one day to the next. It's hard for other people to understand. You don't look like you're sick, but you are always in pain.

I still supervise a program for those who live with chronic spinal pain. As of last fall, almost 200 people have benefited from this experience. I intend to continue writing and working with health-care professionals whose field is chronic pain. My goal is simple: to help as many people as possible get control of their own lives.

18

Massage: There's the Rub!

From 1984 until 1987 I swam every morning — well, *almost* every morning — at a downtown Toronto women's club. The pool temperature was 84 degrees Fahrenheit, which for a cream puff like me is on the cool side of acceptable. But because it was a club for women exclusively, I could swim in the buff, and that went a way toward warming my heart. Best of all, it allowed me to save money on bathing suits, which, in chlorinated pools, disintegrate at the speed of light. Whenever I estimated that I'd saved fifty dollars — about four times a year — I would treat myself to a massage. I recall every moment of those four sessions; they were pure and unadulterated heaven. While I would never try to convince anyone that massage is a miracle cure for back pain, I can certainly say that each session reduced the level of my pain for several days. Besides, having a massage always makes me feel great.

I used to think about this while swimming my daily lengths, and over the years I conjured up an excellent fantasy, which had three parts. First I would write a best-selling novel. Next I'd buy my family a house with an indoor pool; my one selfish act would be to keep the thermostat at 87 degrees even when my beloved daughter complained it was like swimming in a hot tub. But the third part was the best: every morning after my swim I would have an hour-long massage. That would set me up for a pain-free, eight-hour stint at the computer, where I'd pound out several pages of my next best-seller so I could pay for the lifestyle of which I'd grown extremely fond!

Unfortunately, a number of things have always managed to come between me and this excellent fantasy — and, to be honest, I dream more about the back-rubs than the swims.

But I like to look reality in the eye. And so I know that my fantasy is unlikely to come to fruition. At least in this country; the massage part might be possible if I immigrated to Germany. In that country, family physicians write as many prescriptions for massage therapy as for painkilling drugs and the German national health-care plan pays.

The health policy makers of Germany have known for years that massage (used in conjunction with therapies such as exercise, education, and ergonomics) is a cost-effective method of helping back pain sufferers cope. But with my luck, it will take OHIP ten decades to catch on to this wisdom, by which time I will have no need for any type of therapy!

I find it interesting that Germany was able to forge such a prudent policy back in the days when there was very little other than clinical evidence to support the merits of massage. Over the past decade, quite a number of acceptable studies have shown its efficacy, yet not one of Canada's provincial health-care plans is willing to fork out a cent for this therapy, which has been around for thousands of years. (I use the word "acceptable" rather than "excellent" simply because massage therapists have virtually no money to conduct studies, so most of these studies have been done by members of the medical profession. In my opinion, physicians would be able to ask more provocative questions if they had clinical experience with massage.) A number of private insurers will contribute on the order of $130 per year — the clients pay the rest. But $130 is peanuts when you're talking about a treatment that takes at least an hour and works best when it's done fairly often (at least twice a week) during an acute phase. On average, massage therapists charge between $50 and $70 per session. While that may sound like a lot of money to hand over, I have yet to meet a masseuse who is rich. Five massages a day is about all a strong and dedicated therapist can provide, and of course there's massage oil to buy and a well-heated office to run.

THE HISTORY OF MASSAGE

In January of 1993, the prestigious *New England Journal of Medicine* published a survey on the usage of alternative therapies in the United States. (I mentioned some other results of this survey in Chapter 14.) Back pain was the number one reason why Americans consulted alternative therapists and massage was one of the three most frequently used therapies. (The other two were relaxation techniques to help cope with stress, and chiropractic.) I could have told them the same thing, and saved them a bundle of money!

In fact, massage has enjoyed good press since Homer wrote over three thousand years ago about warriors being "rubbed and kneaded" when they returned from battle. In 400 B.C., the great Hippocrates himself (for whom the doctors' Hippocratic oath is named) wrote about massage: "The physician must be experienced in many things but assuredly also in rubbing."

Not much is known about massage during the Dark Ages, but then, not much is known about anything that occurred during that period of time — after all, that's why it's referred to as "dark!" But by the sixteenth century notable European medical writers were again praising the treatment's merits. During that era, the emphasis also changed from kneading to the application of heavy pressure.

Early in the nineteenth century a Swedish masseuse began to advocate the use of yet another variation — the combination of light stroking in one direction with deep pressure in another. This concept gained acceptance and became known as Swedish massage, which is what the majority of North American massage therapists practice today. (A smaller number of massage therapists practice other types of manual therapy, such as shiatsu and reiki.)

Shiatsu and Reiki

Two of the popular forms of "alternative" hands-on therapy blend physical touching with Eastern philosophy to create holistic approaches to healing.

Shiatsu

Some back pain sufferers find relief in **shiatsu**, which is also known as **acupressure**. Related to acupuncture (see Chapter 5) as much as to massage, this oriental therapy involves pressing firmly on the skin at certain precise points. It is based on the theory that the energy of life, or **chi**, flows through the body along fourteen main **meridians**, or channels. If the flow of energy along a meridian is disrupted, the organs and bodily functions associated with that meridian (which, as with an acupuncture point, may not be located nearby) experience problems.

Shiatsu, adherents believe, can help a wide number of disorders. The therapist "contacts" the energy at various points along the meridian, restoring its flow and its yin/yang balance. Shiatsu points for relieving sciatica are located on the small of the back, the buttocks, and the thighs.

Reiki

A Japanese theologian, Dr. Mikao Usui, did not invent the healing system known as **Reiki**, but is credited with discovering it among ancient teachings from the Tibetan sutras. *Rei* means "universal" and *ki* refers to the life force flowing through all living things; the word thus means "universal life force energy." The Japanese character also connotes "balance."

Considered a natural mode of healing based on channeling energy, reiki involves a very gentle laying on of hands combined with certain other noninvasive techniques. Reiki practitioners do not consider themselves to be healers, but only "instruments" of energy flow, guided by intuition as well as experience.

No two people experience reiki exactly the same way. During a typical sixty- to ninety-minute reiki session, the client may experience various sensations, including heat, coolness, tingling, floating, and dreaming. Its proponents claim it can help with everything from physical trauma to life transitions to stress; some back pain sufferers find reiki brings them relief.

The Healing Power of Touch

Whichever theory their technique is based upon, all the massage therapists I know say that (among other things) massage helps contracted muscles to relax. When muscles are relaxed, blood circulation increases, which in turn increases the elimination of toxic waste products, including lactic acid. Muscles in spasm produce lactic acid, and a build-up of lactic acid causes pain.

Massage therapists also maintain that a chronically tight muscle sometimes requires a number of massages in order to permanently relax. This makes enormous sense to me. Muscles go into spasm to protect an injured or strained area, the spasm acting like a natural splint. For one reason or another, however, the mechanism that allows spasm to relax once the injury has healed often breaks down. Sometimes, especially when back muscles are involved, such a spasm can last for months, or even years, particularly when people stay in bed rather than starting gentle stretching exercises as soon as they possibly can. But all this is explained in great detail in Chapter 12, where I also mentioned that stretching can be done passively — i.e., with massage. In a perfect world, back pain sufferers would be able to combine active and passive stretching techniques as soon as possible after an injury.

But the bottom line is that massage therapy is not, in fact, totally passive. While it's true that when you are being massaged you are not moving, there should ideally be some amount of interaction between the giver and recipient of the massage. "It's wonderfully relaxing to 'bliss out' now and then," says one massage therapist I know, "but by doing so, you miss the chance to learn what it feels like when tension, or muscle spasm, lets go." Clients who experience this release also learn how muscle tension in one part of the body can affect another part of the body, even another part quite far away.

The ideal state to be in for this to happen is called the **alpha state**. It's a difficult concept to describe because when you're in it you're both relaxed and alert. You observe your body and how it feels, but without trying to dissect or figure things out logically. The problem with being logical — an enormous problem for me! — is that it distances you from the experience, which means that one of massage's many dimensions is lost.

But apart from reducing muscle tension, being touched has come to be regarded as an instrument of pain relief in its own right. Some researchers talk about how massage works in a way similar to acupuncture or TENS — by modifying the transmission of pain, as described by the gate-control theory. (See Chapter 5.) The 1987 Quebec task force on spinal disorders suggested that massage may increase the body's level of endorphins.

Other studies indicate that massage may shorten the recovery time for surgical patients, and that cancer patients experience less pain merely as a result of being touched by a family member or a close friend. A massage therapist I knew decades ago put it this way: "There is an exchange of energy when someone touches you, and apart from everything else it can help you feel less alone and/or more connected to the world."

Christine Sutherland (whom I quoted in Chapter 3 regarding massage in diagnosis) agrees: "Touch is the most powerful stimulus for relaxation. It's the unspoken language which can provide crucial emotional support for people who have to deal with chronic pain."

These statements lead to an interesting question, one on which massage therapists tend to disagree: in order to be effective, is it necessary for a massage to be given by a trained, board-certified massage therapist?

Some of the literature put out by the American Massage Therapy Association suggests that the answer is yes, and on one level I agree that it's often important for a masseur or masseuse to understand anatomy and physiology, especially when it comes to the human back. But on another level I disagree. Christine Sutherland points out that by the time you leave the office with a stiff neck after a long day, your massage therapist has probably called it quits for the day. She suggests that it's better to get your neck massaged that evening by whatever friend or relative you have available than to wait until the next day for board-certified help. I couldn't agree more. As well, massage is an art as much as a discipline; while it requires both book knowledge and experience, the fact remains that some massage therapists are born with a special ability to heal by the power of touch.

In fact, I personally have taken this philosophy a step further. When I can't find a good friend to rub my back in the evening, I consult my young daughter Atalanti. At the time of this writing, she weighs fifty-six pounds, and a selfish part of me wishes she would stay that size for eternity, because it's the perfect weight when you need someone to walk up and down your back.

If Atalanti agrees to give me a walking massage, I'll agree to turn my fantasy pool temperature down from 87 degrees. But not by very much.

A Few Notes for the Massage Rookie

- Watch out for rashes. My skin is not all that sensitive, but I have been known to develop a rash on my face and occasionally even my arms after a massage. Generally it's a reaction to the massage oil; if you have this problem, ask your massage therapist to try a different kind of oil next time.
- Some soreness may follow a very deep massage. I've experienced a bit of soreness and even bruising. The soreness usually lasts for a day; if it lasts for more than a few days, I'd question the skill of the masseuse.
- The worst part about getting a massage at the massage therapist's office is having to go home when you're done. If possible, don't drive. For one thing, driving is too demanding when you're on Cloud Nine. For another, it's terrible for your back. If you can afford it and find someone to do it, have a massage at home.
- After a massage it's a very good idea to take an Epsom salt bath and go to bed.

- A number of nifty products exist to help you give yourself or someone else a better massage. Some of these widgets are standard — others look pretty peculiar. Many are available from the stores listed in Chapter 11.

VI

BACK IN THE FUTURE

19

A Pain in the Neck!

N eck pain is not quite as common as low back pain, which affects more than 80 percent of us during the course of our lives. Nevertheless, the number of people who suffer from problems of the cervical spine is staggering. Between 38 and 50 percent of adults will have to cope with a neck problem at least once during their lives. According to some studies, 9 percent of men and 12 percent of women suffer from neck pain on any given day. And the numbers appear to be rising; neck pain, I predict, will be an increasingly hot topic in the near future.

TREATMENT: A CHANGING VIEW

The most depressing news about neck pain, however, is that until recently the cervical spine was largely ignored by world-class researchers. Why? Because, while millions of people are driven around the bend by pain in their necks, it has caused far less disability and absenteeism than other medical problems, including low back pain.

For example, a Scandinavian study done back in the 1950s showed that, while approximately half of 1,200 men who worked in heavy industry had experienced neck problems, fewer than sixty-five had ever missed work because of it. Other studies indicate that, in the past, most people with sore necks didn't even bother to consult a health-care professional about their sore necks. Nor did they try to correct their postures, do neck exercises, or examine their lifestyles to see if a few simple changes might help. Basically, most neck pain sufferers simply toughed it out and waited for the pain to subside.

The bottom line is that since ordinary neck pain does not usually prevent people from functioning, and has had less impact on the economy than low back pain, only a handful of researchers have devoted their time and energy to the science of so common a problem.

But times are beginning to change. Says Anita Gross, a physiotherapist who is both a researcher and a clinician at the McMaster University Medical Centre in Hamilton, Ontario, "In the last few years, necks have definitely started to attract the attention of researchers." There are two reasons behind the change: the huge increase in car accidents, which are the main cause of whiplash injuries; and the increase in jobs that require people to work at video display terminals for long periods of time. When workers in such jobs develop a severe neck problem, they *do* become occupationally disabled. And so it is becoming clear that neck pain, like low back pain, is worth investigating in the interest of increasing productivity as well as decreasing human suffering.

As health-care professionals started to look more carefully at the human neck in recent years, they began to realize that there are extremely important differences between the neck and the lumbar spine in terms of anatomy (see later in the chapter for more detail). They began to ask whether neck pain developed in the same way as low back pain — and whether it should be treated the same way.

"Traditionally, neck pain was always lumped together with low back pain," explains Anita Gross. "Now we realize that we made this assumption without knowing whether or not it was based on sound scientific data."

Flip through any number of the back books written for the layperson over the past decade; most of them don't even contain a separate chapter on necks. Subjects such as how the neck is constructed, how it functions, what causes it to stop working properly, and what should be done are usually simply tacked onto the end of corresponding chapters dealing with low back pain. We have always acknowledged that some of the vertebrae of the neck look different, and are more mobile, than the vertebrae of the low back, but the overall outlook has been that a neck problem is simply a back problem that happens to occur higher up.

Once these basics began to be questioned and researched, some interesting findings started to emerge. For instance, the discs between the vertebrae of the cervical spine appear to deteriorate differently than do the discs of the lumbar spine. In the low back, most problems are thought to start in the nucleus, or center, of the disc, then move toward the annulus, or outer casing. In the neck, the process may be different; some evidence shows that the annulus deteriorates first and the process moves inward.

"Logically," says Anita Gross, "if neck problems develop differently from low back problems, then the kinds of conservative treatments that are effective may be different as well."

Not that health-care professionals who treat patients with sore necks have been choosing therapies blindly over the decades. Quite the contrary. Clinicians observe what works for their patients who are suffering from a certain condition; they share their experiences with their colleagues, and if the same method works for them, it will become more popular. This kind of "clinical" research has been going on since the beginning of health care. In the case of sore necks, it accounts for the fact that manipulation and the similar but gentler mobilization have, in recent years, been added to such traditional therapies as medication, heat, exercise, and education. But recently, researchers have begun to move the treatment of neck pain to a scientific level.

Chapter 12 outlined how the treatment of low back pain has evolved over the past decade: researchers such as Dr. Gordon Waddell began to wonder about the validity of long-term bed rest for low back pain; they examined the studies that had already been done, and began to realize that the rationale for long-term bed rest was not based on solid scientific evidence. Clinicians who were also researchers began to delve further, designing and conducting studies on early active treatment; as a result, the philosophy of how to treat low back pain underwent an about-face. "With neck pain," says Anita Gross, "that story line doesn't yet exist."

In order to help develop a story, she formed a research team with several other health-care professionals — a chiropractor, a statistics specialist, and a rheumatologist — and began the long, complicated process that will ultimately provide some scientific data. Several other research teams have been plugging away as well.

Surgery for neck problems is very rare (it is discussed separately at the end of the chapter). For this reason, Anita Gross and her coresearchers decided to limit their study to conservative methods of treating neck pain. Then they worked out the basic question they wanted to answer: which treatment, or treatments, for neck pain are the most effective?

With this question in mind, they began what health-care professionals call a **meta-analysis**. Basically, this is a study that systematically reviews the material that has already been published on a certain subject throughout the world. By analyzing these data carefully, some universal conclusions can often be made. If one study — especially one that looks only at a small number of subjects — says that a certain treatment is more effective than another, it may not mean very much. But if several studies show the same thing, health-care professionals can feel more confident about the conclusions.

If you think doing such a systematic review sounds easy, think again! Anita Gross's team collected and pored over about two hundred studies from around the world. But the exercise turned up a number of interesting points.

First of all, in many of the studies where patients had been divided into two groups and the outcomes of different treatments compared, more than one treatment was used on every patient. Therefore, all the team could really say was that a certain *combination* of treatments appeared to work better than another combination; in fact, it was possible that only one of the treatments was actually doing the trick. The team tried comparing various treatment combinations and came up with some clues, but, as Anita Gross points out, "Clues are not the same as scientific evidence."

Another finding was that, while most of the studies concluded that a particular treatment worked better than another treatment (or, in some cases, no treatment), they often didn't say *how much* better the treatment worked. There was no way to know whether the patients felt 20 percent better or 80 percent better.

Then there was the question of how well each study was designed. Were the researchers objective, or were they perhaps trying to show that the treatment method they subscribed to personally was better than one they were philosophically against? Was the number of patients in the study large enough to give the conclusions some weight? Was there enough follow-up to ensure that an apparently successful treatment didn't stop working a few days later?

The last issue was a particular problem for the research team; the longest follow-up time — after treatment — in the studies they came across was a mere three weeks.

Using these criteria, the research team selected thirty-two studies that they felt were worth analyzing with a fine-tooth comb. They decided to compare therapies rather than disciplines, since health-care professionals from different disciplines often use the same techniques. (In Holland, for example, manipulation is performed mostly by physiotherapists, since there are few chiropractors.)

The researchers divided neck pain treatments into four categories:

- physical modalities, such as exercise, heat, ice, ultrasound, laser treatment, biofeedback, acupuncture, transcutaneous nerve stimulation (TNS), and electromagnetic therapy;
- manual ("hands-on") therapies, such as massage, mobilization, and manipulation;
- education, for instance, advice on ergonomics and good posture; and
- drug therapies, such as analgesics, anti-inflammatory drugs, muscle relaxants, and antidepressant medication.

Two and a half years after they started, Anita Gross and her team of researchers had reached some very general conclusions: Over the short term (a few weeks), manual therapy, manipulation and mobilization in particular, appears to relieve neck pain when it is used in conjunction with some other type of therapy. Such "other" therapies include medication, particularly muscle relaxants, and physical medicine modalities, particularly **electromagnetic field therapy**, which stimulates cells to take in oxygen and expel waste products.*

While these findings were exciting, Anita Gross has always stressed that the results of her team's work must be interpreted cautiously. For one thing, there were fewer than a hundred patients in most of the studies they analyzed; studies on people with heart problems, for example, usually include thousands of patients. Furthermore, it's hard to draw solid conclusions from only thirty-two studies. Still, it was a beginning.

At about the same time, the RAND Corp. (which we met in Chapter 17) published its findings on the appropriateness of manipulation and mobilization for neck pain. With much greater funding, the RAND researchers based their analysis on 362 articles. Their findings were not dissimilar.

They found that where human necks are concerned, manipulation and/or mobilization may provide at least short-term pain relief and increased range of motion for people suffering from "sub-acute" and chronic neck pain. (Most — but not all — researchers define sub-acute as neck pain that has gone on for longer than three weeks and chronic neck pain as neck pain that has gone on longer than three months.) The RAND researchers reported that there was not enough data available to draw any conclusions about the efficacy of manipulation on acute neck pain. Mobilization, the "limited" data suggest, may be beneficial for acute neck pain, at least compared to rest or wearing a collar. On the other hand, other therapies such as exercise are probably of equal value.

Many people worry about the risks of manual therapies for neck pain, manipulation in particular. Anita Gross's analysis found no evidence of serious complications. RAND's analysis of 145 articles on complications resulting from manipulation and mobilization of the cervical spine did

---

* The study was published in the August 1996 issue of *Clinics of North America Rheumatic Disease Clinics.* Its title is "Manual Therapy in the Treatment of Neck Pain" and the authors are A. R. Gross, P. D. Aker, P. H. Goldsmith, and P. Peloso.

find some evidence of serious complications but they were very rare. Even minor complications were rare; examples of those that sometimes occurred include severe dizziness or nausea, increased pain, and numbness, or a feeling of pins and needles, sometimes in the arms and hands.

These conclusions about the best way to treat neck pain may sound disappointingly vague. But if you bear in mind that, less than a decade ago, research into treatment for low back pain was at a similar stage, there is good reason for hope.

In the meantime, here are a few rules of thumb about neck pain treatment:

- Try to pick a health-care professional who treats a fair number of neck patients.
- If you are going to try manipulation or mobilization, talk to your health-care professional about the risks and benefits and be aware that, because of other medical problems, or your age, you may be at risk.
- Realize that there are risks and side effects to every medical treatment. If you get good results, it's probably worth it if the only negative side effect you have to cope with is soreness that lasts for a couple of hours, or even for a day. This can happen with any kind of manual therapy: massage, exercise, mobilization or manipulation.

The View from the Top: Anatomy of a Neck

The bones of the neck, you will recall, are called cervical vertebrae, and every mammal on earth, even the giraffe, has seven of them. Of course, in humans, the cervical vertebrae are obviously a lot smaller than in giraffes. In fact, in humans, they are smaller than the vertebrae in the other areas of the spine. Cervical vertebrae are also different in that they have an opening in the transverse process; nerves and blood vessels pass through these "holes." (See Figure 19.1.)

The top two cervical vertebrae — C1 and C2 — are called the **atlas** and the **axis**. If you compare them to the other five bones of the neck, you'll see that their shape is quite different. As well, there is no disc between them.

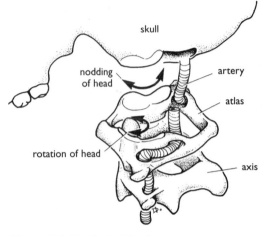

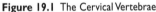

Figure 19.1 The Cervical Vertebrae

The atlas gets its name from the giant in Greek mythology who had to support the entire world on his shoulders. In our case, the world is a twelve- to sixteen-pound head! On either side of the atlas are two flat surfaces, which support the skull. When you nod your head to say "yes," your skull rocks back and forth on your atlas.

The next vertebra down is called the axis. Its most interesting feature is a large post that projects upward and fits into a ringlike opening in the atlas. When you shake your head to say "no," the atlas swivels around this post.

Eight pairs of nerves emerge from the spinal cord at this area. The lower four merge to form the major nerve branches to the arms. In the same way as pain from the lumbar spine sometimes radiates down into a leg, pain that starts in the cervical spine is sometimes referred into the arm. One reason that the diagnosis of neck pain is so difficult is that pain radiating into an arm can also be caused by a wrist problem, a shoulder problem, or a jaw joint problem.

In many cases, a tough-to-diagnose neck problem can be narrowed down with the help of a test that can show which nerves, if any, are not conducting impulses properly. But, as is true of low back pain, the precise cause of neck pain frequently remains a mystery. For some people, not knowing exactly what's wrong causes stress, which causes more neck pain, which causes more stress. . . . Fortunately, a neck problem can generally be treated successfully even when the exact cause is unknown.

There are several layers of muscles in the neck. The one that tenses up most often is the triangular-shaped **trapezius**, which is closest to the surface (see Figure 19.2). When you see people reaching back to massage their shoulders, it's the trapezius muscle that they are trying to loosen up.

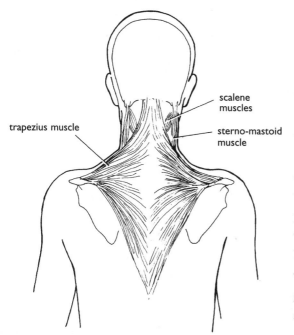

scalene
muscles

sterno-mastoid
muscle

trapezius muscle

Figure 19.2 The Muscles of the Neck

The other two muscles of the neck region that have a tendency to tighten up are the **sternocleidomastoid** (often referred to as the sterno-mastoid) and the **scalene muscles**. It's the spasm in these two muscles people are trying to undo when they probe the backs of their necks with the end of a finger after long hours sitting at a desk.

What Goes Wrong?

Like the low back, the neck is subject to sprains and strains, joint problems, and disc problems.

When younger people develop acute neck strain it is usually a result of turning awkwardly during the night, or playing a sport such as squash, which requires jarring movements. They may also strain the trapezius muscle lifting things improperly.

Middle-aged people are more likely to develop neck pain as a result of the normal degenerative changes of the discs and facet joints of the cervical spine. (See Chapter 2 for a detailed discussion of this process.)

Whiplash — sprained, or torn, ligaments and/or muscles — can affect people of any age. In most cases, whiplash is caused by a car accident; when your car is hit from the rear, your head is snapped backward as your body is thrown forward.

Over the last few years, a new category of neck patients has been emerging: people whose jobs require them to sit for long periods in a position that stresses the cervical spine. The most common example is computer work. By adjusting their work stations, and changing a few of their work habits, many of these people can eliminate, or at least reduce, their neck pain.

COMPUTER TALK

When personal computers were first developed, many employers started to dream about productivity curves that went off the top of the chart. But, as is true about most things in life, when you gain something, you generally lose something. It soon became apparent that people who sat in front of video display terminals (VDTs) for long hours were developing low back, wrist, eye, and neck problems.

Chairs, which were mostly responsible for the rapid increase in low back problems, were tackled first. Over the past decade, a huge amount of information has been published about the importance of ergonomic chairs, which accommodate the needs of your body, rather than forcing you to fit into a contraption that strains your muscles, ligaments, and joints. Most bosses are now knowledgeable enough to know that money spent on ergonomic chairs for employees is a sound investment. Compared to the cost of lost productivity and the treatment of back

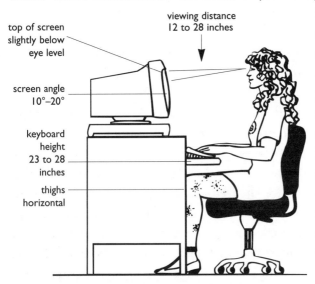

Figure 19.3 An Ergonomic Work Station

top of screen slightly below eye level

viewing distance 12 to 28 inches

screen angle 10°–20°

keyboard height 23 to 28 inches

thighs horizontal

pain caused by sitting in a badly designed chair, the initial outlay is peanuts.

But research also indicates that almost a third of "work station" problems cannot be blamed on the chair. Eye problems caused by poor lighting are becoming more common among VDT users. So is carpal tunnel syndrome. And, most recently, ergonomists have started to pay attention to the millions of human necks that ache at the end of the day.

If you work at a computer, try to keep two basic principles in mind:

1. Your cervical spine has a natural lordotic curve much like the lordotic curve in your lumbar spine. You should maintain, but not exaggerate or decrease, this curve.
2. Your neck has the ability to be extremely flexible and it likes to use that ability. (If you don't use it, you lose it!) If you work at a computer, you must figure out ways of giving your neck a chance to change positions, even if it's only for a ten-second stretch break. Some people program a "take a break" reminder right into their software; every twenty minutes or so, a message appears on their screen!

Here are some specific pointers to watch for in the interests of your neck. (See Figure 19.3.)

- Your keyboard should be between twenty-six and thirty-two inches from the floor.
- Arrange your computer screen on your desk so that the top of the screen is just at eye level when you are sitting comfortably. If your computer screen is too low, for instance, your neck will be forced into an overly flexed position. Unfortunately, most of us spent endless hours in this position when, as students, we sat at desks reading textbooks and writing essays.
- Tilt the screen slightly backwards — but watch that this does not create glare. Most people find that their necks are most comfortable when their normal line of sight is about 15 to 20 degrees below horizontal. (Not sure? Try this. Look at the top of the screen. Now

close your eyes. Get comfortable. Now open your eyes slowly; this is your natural angle of vision. If you aren't focusing on the center of the screen, trying raising or lowering the screen slightly.)

- Most people find that their necks and eyes are most comfortable if they are sitting twelve to twenty-eight inches from their screen. If you are typing from a document, it should be set up at the same distance. These recommended numbers have been changing over the past few years, however, so if this distance feels wrong to you, have the confidence to use your own judgment.

KEEP IT MOVING!

The neck is by far the most mobile portion of the spine. Its range of rotation is generally 70 to 90 degrees, while the lumbar spine can only rotate 3 to 18 degrees. (See Figure 19.4 A.) The neck can tilt to one side or the other about 45 degrees, while the low back can only tilt to between 15 and 20 degrees. (See Figure 19.4 B.) The neck can extend (bend backwards) about 70 to 90 degrees, while the low back can only extend 20 to 35 degrees; similarly, while the neck can flex (bend forward) about 80 to 90 degrees, the low back can flex only 40 to 60 degrees. (See Figure 19.4 C.)

A simple but important question is, what kind of lifestyle would our necks pick if we were to give them a choice?

"Necks like to move a lot," says physiotherapist Anita Gross. "And they

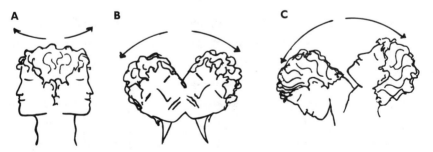

Figure 19.4 The Range of Motion of the Neck

like to move into and out of their full range of motion . . . but gently rather than in a jarring way."

The problem is trying to translate that bit of sensible information into day-to-day reality. Yet most of us take very little advantage of the neck's amazing powers of mobility. For example, you rotate your neck fully when you look over your shoulder, then back your car down the driveway. But how often do you do that? You also extend your neck fully when you look up at the ceiling; most of us do that even less frequently. The point is, most of us live lifestyles that our necks would not choose. I, for one, intend to smarten up . . . and that should be soon since there are only two chapters to go!

Neck Exercises

The beauty of neck exercises is that many of them can be done while you're sitting. This makes it kind of tough to come up with an excuse for not doing them! On days when your neck is particularly sore, you may find it more comfortable to do **isometric**, as opposed to **isotonic exercises**. (When you work a muscle isotonically, you shorten the distance between the muscle's two ends. When you work a muscle isometrically, the contraction is static, which means that no shortening is involved.)

Here are a few basic neck exercises to get you started.

Chin Tuck Stretch
This is an isometric contract-relax technique for relief of a tight trapezius muscle.

This exercise can be done while sitting or standing. Place your left hand on the left side of your forehead. Then, without straining, let your head drop forward to the end of its range of motion. (See Figure 19.5.) Tilt your head slightly to the left, turning your chin a little to the right. Now, while resisting with your hand,

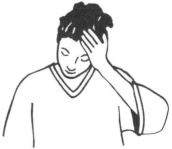

Figure 19.5 The Chin Tuck Stretch

push your head down into your hand and hold this contraction for five seconds. Relax. Let your head fall forward again, then repeat the exercise several times. After three or four repetitions, you will find that your range of motion has increased and that the right side of your trapezius muscle feels looser. To loosen the left side of your trapezius muscle, repeat the exercise with your right hand on the right side of your forehead and with your head tilting to the right. Remember to do this exercise gently.

Side Bend Stretch

This is an isometric contract-relax technique for relief of tight scalene muscles.

This exercise can be done while sitting or standing. To stretch the right scalene muscles, position your head so that your face is vertical and your eyes are focused straight ahead. Then tilt your head to the left side as far as possible without strain. Place the heel of your left hand on the left side of your head just above the ear. (See Figure 19.6.) Push your head sideways into your left hand while resisting movement with your hand. Relax and repeat three times. Then repeat the exercise in the opposite direction using your right hand to resist movement.

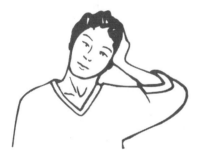

Figure 19.6 The Side Bend Stretch

Side Bend Stretch (alternate version)

This isometric hold-relax technique for tight scalene muscles is a variation of the previous one. Try both and pick the one that works better for you.

As in the previous exercise, tilt your head to the left until you feel your right scalene muscles stretch to their maximum without discomfort. Place your left hand just above and slightly behind your right ear, then push your head sideways against your left hand, using the hand to resist the movement. Relax and let your head stretch farther. Repeat three times, then switch sides.

Neck and Shoulder Relaxers

- Sit or stand with your arms hanging loosely at your sides (see Figure 19.7). Shrug your shoulders up as high as you can. Count slowly to ten and relax. Repeat a minimum of ten times.

- In the same position, pull your shoulder blades back together as if you are trying to create a furrow in the middle of your back. Hold for a count of ten and relax. Repeat a minimum of ten times.

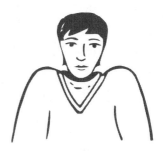

Figure 19.7 Neck and Shoulder Relaxers

- In the same position, bring the shoulders forward into a hunched position. Hold for a count of ten and relax. Repeat a minimum of ten times.

- Sit in a chair with proper back support. Stretch your arms above your head with your fingers interlocked and your palms up toward the ceiling. Hold for ten seconds. Repeat as often as you like.

NECK SURGERY

Surgery for neck pain, as I have said, is extremely rare. But it is on the rise; a 1994 study showed that hospitalizations for cervical spine surgery increased 45 percent in the United States between 1979–81 and 1988–90. Reasons proposed for this rise include the increasing use and acceptance of magnetic resonance imaging (MRI) to diagnose problems early; the emergence of a number of new cervical surgery treatments; and the increase in the ratio of surgeons to patients — all those orthopedic and neuro-surgeons need something to do!

The small number of patients who are candidates for neck surgery should be aware of the additional risks posed by the presence of the spinal cord running through the cervical vertebrae. (Remember, most lumbar surgery is below the spinal cord, which ends at the conus medullaris.) Damage to the spinal cord at the neck can leave a person a quadriplegic

— this is why neck surgery is usually performed by a neurosurgeon. I know if I needed neck surgery I'd get the best neurosurgeon in town, and I'm not sure I'd let even him or her touch my neck. An orthopedic surgeon I interviewed told me he never operated above C3, and rarely did necks at all.

The most common neck surgery procedure is **cervical fusion**, which can relieve neck pain caused by a badly degenerated cervical disc, or arm pain caused by a bulging disc putting pressure on a nerve root. Similar to a discotomy/fusion performed elsewhere on the spine (see Chapter 17), this procedure basically involves removing the damaged disc and replacing it with a small wedge of bone taken from the pelvis. In about 80 percent of cases, the bones fuse in about eight to twelve weeks.

20

Back to Work

There's a concept I've touched on in various chapters of this book but now I'd like to drive its importance home. To suffer from back pain is one thing. But to suffer from back pain and to be disabled to boot is quite a different kettle of fish.

Some researchers believe that the actual number of low back pain sufferers has not increased all that much over the years.* What has, of course, increased — *dramatically* increased — is the number of people who become disabled because of their sore backs. As I pointed out in Chapter 12, this group costs our society a fortune. This group is also the reason why, over the last decade or so, so many billions of dollars have been spent on back pain research, some of the best of which has been done in Canada. We must find ways of identifying who is at risk of becoming part of this notorious group . . . or the insurers who pay for treatment and long-term disability will go bankrupt.† It's that simple.

Here are a few statistics that will blow you away:

---

* Because of motor vehicle accidents and computers, neck problems have increased in terms of actual numbers (see Chapter 19).

† The Ontario WCB, with its unfunded liability of billions, is already, in my opinion, bankrupt.

- I mentioned this in Chapter 12 but I think it's worth repeating. Back pain accounts for approximately a third of all workers' compensation board (WCB) claims. Studies also indicate that, once an injured person has been off work for six months, the chances of his or her *ever* going back to work are only 75 percent. After a year, those chances decline to 50 percent; after two years, they are more or less zero.

- Canadian statistics on the costs of treatment are hard to come by and, of course, are quite a bit less than they are in the United States. Nevertheless, according to Dr. Rowley Hazard, who does research at the Vermont Back Research Center, the average bill for a single work-related back injury is in excess of $8,000 (U.S.). The total cost of work-related back injuries in the United States, if you include lost work time and wages as well as the cost of treatment, is $50 billion (U.S.). Obviously, those people who never work again for the rest of their lives account for the bulk of this money.

The best way to eliminate these costs would be prevention; if no one were to develop back pain in the first place, this disabled group would cease to exist. However, nipping all debilitating back pain in the bud is not realistic. Back pain cannot be wiped off the face of the planet like smallpox or the plague, since it's a complex condition as opposed to a disease. Instead, the crème de la crème of today's back pain researchers are concentrating their efforts on finding what the medical profession calls "risk factors." In other words, the push is on to find out why 10 percent of back pain sufferers become disabled while the rest do not.

Obviously the physical severity of a back problem has something to do with whether or not a person becomes disabled. But not as much as we used to think. (I've talked about this fact in various parts of this book already; see, for example, in Chapter 3, which deals with diagnosis.) For instance, recent research is beginning to indicate that how much a person likes his or her job is right up there among the important risk factors. So is how a back pain sufferer is treated by his or her employer — which, of course, is part and parcel of how much a person likes the job. It's also recognized that how well a person gets on with coworkers can make a huge difference. And, of course, there are some basic risk factors such as cultural attitudes toward pain, which I've discussed in Chapter 5. This risk factor research is still in its infancy, however; I can only hope that progress is made before we go bust.

PHYSICAL RISK FACTORS FOR DISABILITY

Physiology does play an important role in one's risk of disability, and some world-class researchers are devoting their careers to studying this role. For instance, some researchers are working in the area of general fitness, which has to do with lifestyle. Others are concentrating on the specific risks that go along with various jobs.

Lifestyle has to do with the way you spend your leisure time. For instance, if you're an overweight couch potato — and especially if you are a couch potato who has a physically demanding job — you are at greater risk of injuring your back than someone who is physically fit.

Other, more specific, risk factors have to do with the requirements of your job. If, like me, you have to sit at a computer for long periods of time, the risk of developing a back problem increases. It also increases if you have a job where there tend to be accidents such as slips and falls. But many researchers still believe that the biggest risk factor is overexertion while moving things around; they call this **manual materials handling,** or **MMH** for short. Some fascinating research about prevention has been done on this subject.

MMH, which may involve lifting, lowering, pushing, pulling, carrying, and/or handling objects, causes back pain in about 75 percent of Canadians whose jobs require it, although it does not always result in disability. It has been estimated, however, that MMH does account for about a third of the lost work time caused by back pain.

In an attempt to reduce the number of back injuries caused by MMH, three main areas have been studied:

- training — i.e., teaching people to lift properly;
- job selection — i.e., making sure that people are capable of doing the MMH job to which they have been assigned; and
- ergonomics — i.e., making jobs fit the needs of workers, rather than the other way around. (For more on ergonomics, see Chapter 11.)

All three approaches have their place when it comes to preventing back injuries, but the experts agree that, in most cases, ergonomics is the most important of the three. (The training and selection approaches tend to make more sense in jobs like nursing or firefighting, whose very natures make them harder to control than, say, assembly-line jobs.) Rather than placing the burden on the worker in terms of skill and/or strength, jobs should be designed so that, in all but the most exceptional circumstances, the general population can do them without undue risk of injury to their backs.

For one thing, it's less expensive — not to mention more ethical — for companies to take care of the people they've got. As well, research shows that the cost of modifying many jobs is far less than most employers believe. Several American studies have shown that 80 percent of jobs can be modified for under $500; the average cost is a mere $300.

Dr. Stover Snook is an American researcher who has devoted his career to this subject. He works as an ergonomist for Liberty Mutual Insurance, which insures the workers of hundreds of U.S. companies; only six states have government-operated insurance like Canadian provincial workers' compensation boards. (Liberty Mutual recently bought the Canadian Blue Cross.) Dr. Snook believes that, if properly applied, ergonomics could reduce workplace injuries by a third. Using the other two approaches in addition to ergonomics, he believes that this figure could be increased even further. On the other hand, a number of studies have shown that training and job selection, used on their own without ergonomics, don't work very well.

This raises an interesting question. How can we, as a society, make sure that jobs are ergonomically designed? In Canada, the federal Labour Code legislates that workers can handle 10 kilograms with no restrictions, but that when the load is more than 45 kilograms, written instructions must be provided. In between, verbal instructions will do. This legislation, however, only applies to people who work for federal agencies.

Most provincial labor codes, however, say only that MMH must be done in a "safe way," which means very little. Remember, however, that we have only recently learned enough about MMH even to consider the idea of legislating safety. As well — and this makes the issue even more difficult — the main thing we have learned is that MMH is very complex. Simply telling workers to lift no more than a certain number of kilograms is not very helpful. As important as how much a person lifts are the kinds of things I discussed in Chapter 11: the distance the load is held from your body, whether you must twist and lift at the same time, etc.

In the United States, standards are set by the Occupational Safety and Health Administration (OSHA). Another organization, called the National Institute for Occupational Safety and Health (NIOSH), conducts research and sets MMH guidelines. These guidelines — which take the form of a mathematical equation — are so precise they can make a layperson's head spin. Guidelines, of course, are not the same as legislation. But more and more companies are finding that following them reduces injuries without lowering productivity.

THE NIOSH EQUATION

In 1981, NIOSH published its first MMH equation, a mathematical formula that can help design or fix jobs ergonomically. In those days, ergonomics was in its infancy, and we knew less about human body mechanics. The equation, as published in the U.S., looked like this:

$$AL = 40(15/H)(1-.004[V-75])\ (.7+7.5/D)(1-F/Fmax)$$

A few years later, however, our knowledge of body mechanics increased, and the people at NIOSH began to work on the equation again. They added more information, for example, the consideration that many lifts are done while twisting, which increases stress dramatically. They realized that people are not able to hold objects as close to the body as was originally thought. They worked out what would happen if handles were added to a box, which makes lifting easier. And they worked in the fact that women now make up a large portion of the workforce. The result was an even more complex equation, which I won't try to dazzle you with here.*

Many laypeople, myself included, would have a hard time using the NIOSH equation, but grasping its spirit is fairly simple. Basically, it offers a number of possibilities to work with. You start with a base weight — forty pounds was used for the 1981 equation — and then reduce that amount when concerns like distance from the body, or frequency, make the lift more stressful.

But the equation also offers choices. For instance, one aspect of a lift may be easier (or less expensive) to change than another. Maybe the weight itself cannot be reduced, but how high — or often — it has to be lifted can. Let's say, for instance, that you have a bulky, twenty-two pound box that you are holding sixteen inches from your body. You need to move it from point A, at floor level, to point B, at shoulder level, four times every minute. There are a number of ways to make this lift safer: You can put the contents into two lighter boxes (this will also make the load less bulky, but you must be careful not to raise the frequency too much for the sake of productivity). Handles may be added to the box. It might be possible to figure out a way for the worker to hold the box closer to the body. Or, if no other solution is possible, the frequency of the lift might be reduced.

An experienced ergonomist can use the equation to play around with the various possibilities and come up with the best combination: the safest, most efficient, least expensive way of getting the job done.

While most experts agree that the revised NIOSH equation is pretty amazing, it's not perfect by a long shot. For one thing, its complexity limits its use to large companies that have an ergonomist on staff, or can hire one from time to time. Between 60 and 70 percent of Canadian businesses are small ones where — at least at the moment — ergonomic principles are not well understood. In addition, the NIOSH equation does

---

*   If you're interested, it was published in the journal *Ergonomics* in July of 1993.

not specifically address people who have already had an injury and may be at greater risk of having a second injury than people who have not. More research must be done in this area.*

On the positive side, ergonomists who use the equation in the real world have found that it is no more expensive to design jobs based on good ergonomic principles. And, as I have mentioned, the studies that have looked at the cost of fixing high-risk MMH jobs show that making changes is far less expensive than most employers assume it will be. In virtually all cases, the cost is definitely a lot less than the cost of just one serious injury. This is the message top management must come to believe.

What does seem clear, however, is that we are at an important crossroads where prevention is concerned. The decisions we make today will have an impact for many years to come. Unfortunately, hard economic times are making a tough challenge even tougher.

Some workers' compensation boards are offering incentives: if they can reduce their claim costs, companies get money back. Legislation will likely become tougher, and more specific. But attitudes must change as well. Canadian industry must begin to look at human resources as its most valuable commodity. It must realize that, in the long run, replacing a person costs more than replacing a machine.

SOFTWARE FOR THE FUTURE

The NIOSH equation is one tool professional ergonomists can use to make the process of preventing injury more precise. The computer is another — and at the forefront of new technology in this area worldwide, is a Montreal company called Promatek. Promatek's computer software, Vision 3000, interfaces with a simple video camera and a personal computer to produce reports on repetitive lifting that boggle the mind. Many therapists believe that, within a few years, this technology will become commonplace.

---

* The Canadian Centre for Occupational Health and Safety has a simplified form of the NIOSH equation, with some simple examples on how to use it. If you're interested, call the charming genius who came up with it, Andrew Drewczynski, at 1-800-263-8466.

In order to decide if someone can lift a certain weight, in a certain way, over a particular period of time, without risk of injury, you need to know how much stress that lift places on the person's joints: the back, the knees, the shoulders, etc. You should also know if the lift strains the person's joints by requiring them to move beyond what is comfortable — in other words, beyond their range of motion. If the lift is very difficult (or very easy), a skilled therapist can probably eyeball it. But most lifts are not so obvious.

For instance, lifting a box may take two or three seconds, but the problem may occur for only one-tenth of a second, which is easy for the eye to miss. If someone loads a pile of boxes from a pallet onto a shelf, it may only be the very lowest box that is causing the problem. In theory, a skilled physiotherapist could calculate the risk of even the most complicated job. But doing it would involve thousands of measurements. Analyzing them would take weeks! A computer can reduce these weeks to minutes.

To use the Vision 3000 program, for example, the therapist tapes a reflective marker or even a small piece of plain white paper to the person's joints, right over his or her clothes. The video camera can now "see" the position of each joint during each phase of the lift. The person performs the lift, recorded by the camera, which then sends the data to the computer. The Vision 3000 software calculates the joints' angles and analyzes the stresses on them. It then produces a report (see Figure 20.1), using the new NIOSH lifting guidelines or one of two other models: the University of Michigan's 2D Static Strength Model, or the University of Waterloo's

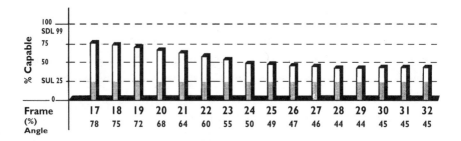
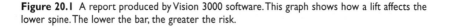

Figure 20.1 A report produced by Vision 3000 software. This graph shows how a lift affects the lower spine. The lower the bar, the greater the risk.

WATBAK guidelines. The report compares the stresses on the person's joints to what is considered to be safe for the average worker.

But like most computerized technology, what comes out depends largely upon the creativity and expertise behind what goes in. Physical therapist Linda Woodhouse, who uses Vision 3000 for research, explains how it is used for rehabilitation: "These days most patients arrive at rehab with a Physical Demands Analysis of their job. So we know what we want to accomplish and we can test the person to see how far he, or she, is from that goal." With the Vision 3000 program, a therapist can also tell exactly what aspects of the job — if any — are likely to cause problems; with this knowledge, he or she can design a suitable program that includes strengthening and education regarding posture and lifting techniques. At that point, the therapist can also decide how realistic it is to expect full recovery over the course of several weeks. "If you think the person can recover fully, fine. If not, you can begin to negotiate for a modified job," explains Linda Woodhouse.

Just a few years ago, a modified job would likely have meant that the person's lifting capacity would be restricted. For instance, he would be told not to lift more than five pounds, period. "In effect, he didn't lift anything," says Linda Woodhouse. "Instead, he was put on a desk job for a couple of months, by which point he would be completely out of condition. Then someone would decide he should return to his preinjury job, which might involve heavy lifting. Since he had no chance to improve his physical fitness, he would be at risk of injuring himself again."

With the Vision 3000 report, a job modification can be very specific. For example, someone might be able to lift twenty-pound boxes from the floor to the table, but not from the table to the top shelf — or the other way around. In other situations, lifting the boxes from a pallet, rather than from the floor, might solve the problem. Or a person might be able to do the lift forty times a day instead of sixty.

Most people now agree that it is the rare individual who would rather stay at home than return to the job. The hot topic is *how* to get injured people back on the job as soon as possible, in a way that is safe and benefits everyone: management, labor, and industry as a whole.

BE NICE!

One of Dr. Stover Snook's most interesting articles was published in 1989 as a chapter of a book called *Manual Materials Handling: Understanding and Preventing Back Trauma*. As you can imagine, the article talks about the three main methods that are used to reduce workplace injuries: ergonomics, training, and selection. But it also talks about the positive role that management should play.

Dr. Snook agrees with those who say that all back pain cannot possibly be prevented. But he does feel that employers can reduce, and sometimes

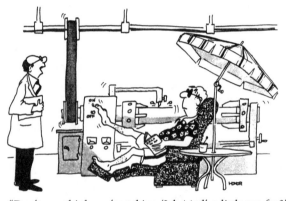

"Don't you think you're taking 'Job Mod' a little too far?"

prevent, low back disability by being understanding and accepting when people injure their backs. He believes that management should promote early treatment and early return-to-work programs. Employers must also learn to communicate well, and to respond supportively to people with back injuries. Recovering workers are sometimes accused, either directly or by implication, of malingering. This, he feels, just causes them to look for ways to get back at their employers, and lengthy disability — which is bad for everyone — is the most common result. Comments from a supervisor such as "He just wants some time off," or "It's his own fault for not lifting properly," make the situation worse and are usually wrong in any case. Management (from the supervisor all the way up to the president) needs to be trained about the true nature of back pain. It is:

- a disorder of unknown cause;
- a disorder that happens to practically everyone;
- a disorder that usually develops gradually and insidiously;

- a disorder that is not always precipitated by an unusual or strenuous activity;
- a disorder that does not respond well to treatment;
- a disorder that recurs frequently; and
- a disorder that resolves itself in a few days or weeks about 90 percent of the time.

The best way for managers to respond? According to Dr. Snook, they should show concern and avoid making judgments. They should encourage their employees to seek immediate medical treatment — in-house, if possible — and, if at all possible, modify the job so that the worker can keep on working. When employers follow this advice, workers' compensation costs for low back pain generally decrease by astounding amounts.

The moral of this story is, if you're a manager, be positive and supportive! Like Dr. Snook says, be nice!

CONSIDER THE PACKAGING

Wonderful things often come across my desk, although sometimes the packaging is pretty boring. Take, for instance, *The Disability Management Sourcebook*, which someone sent me from Washington, D.C. Neither the name, nor the cover — gray, blue, and purple — inspired me to stay in bed with a trumped-up backache so I could devour every word without interruption.

Which is a pity — and kind of amusing as well, because one of the things the sourcebook talks about is the importance of packaging in reports describing the abilities of not-yet-fully-recovered workers. The authors suggest that these reports be written in what they call "Positive Speak" rather than "Negative Speak." Here's an example:

Dear Ms. Manager,

Joe Brown is returning to your department on Monday. I'm sure he'll make a full recovery within about two weeks. In the meantime, Joe:

- *can lift up to 40 pounds;*
- *can stand for up to 30 minutes;*
- *can sit for moderate periods;*
- *can work for extended periods with breaks; and*
- *needs your help to find alternate methods of working that don't require bending.*

Yours sincerely, etc.

Here's the same thing in Negative Speak:

Dear Ms. Manager:
Joe Brown will be returning on Monday. He:

- *cannot lift over 40 pounds;*
- *cannot stand for more than 30 minutes;*
- *cannot sit for long periods;*
- *must take frequent breaks;*
- *cannot bend . . .*

You get the picture.

The message, of course, is obvious — so obvious that common sense makes it hard to imagine that anyone would dream of using anything but Positive Speak in an early-return-to-work report. (Just for openers, Negative Speak couldn't help but increase a person's stress!) And yet, when I told a few health-care professionals that I was thinking of writing about this topic, they all thought it was a super idea. Apparently, common sense is not as common as I'd like to believe.

JOB MODIFICATION: A TEAM EFFORT

Positive Speak, while extremely important, is only one part of the issue. Making a person's early return to work successful also depends on trust, cooperation, humor, and knowledge, on all sides. Whether a workplace has an official Job Modification Program or everyone is winging it informally, both managers and employees must be accountable to one another for "job mod" to work. And it can work very well indeed. I've included below two women's stories, in their own words, of successful job modification efforts, one from a program manager's and one from an employee's point of view.

Job Mod at Mount Sinai
JOANNE MALVERN

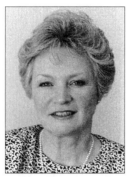

Joanne Malvern

In 1988, Joanne Malvern laid the ground-work for a Modified Work Program for injured employees at Mount Sinai Hospital. By the time she left in 1996, she and her staff — particularly occupational health nurse Lina DiCarlo — had helped more than 800 people return to work before they were fully recovered. Today the program, which includes restricted duties and/or shorter hours, is still going strong. And the hospital is still reducing its WCB claim costs enough to receive a rebate of $500,000 a year. She tells how this was accomplished.

One of the keys to managing a WCB claim successfully is to get the injured person functioning as soon as possible. But if you're going to put people back to work before they are 100 percent better, then your whole way of thinking has to change. The people at the top — that is, senior management — have to believe that modifying jobs for injured workers is the right thing to do.

At first, some people worried a lot about "what ifs." What if we let this person come back to light duties and then everyone wants light duties? What if Nurse Jones comes back before she is completely recovered and is walking down the hall with Patient Brown, who suddenly falls? What if someone comes back too soon and gets injured again? If you're not careful, these "what ifs" can act as mountains.

You have to focus on people's abilities, rather than on their disabilities. You have to say that we'll deal with the "what ifs" when and if they happen and, by the way, they very rarely happen. You also have to realize that employers can't afford not to do this. It's not only a matter of what's morally right. It makes sense from a financial point of view.

At Mount Sinai, as with other hospitals, over 70 percent of the global budget is related to salaries and benefits. Either these people are our biggest asset, or our greatest liability. If you lose experienced workers, orientating new ones costs a great deal and affects patient care. So it makes good business sense to take care of the employees you have.

Usually, the Modified Work Program runs pretty smoothly. But, when you stop to think about it, there are a lot of people to satisfy when you're trying to modify a job. There is the injured employee. There's the doctor, who may be used to sending patients to bed. There's the supervisor and, sometimes, a caseworker from the WCB. If a worker is going to return to a position that crosses union boundaries, Human Resources gets involved to smooth the way. We've been very pleased that the unions have supported this program.

The occupational health nurses who manage these claims are working for, and on behalf of, the injured worker, as well as for, and on behalf of, the employer. The goal is to do the best for everyone involved, and sometimes this can be tricky. An injured man, for instance, may be fearful about getting reinjured if he comes back to work too soon. He might become very dependent for a time — much more needy than usual. He may be having problems at home because the roles have had to change. Maybe he can't make love to his wife. Or play with his young children.

Or do the grocery shopping. And so, the counseling that occupational health nurses provide is important.

We also had to work closely with supervisors, some of whom have a tough time juggling jobs in a creative way. Let's say, for example, that a nursing supervisor decides she needs the normal number of nurses on a shift. In that case, the injured nurse who is doing lighter duties will be an extra person. This makes life easier on the unit, but the salary for the extra person will show up on the supervisor's budget. So the supervisor has to know that those above her believe that, in the end, the hospital's budget will be healthier.

On the other hand, if the injured person is not an extra, but part of the team, the other nurses on the shift are going to have to be flexible. Whether this works well or not depends a lot upon what kind of relationship these coworkers had before the injury. If the injured person is someone who would have extended herself to help a colleague, then it's a good bet that her coworkers will do the same for her.

But I'd like to stress that my experience was mostly positive. When they were asked to support the program, our supervisors generally found out how well it works when they get a valuable employee back. Then it was a lot easier for us to approach them the next time.

As a hospital with an excellent rehab department, Mount Sinai does have an advantage over businesses that cannot offer physical and occupational therapy to their injured employees. This works well for a variety of reasons. For instance, most people who are injured at work go through a stage of being angry, and it's normal for some of this to be directed at the employer. In a hospital, it's possible to offer help, so it's easier for injured people to realize that their employer cares.

As well, having rehab at the site of employment means that injured people can visit their work area and friends soon after the injury. This is something we encourage. It's great for an injured nurse to be able to have coffee with her friends, to have people say they miss her and hope she'll be better soon. It keeps the link going, both mentally and physically.

But a program such as ours doesn't start after a couple of months. It's a concept that we bring up right on the day of the injury.

At the outset, we explain that the Modified Work Program is part of the healing process. The goal, we tell people, is to get them back to work as early as is safely possible so that they don't lose their ability to function — in other words, they don't become deconditioned. We also keep in touch with people while they are at home resting, or while they are having therapy some place else if, for some reason, they have been sent to a clinic near home. And when I say we keep in touch, I mean that we talk to an injured employee at least once a week.

I feel we offer comprehensive support. After all, an injury affects the whole person, not just a back or an arm. We help people link themselves up to other services, if needed. If someone is feeling depressed, or has a pain management problem, or is deconditioned, we'll help him, or her, to find the resources they need.

Not all employers will agree to offer all this. It takes people with a lot of skill and it takes time. If a business with 3,000 employees has one occupational health nurse, that nurse will scarcely be able to keep up with the headaches and the colds. We have four occupational health nurses, plus myself, a part-time medical director, and support staff. The trouble is that developing a department like this can be a chicken-and-egg thing. Management wants proof that it will work before they'll make the commitment, but you can't prove it until you have the resources. So you stretch a little in between.

When we feel that a person may be able to return on an early re-entry basis, we look at the physical demands of the job and the kind of injury the person has had. We work with the person's physician and our rehab department to streamline the job in terms of lifting, pushing, and carrying. Sometimes, we send the physician a "Physical Demands Analysis" of the job, which is like a detailed job description. And, in some cases — with the permission of the injured person — we'll contact the doctor and suggest that the time is right, rather than waiting for that physician to call us.

In addition to all this, Lina DiCarlo has developed a new support group for injured workers, which meets for an hour each month. People in the group tell us what has worked for them and what hasn't. Many of them are very open about their fears and find it helpful to share their experiences and air their frustrations. Again, supervisors cooperate by supporting their workers during this down time. Sometimes, we bring in a guest speaker.

The hospital has also created a position especially for people on the Modified Work Program. It's a very useful job: operating the elevator that moves patients to and from the operating and recovery rooms. When a supervisor has a problem accommodating an injured worker, the elevator job can be used until more suitable work can be found in the regular work area.

I'd also like to mention something about the myth that all injured employees want to abuse the system. It's simply not true. Not in my experience. Quite the contrary. The biggest challenge is to help injured people to find ways of taking responsibility for themselves. To gain the confidence to put their best foot forward — through the good times and the bad times, because there are bound to be some tough days. But my experience is that 99 percent of people want to come back to work as soon as they can. They put their hearts and minds into the Modified Work Program, and they make it work.

The Worker's Word
DOROTHY MCALAND

Dorothy McAland injured her back on the job and was off for six weeks. When she returned to work she was much better, but she was certainly not operating at 100 percent. With the support of her

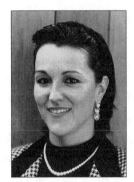

Dorothy McAland

manager and the help of her coworkers, she modified her job for a couple of months to accommodate her limitations. Everyone was glad. Here's Dorothy's story in her own words, from an interview with Back to Back *several years ago.*

I'm a sales rep for a company called Tremco. I sell rust paint, caulking, and roof repair products in Toronto and as far north as Huntsville, which means I sometimes do a lot of driving. As well, part of my job involves setting up displays, and many of the items I handle are heavy.

When you do a display, you don't just pick up a can of paint and stick it on a shelf. First you clear the shelves. Then you take them off the backboard, change the spacing, and put them back up. *Then* you figure out where the products should go. Believe me, moving four-foot shelves is not always so easy.

In the spring of 1992 — during paint season — my back started to hurt. At first it was an "off and on" kind of pain and, basically, I tried to ignore it. By the end of May, however, I had a lump on the left side of my lower back and pain in one leg.

My doctor diagnosed it as a bad strain and gave me anti-inflammatory medication. The sales rep who has the territory next to mine helped me out with my displays and I tried to take it easy. But at the end of the week, I didn't feel any better. So my doctor told me to stay home and rest. I also went to physiotherapy, where I got heat and a few stretching exercises. After two weeks of that, I'd had it. My little boy was four and I couldn't pick him up. I couldn't take him to the park. I couldn't do anything.

Then someone in personnel told me about a community clinic called the Physiotherapy Wellness Institute, an early active treatment center for injured workers. And that's when things started to change.

The first thing they had me do was set some goals. The physio-therapist asked me when I wanted to go back to work and I decided on one month. So I had four weeks to get myself ready. Every morning, I went to the stretching exercise class, and afterwards I worked out in their gym. Every afternoon, I swam at a public pool. I was constantly checked and monitored, but the goals were my own. For instance, when I started, I was able to swim for twenty minutes. The next week, I increased it to half an hour, and by the end, I was up to sixty minutes. I started off riding the exercise bike for five minutes and ended up being able to manage twelve minutes.

I think I knew that, at the end of the month, I wouldn't be ready to pull my own weight 100 percent. But I also knew that I had the support of my manager and that I was going to get help from my coworkers. The term "job modification" wasn't used specifically — probably because I don't have a structured job, like someone who works on an assembly line and is given lighter boxes to lift for several weeks. I had to figure out what I could do and what I couldn't do on my own.

My point is that I wanted to get back to work as soon as possible and start feeling like I was making a contribution; I didn't want to lose my place as part of the team. From Tremco's perspective, they wanted me to come back and stay back, rather than try to do too much and injure myself again. Their philosophy was to support me in any way they could. If I had to take off some time during the afternoon to swim, that was just fine. They never made me feel that I was letting them down.

The first day, I met with the people who had been covering my accounts. We went through them, store by store, so I wouldn't have to walk in cold. My customers had been told why I was off work and they didn't expect me to be able to do everything — at least not right off the bat. And my coworkers pitched in whenever I had to set up a heavy display.

The first couple of weeks were brutal. I had a lot of doubts about what I was capable of doing. Even when I was more or less back to full tilt, there were days when I woke up feeling just awful. On those days, if I needed help, I asked for it; if there was no one to help me, I rescheduled the heavy work for another day.

I think it's really important to make sure that the people who are helping you out know how much you appreciate their effort. As well, I always wrote a memo to my manager, so he'd know too. Earlier in the year, I helped out one of my coworkers who was off sick. That's just how we do things here. We're a team; we want to meet our regional objective, and we're all happy to jump in. Everybody's not just in it for themselves.

I also work a lot smarter than I used to. I use my body more efficiently and I'm better organized. For example, before my injury, I would rush around and try to do everything as fast as possible. Now I realize that it makes a lot more sense to stand back for ten minutes and plan what you have to do, so you don't end up moving and lifting things four or five times. At first I thought all this planning took more time. But it's better for me and better for my back — and the truth is, it doesn't take any longer. It's just a lot less frustrating!

I've also found that, if I incorporate some of my back exercises into my life, it seems like less of an effort. For instance, in the evening, I often lie in a passive extension posture and read my son a book at the same time. I also try to pace myself. I don't come home from the grocery store and whip the cans into the cupboard; I take twenty minutes to catch my breath.

But I think there's something else that's important to remember: people give back what they get. The people in my company have been very good to me. They've always made me feel valuable and that has been a great source of motivation. For instance, there aren't a lot of women in sales jobs. When I injured my back, I worried people would say that women shouldn't be doing this job. You know — "We were right all along" type of thing. But I found quite the opposite. One guy actually phoned me up and told me that he has been doing this job for twenty-five years and, every year during paint season, his back hurts. He told me it doesn't make any difference that I am a woman — that if that was what I was thinking, I should forget it. No one at Tremco was expecting me to be Superwoman.

Before all this happened, I was very busy trying to be Superwoman. That was my problem. Now I understand a lot more about balancing my life.

HELP FOR REHABILITATION: BACK BELTS

Back belts — wide, thickly padded belts, tightened with Velcro or buckles, that cover the area between the midriff and the hips — are becoming increasingly popular among employers both for injury prevention and for rehabilitation purposes. The jury is still out on their effectiveness, however.

When properly worn, the belts are said to increase the stability of the wearer's spine by increasing **intra-abdominal pressure** (IAP — the pressure within the abdominal cavity). Experts disagree, however, as to the effectiveness and benefits of increasing IAP.

What can I tell you about the debate so far? Well, to date, study results have not provided conclusive evidence that back belts prevent injury. Medical associations have yet to offer a recommendation. For the time being, the use of back belts by healthy workers whose jobs involve heavy lifting is still controversial, and caution is advised.

On the other hand, research results seem more favorable regarding the effectiveness of back belts during rehabilitation. Studies suggest that, used as a temporary measure following a back injury, a back belt can help reduce pain and increase the wearer's ability to function, particularly for those who suffer from nerve root and disc problems or have hypermobile backs. Besides acting as a stabilizer, a belt may help you to adopt good posture habits and remind you to avoid moves that could harm your back during its healing process.

If you are considering the use of a back belt for rehabilitation, remember these important tips:

- have the belt prescribed and custom-fitted for you by a back practitioner;
- avoid developing a dependency on it — back belts are recommended for short-term use; and
- use your belt in conjunction with a rehabilitation exercise program designed specifically for you.

21

Osteoporosis: Getting Less Dense

O steoporosis is a dreadful disease that strikes little old ladies in particular. The bones of those who suffer from osteoporosis lose calcium and, as a result, become less dense and more brittle, which makes them susceptible to fractures. The vertebrae and hipbones are affected most. Thin, fair-haired, Caucasian women are especially at risk. Each time I flip through the pages of a high fashion magazine, I am reminded that this most at-risk body type is the dream image of so many young girls, and I worry for their future well-being.

WHY OSTEOPOROSIS IS ON THE RISE

Approximately 27 million North Americans — 80 percent of whom are women — currently suffer from osteoporosis. It has been estimated that the disease is responsible for about 850,000 fractures each year.

Worse, in spite of recent research advances, the incidence of the disease is growing by leaps and bounds. In Britain, for instance, the number of hip fractures from osteoporosis has doubled over the past thirty years, and not because people are living longer. Here in North America the figures are less precise, but the number of sufferers is definitely on the rise.

Recently, some old bones dug up from a church burial crypt in London, England, provided researchers with a clue as to why. When Christ Church Spitalfields was being restored, workers had to move the crypt in which eighty-seven women had been buried between 1729 and 1852. Researchers were anxious to examine the remains of the women, all Caucasian, because detailed records had been kept of each woman's age and lifestyle. This gave the scientists a chance to compare the bones to the bones of women who are alive today, taking lifestyle factors into account. Such an opportunity had never before arisen.

The dead bones, of course, could not provide any information about muscles and fat, which also play a role in osteoporosis. But bone density is the major issue and they could certainly measure that.

When they examined the bones of women who were past menopause — the little old ladies of two centuries ago — the scientists found them to be definitely denser than the bones of women of this age group who are alive today. When they looked at the bones of the young women who had been buried in the church, there was no sign of bone loss at all. Today, many women have signs of bone loss years before they reach the age of menopause.

On average, the women who had been buried at Spitalfields had given birth to 3.4 children. They didn't smoke and probably didn't drink much (if any) alcohol. They also seemed to have had a fair amount of calcium in their diets from milk and certain kinds of green vegetables. These aspects of their lifestyles may have contributed to the higher density of their bones, but this was not what grabbed the attention of the researchers.

What stood out was physical activity. The women who were buried at Spitalfields had various occupations, but the most common job, by far, was silk-weaving. These weavers worked hard, often fourteen to sixteen hours a day. They also walked a great deal.

For a long time, researchers have tried to figure out what causes osteoporosis. The reasons appear to be complicated, but many scientists believe that, along with nutrition, physical activity — the kind of physical activity that puts stress on the long bones of the body and builds up muscle mass — plays an important role. The research from Spitalfields appears to confirm this theory.

HOW OSTEOPOROSIS AFFECTS THE BONES

To understand how osteoporosis affects the bones of the spine, you need a basic understanding of how bone forms, or ossifies.

Most of us tend to think of bone as inert. On the contrary, it is very active. Our bones produce blood cells and store minerals — mostly calcium, which gives bones their strength. As well, bone is constantly dissolving and being generated. If you could monitor the composition of a bone in the body of an active person, you would see that all of its cells and all of the bone minerals are replaced over a seven-year period.

The cells in bone responsible for production are called **osteoblasts**. Other cells, called **osteoclasts,** reabsorb bone cells that have either died or are no longer functioning. Osteoclasts are also thought to be responsible for maintaining normal calcium levels, required by nerves and organs in the blood.

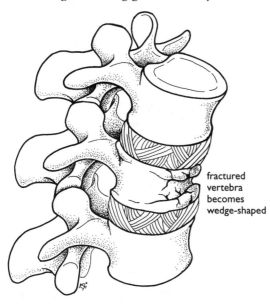

fractured vertebra becomes wedge-shaped

Figure 21.1 Osteoporosis

Normally, a balance exists between the activity of the osteoblasts and that of the osteoclasts. Enough new bone is produced to make up for the amount that is reabsorbed. However, when the osteoclasts reabsorb more bone than the osteoblasts can produce, the net amount of bone decreases. The result is called osteoporosis. An easy way of visualizing the process is to think of the bone tissue as a slice of Swiss cheese. As osteoporosis develops, the holes in the cheese become bigger and bigger. The result is less cheese, or in the case of the body, less bone. In fact, once the disease has progressed to a severe stage, bone density can decrease to such an extent that a fracture can occur spontaneously. In extreme cases, the weight of the upper body can literally crush the vertebrae of the lumbar spine (see Figure 21.1 on the previous page).

Most fractures caused by osteoporosis eventually heal in the sense that the two lines of fracture "knit" together, but if the vertebra has been crushed into a wedge shape, it remains that way, causing the spine to hunch forward. If several fractures have occurred, a person can lose up to several inches in height as a result.

WHY THE SPINE?

Exactly why osteoporosis develops, doctors do not know. They are not even certain why osteoporosis tends to affect the bones of the spine more frequently than the other bones of the body, an exception being the bones of the hips. But there are theories.

The most widely accepted theory is based on the fact that all bones are composed of two kinds of tissue: cancellous and cortical.

Cancellous tissue is often found in the interior of the bone and has a mesh-like structure. **Cortical tissue**, which is hard, forms the exterior portion of the bone. Cancellous tissue is responsible for the production of the blood cells; it is also where the many items that move in and out of the marrow are stored. Because it is more active, the cancellous portion of any bone is thought to be more sensitive to metabolic changes in general, some of which have been linked to osteoporosis. Most doctors explain the high susceptibility of the vertebrae and hipbones to osteoporosis by the fact that these bones contain more cancellous tissue than most other bones.

Risk Factors

Osteoporosis is in part attributable to the aging process — this much seems clear. It is logical that less tissue is generated as our bodies get older. But osteoporosis, say world-class researchers, is a multi-causal condition, and some of the links to other risk factors are less obvious.

For instance, osteoporosis has been linked to genetics, low body weight, eating disorders such as anorexia and bulimia, small bone structure (found in many Asians), the use of certain medications and drugs, and estrogen deficiency as well as other menstrual irregularities. Diet and inactivity, however, are at the top of the list.

Inactivity

Activity contributes to the production of bone mass. When they are under strain, the osteoblasts increase their production of bone tissue. The greater the amount of strain that is placed on a bone and the heavier the load it has to carry, the more bone it produces.

The bones of athletes, for example, are significantly heavier than those of people who do not engage in sports. An American study compared a group of women who exercised for an hour, three times weekly, to women who did no exercise. At the end of a year, the women in the active group had increased their total body calcium by 2.6 percent; those in the inactive group found that their total body calcium had *decreased* by 2.4 percent. That's a 5 percent difference in only a year! While more long-term studies are required in this area, there is no doubt that exercise should be a part of your life.

On the other hand, too much exercise can cause harm. Studies have shown that women runners who run more than fifteen miles per week have a tendency to lose bone because of a decrease in estrogen. Moderation is the key.

Diet — Calcium Deficiency

In some cases, osteoporosis is thought to be caused by a calcium deficiency. Either an insufficient amount of the mineral is being consumed, or, in some instances, the body is not able to absorb the calcium it takes in.

Recent studies have shown that North Americans, particularly women, tend to consume insufficient amounts of calcium. Many researchers blame our society's preoccupation with slenderness for the fact that our diets tend to be so low in calcium-rich foods; many women diet constantly.

Unfortunately, many women are unaware of their calcium needs.

Premenopausal women should take in at least 1,000 milligrams of calcium daily. As well, during pregnancy and while they are breast-feeding, they ought to increase their calcium intake substantially. Many women find it difficult to get the required amount from dairy products and other calcium-rich foods, so they take calcium supplements. If you take calcium supplements, be sure it's elemental calcium that is lead-free. It's a good idea to have your calcium levels periodically checked if you are taking supplements.

There are a number of reasons why some people's bodies are not able to make use of the calcium they consume. First of all, various nutrients, including vitamin D and phosphorus, are essential in the absorption process of calcium. Once absorbed and transferred to the bones, calcium and phosphorus combine chemically. Both are essential. The proper calcium/phosphorus ratio is 2.5 to 1, together with approximately 400 milligrams of vitamin D daily. Generally speaking, North Americans do not suffer from a deficiency of either vitamin D or phosphorus. In fact, North Americans tend to consume more phosphorus than calcium.

Diet — An Excess of Phosphate and Protein

In studies on animals, an excessive amount of phosphate was found to increase the risk of osteoporosis. This evidence has never been substantiated in humans, however. On the other hand, diets extremely high in protein have been linked to osteoporosis in humans. One study has shown that people who increase their daily protein intake from 70 grams to 100 grams increase their annual bone loss by 1 percent.

Diet — Coffee and Alcohol

Some studies have shown that people who drink large amounts of coffee tend to lose more calcium than those who do not. The mechanism for this phenomenon, however, is not well understood.

Heavy use of alcohol increases the amount of calcium that is excreted by the body. But in these studies, too, the mechanisms are not clearly established, and researchers point out that calcium deficiency among alcoholics may be mainly due to the fact that their diets are poor.

The Decline of Estrogen Production in Women

The ovaries of postmenopausal women produce far less estrogen than the ovaries of women who are still menstruating and, eventually, they stop producing estrogen completely. Studies have shown that, shortly before menopause, the average woman loses approximately 0.3 percent of bone mass per year. For five to eight years after menopause begins, the average yearly loss is nine times that amount (2.7 percent); then it levels off.

The incidence of osteoporosis is much higher among postmenopausal than premenopausal women. Most researchers believe that estrogen plays an important role in the development of the disease, but the exact nature of this role has yet to be determined. Some studies have indicated that a high level of estrogen decreases the amount of calcium excreted by the kidneys; from this, researchers have concluded that postmenopausal women may excrete more calcium than women who are still menstruating.

The presence of estrogen is also thought by some researchers to keep the amount of calcitonin produced by the thyroid glands at a high rate. A high level of calcitonin is thought to stop the osteoclasts from reabsorbing calcium. When estrogen levels are low, little calcitonin is produced and, so the theory goes, the osteoclasts reabsorb greater amounts of calcium from the bones.

For reasons which are not well understood, overweight women produce more estrogen than slender women and develop osteoporosis less frequently. Some studies indicate that, after menopause, fat cells may produce estrogen.

Drugs

Osteoporosis has been cited as a side effect of corticosteroids, drugs that have a tendency to inhibit calcium absorption and promote the excretion of calcium in the urine. Other drugs that have been likened to osteoporosis are Heparin and aluminum-containing antacids. If you are taking these drugs, especially if you are also female and over the age of forty, you should discuss the increased risks of osteoporosis with your family physician.

DIAGNOSIS OF OSTEOPOROSIS

The challenge with osteoporosis is early detection. Bone loss can be arrested, but it is extremely difficult to replace bone that has already been lost. The key is to measure bone density — several methods have been developed in recent years to do this. **Dual Photon Absorptiometry (DPA)** has been in use for many years, but has more recently been replaced as the "gold standard" of densitometers by **Dual Emission X-ray Absorptiometry (DEXA)**, which is more precise.

TREATMENT OF OSTEOPOROSIS

The main treatment — which really can only prevent the disease from progressing — is a combination of calcium supplements and exercise. In some instances, estrogen supplements are also prescribed for post-menopausal women. Recent avenues of research include the use of sodium fluoride and several other types of drugs.

Calcium Supplements

For both men and women suffering from osteoporosis, a dose of 1,500 milligrams of elemental calcium per day is generally prescribed, along with as much exercise as possible. On rare occasions, when a patient's body may have difficulty metabolizing calcium, approximately 400 units of vitamin D per day will be prescribed as well. (In the past, much larger doses of vitamin D were prescribed for patients with osteoporosis, but its use has become less common in recent years.)

Calcium supplements, however, do not increase bone formation. They can only act to suppress the mechanisms by which bone is reabsorbed.

Furthermore, calcium and vitamin D in extremely high doses can some-times cause adverse side effects. Megadoses of calcium have been linked to constipation and kidney stones; overdoses of vitamin D can also lead to kidney stones, as well as abnormally high levels of the vitamin in the blood. (Generally speaking, however, a person who is taking calcium sup-plements need not worry about overdosing; moderately excessive amounts of calcium are merely excreted by the body, or stored in the long bones for future use. Most doctors believe that painful calcium deposits such as those of bursitis and scleroderma are not caused by an excess of dietary calcium.)

Exercise

On the other hand, exercise can increase bone formation, although it cannot reverse the toll taken by bone mass that has already been lost. The difficulty is, of course, that osteoporosis patients who have suffered a painful bone fracture are hardly in the mood to exercise. Nevertheless, once a fracture has healed and the pain has subsided to some degree, most doctors recommend that their osteoporosis patients try, at least, to walk as much as possible. Many experts recommend a minimum of twenty minutes of brisk walking at least three times a week.

Estrogen Replacement Therapy

Like calcium supplements, estrogen supplements can suppress bone reabsorption, at least in some women. The still-unanswered question is, which women? For a number of years, in the late 1960s and early 1970s, estrogen was frequently prescribed to women in their fifties suffering from hot flashes and other symptoms that frequently accompany the onset of menopause. The drug worked in that it decreased these symptoms and, although researchers didn't realize it until some years later, it also prevented osteoporosis in many cases.

However, since the discovery that estrogen also increases the risk of cancer of the endometrium, the lining of the uterus, its use for both the symptoms of menopause and osteoporosis has been controversial.

Some researchers believe that if progesterone — which brings on a "period" during which the endometrium is shed — is added for the last ten to fourteen days of the cycle, the risk of endometrial cancer becomes significantly reduced. Others disagree, saying that unless a woman has had a hysterectomy (in which case there is no uterus in which cancer can develop), estrogen therapy can be risky. One thing is certain: if you are taking estrogen supplements, it is advisable to take progesterone as well. In addition, your doctor should be monitoring you frequently for precancerous changes in the cells of the endometrium.

Sodium Fluoride

In 1987, a study conducted at the Bone and Mineral Metabolism Unit of the University of Toronto on the use of sodium fluoride showed it to be promising as an agent that could increase bone mass. Dr. Timothy Murray, director of the Metabolic Bone Clinic at St. Michael's Hospital, put it this way: "The current status of sodium fluoride is that it is still in the research stage . . . I think it is going to turn out to be a useful treatment in the future. But the really exciting thing about this fluoride research is that it has shown that it is possible to take an osteoporotic skeleton and get it to form new bone. Until now, there was nothing that could do this."

Just a few years later, however, a major American study conducted at the prestigious Mayo Clinic came up with negative results, and sodium fluoride was more or less consigned to the scrap heap. Dr. Murray complained bitterly, saying that the poor results were due to the design of the study and in particular the dose of sodium fluoride that was used. But no one in the lay press gave him the time of day.

In fact, the results of two new studies suggest that Dr. Murray was right all along. One was done in Europe and the other in Texas, where slow-release sodium fluoride was used along with calcium. Meanwhile, the Mayo Clinic researchers mentioned above have now concluded that Dr. Murray had a good point. It appears that there is a very narrow window in terms of dosage: less than 50 milligrams of sodium fluoride per day is ineffective, and more than 90 milligrams per day may result in the formation of poor-quality bone. But that's only one issue in a complicated story. Hopefully, research over the next few years will bear more fruit.

Other Drugs

Etidronate, a biphosphonate, appears to be useful in increasing bone mass and reducing the incidence of vertebral fracture in primary osteoporosis if it is given cyclically, alternating with calcium; etidronate is well tolerated with very few side effects, but there have been some concerns about mineralization problems seen with the drug. Over the next few years we will hopefully learn more. Studies have also shown that calcitonin, a hormone secreted by the thyroid gland (it is derived commercially from salmon), may help maintain bone mass and reduce the rate of fractures in osteoporosis patients. Calcitonin has also been shown to be useful in alleviating the pain associated with fractures. There are side effects, however, which include nausea, rash, and flushing. As well, it must be injected.

Over the next few years, a number of new therapies are expected to become available.

If you are interested in more information, you may want to get in touch with the Osteoporosis Society of Canada, or with Women Against Osteoporosis, a volunteer organization (now a chapter of the Osteoporosis Society of Canada) first formed by a group of Toronto patients to generate funds for research, increase public awareness about this disease, and offer support to fellow patients.*

---

* Osteoporosis Society of Canada: Box 280, Station Q, Toronto, Ontario, M4T 2M1. Toll free information line: 1-800-463-6842.
Women Against Osteoporosis: 63 Springhome Road, Barrie, Ontario, L4N 4S3. Telephone: (705) 726-3623.

Acknowledgments

I have put off the writing of this section for so many weeks that my publisher has threatened to strangle me. The reason is simple: sheer terror. If I were to leave out even one name that belongs in these pages, the egregious omission would mortify me for eternity.

With that said, I would like to make it clear that I alone am responsible for any errors this book may contain; while I pride myself on being a tenacious and thorough researcher, I'm humble enough to realize that, like poltergeists, mistakes do appear. Please also bear in mind that I am a generalist. To unravel the mystery of back pain completely would take several lifetimes and I've been at it for a mere seventeen years. (Some surgeons devote their entire careers to the three lowest lumbar discs!)

First and foremost, I want to thank an institution whose support has made both the writing of this book, as well as the continued existence of the Back Association of Canada, possible: Whitehall-Robins, the makers of Robaxacet. Institutions are nothing but the human beings who make them fly; more than a dozen people from Whitehall-Robins have made commitments to me on the strength of a handshake and my word, and this relationship has now been going on for seven years. I am grateful and honored to enjoy that kind of trust. I would also like to make it clear that, during all these years, Whitehall-Robins has never tried to influence the editorial content of educational information written by BAC, or of this book. My heartfelt thanks to: Greg Cain, Chris Clark, Braden Dent, Pierre Desjardins, Mike Farley, Maria Holjevac, Guy Genest, Cynthia Ha, Pierre McClelland, Karla Minello, Ernie Mulligan, David Postill, Catherine Shand, Karen Small, and Miriam Irving, who propped me up when I was ready to fall over during the fall of 1996.

Next I'd like to thank the people who, in various ways, helped me survive while I wrote the last part of *The Ultimate Back Book*. This took place during one of the most dreadful periods of my personal life. On several occasions I considered abandoning the project but I kept going and finished —only a few weeks late—because of the unfailing support I got from the many fine people at Stoddart but especially Don Bastian, Marnie Kramarich, Jeannine Rosenberg, and Laura Siberry, as well as friends, relatives, and colleagues who read me the riot act when necessary and reminded me that the brave don't lie down and die. I am grateful to: Plato, Atalanti Hoffman, Harold S. Fine, Barry N. Fine, Sharlene Samuel, Susan Blumenstein, Araminta Wordsworth, Bronwyn Drainie, Frank Powell, and Kathy Edwards, as well as Chris Bettencourt, Debbie Black, Seth Blumenstein, Melanie Brown, Grace Bunyi, Obi Bunyi, Samantha Camp, Carl Campbell, Jared Cohen, Laurie Coulter, Randy Davis, Henry Durost, David Edwards, Elliott Fine, Donald Fraser, Malcolm Fraser, Stanley Freeman, Francis Gallant, a passel of Garbers, Cheryl Goldhart, Stephen Grant, Chuck Greene, Lucia Guinomtad, Grant Hinchey, Lloyd Hoffman, Murray Hoffman, Isabel Hornstein, Jon Hursey, Reesa Kassirer, Linda Kelloway, Vincent LaMagna, Alan Levy, Joanne Levy, Jim MacDonald, Cheri Mariotto, Euphemia Masacayan, Sandy McLeod, Rosalie Mednick, Evangelina Papadouris, George Pereira, Rhoda Reisman, Stephen Roselle, Ray Rubin, Morrie Ruvinsky, Ian Saginofsky, Judita Saginofsky, Ahmed Sakoor, Nancy Salem, The Serbian Vixens, Karyn Speisman, Gita Steiner, Les Steiner, Charles Szlapak, Lynn Thomas, Sharon Thornton, Paul Waitzer, Val Waitzer, Andrea Watley, Linda Woodhouse, Caitlin Wordsworth, Robin Wordsworth, Bobby Yudin; and my northern neighbors who have no option but to be brave: Henry Adema, Scott Andreas,

David Apramian, Bonnie Blundon, Liz Bradley, Arden S.G. Brooks, Cathy D'Allaire, Mike D'Allaire, Bonnie Diver, June Halineen, Al Hawthorne, Irene Hawthorne, John Helmond, Gail Henderson, Barb Huntley, Chris Huntley, Lynn Ingham, Tony McCauley, Alisa McComisky, David McComisky, Monica McComisky, Barry Rudachyk, Ron St. Julian, Nancy Vandershea, Doug Winter, and Keith Zehr.

I would like to thank the "professionals" who have contributed to the factual side of this book, including first and foremost the back pain sufferers whose own experiences make this book sing. In addition to those whose names appear throughout the text, this group includes the many members of the Back Association of Canada. I am especially indebted to the members who have also served as directors of BAC: Maureen Armstrong, Susan Blumenstein, Stephanie Bolton, William Curley, Kathy Edwards, Mike Farley, David Herlick, Cheryl Lavine, Eleanor Levine, Joanne Malvern, Sharlene Samuel, Sandra Svatos, and Sarilyn Zimmerman.

My very special thanks to:

Tannice Goddard, with whom I have had the honor to work for eighteen years, is responsible for the text design which to my way of thinking was conceived with love, insight, and an eye for beauty. In return, Tannice, I offer you my loyalty until my dying day — at least!;

Elizabeth d'Anjou, whose name I'd kill for, came into my life as an editor when my brain was functioning at zombie speed. Somehow, she roused me from somnambulance and sweet-talked me into answering hundreds of queries in the name of clarity. She also restructured and rewrote a number of sections so deftly that I defy you to figure out which ones they are. Finally, Elizabeth copyedited *The Ultimate Back Book* with conviction and guts, which was no mean feat for someone who had to cope with the likes of Judylaine Fine during the fall of 1996! God only knows what I would have done without you, Elizabeth;

Dorothy Irwin and her associate Jan Pèrez Vela, whose medical illustrations bring to reality concepts that words alone cannot adequately describe;

Peter Honor, whose cartoons liven up this book and my life.

Finally, I offer my heartfelt thanks to the hundreds of back pain sufferers and health-care professionals who have taught me what I know.

Because they know me and the way I operate, I am sure they will not be offended by my decision to use only their Christian and family names — i.e., to treat them just like the rest of us! Thanks to: Riyaz Adat, Arnold Agnew, Alan Banack, Kathy Bedali, Fadi Bejani, the late John Bonica, Barry Brown, Jeremy Brown, Diane Cachia, David Cassidy, Paul Caulford, Toni Clark, David Corey, the late James Cyriax, Howard Dananberg, Randy Davis, Elvio DelZotto, Elizabeth Dow, Jan Dowsling, Mark Dreschel, Andrew Drewvczysky, David Drum, Margaret Duffy, Duffy Dufresne, Pierrette Ferth, Stan Fettis, Elspeth Finch, Hillel Finestone, Judy Flaschner, James Fox, Donald M. Fraser, John Frymoyer, Mary Gale, Joyce Gordon, David Goulding, Janet Greenbank, Bob Grisdale, Anita Gross, Dick Hasselback, Rowley Hazard, Don Himes, Debby Howe, Geralyn Howell, Elizabeth Kaegi, Harold Kalant, Karen Kelly, Mike Kenny, Elizabeth Kirkaldy-Willis, William Kirkaldy-Willis, Louise Koepfler, Martin Krag, Marta Krywonis, John Lama, Tom Leamon, Chris MacHattie, Dorothy McAland, Todd McKenzie, Robin McKenzie, Rebecca Mueller, Timothy Murray, Alf Nachemson, Craig Nelson, James Nethercott, Margareta Nordin, Sandra O'Connor, David Olson, Glenn O'Reilly, Christine Pavacic, Paul Peloso, Olive Pester, Joanne Piccinin, Linda Rapson, Karen Raybould, the late Beverly Reid, Sheila Reid, Steve Reineke, Carole Renaud, Marcel Reux, Frank Roberts, Eugenia Saganich, Ken Saito, Ahmed Sakoor, Lina Santaguida, Mary Sauriol, Michael Schwartz, Steve Scolfield, Chris Sfatcos, the late Lyman Smith, Stover Snook, Christine Sutherland, Bob Taylor, Marvin Tile, Tinny Van Schoon, the late Capt. J. L. Varma, Molly Verrier, Carl von Baeyer, Gordon Waddell, Tom Waters, Jerry Weisman, Shirley Wheatley, Marjorie Wilson, George Wortzman, and Ellen Yolich.

A Bibliography of Sorts

The bibliography of *Your Guide to Coping With Back Pain* took up seven pages and I doubt if it was useful enough to warrant the trees that went into its making. If I were to provide a bibliography in the same vein for this book, a small forest would have to be sacrificed.

Therefore, I've decided instead just to list, under some general headings, a number of the books and periodicals that I've found edifying over the years. (Most of the journal articles appeared between 1987 and the present.) If you have additional queries, all you have to do is join the Back Association of Canada and I'll help you with the research!

GENERAL

American Medical Association. *The American Medical Association Book of Back Care*. New York: Random House, 1982.

Cyriax, James. *The Slipped Disc*. Epping, England: Gower, 1980.

Delvin, David. *You and Your Back*. London: Pan Books, 1977.

Hall, Hamilton. *The Back Doctor*. Toronto: Macmillan, 1980.

———. *More Advice from the Back Doctor*. Toronto: McClelland and Stewart, 1986.

Imrie, David. *Goodbye Backache*. Toronto: Prentice-Hall/Newcastle, 1983.

Jayson, M.I.V. *Back Pain: The Facts*. 3rd ed. New York: Oxford University Press, 1992.

Keim, Hugo A. *How to Care for Your Back*. Englewood Cliffs, N.J.: Prentice-Hall, 1981.

Kirkaldy-Willis, William H. *Managing Low Back Pain*. 2d ed. New York: Churchill Livingstone, 1988.

Klein, Arthur C., and Dava Sobel. *Backache Relief*. New York: Times Books, 1985.

Zimmerman, Julie. *Chronic Back Pain: Moving On*. Brunswick, Maine: Biddle Publishing, 1991.

Annals of the Rheumatic Diseases

Archives of Family Medicine

The Back Letter (newsletter published by the Sköl Corporation, Newburyport, Mass.)

Consumer Reports

Back to Back (newsletter of The Back Association of Canada)

British Medical Journal

Clinical Orthopaedics & Related Research

Canadian Medical Association Journal

Journal of the American Medical Association (JAMA)

Journal of the Neuromusculoskeletal System

Lancet

New England Journal of Medicine

Nurse Practitioner

Orthopedics

Spine

ANATOMY AND PHYSIOLOGY

Francis, Carl C. *Introduction to Human Anatomy*. Saint Louis, Missouri: C.V. Mosby, 1973.

Guyton, Arthur C. *Basic Human Physiology: Normal Function and Mechanisms of Disease.* Philadelphia: W.B. Saunders, 1971.

Thomas, Lewis. *The Lives of a Cell.* New York: Viking, 1974.

PAIN AND STRESS

Bonica, John J., ed. *Pain.* New York: Raven Press, 1973.

Cheng, Richard Shing Sou. *Mechanisms of Electroacupuncture Analgesia as Related to Endorphins and Monoamines: An Intricate System Is Proposed.* Toronto: University of Toronto, 1980.

Corey, David, and Stan Solomon. *Pain: Learning to Live Without It.* Toronto: Macmillan, 1988.

France, Krishnan, ed. *Chronic Pain.* Washington, D.C.: American Psychiatric Press, 1988.

Goldberger, Breznitz, ed. *Handbook of Stress.* New York: The Free Press, 1993.

LeCron, Leslie M. *The Complete Guide to Hypnosis.* New York: Harper & Row, 1971.

Melzack, Ronald, and Patrick Wall. *The Challenge of Pain.* Harmondsworth, England: Penguin, 1982.

Pribram, Karl H., ed. *Mood, States and Mind.* Harmondsworth, England: Penguin, 1969.

American Journal of Psychiatry
Behavioural Medicine
Journal of Clinical Psychology
Journal of Family Psychotherapy
Journal of Psychosomatic Research
Pain

MEDICATION

Berner, Mark S., and Gerald N. Rotenberg, eds. *The Canadian Medical Association Guide to Prescription and Over-the-Counter Drugs*. Montreal: Reader's Digest Association (Canada) Ltd., 1990.

Brecher, E.M. et al., eds. *Licit and Illicit Drugs*. Boston: Little, Brown, 1972.

Cox, T., et al. *Drugs and Drug Abuse*. Toronto: Addiction Research Foundation, n.d.

Graedon, Joe. *The People's Pharmacy*. New York: Avon, 1976.

British Journal of Clinical Pharmacology

EXERCISE AND FITNESS

Bouchard, Claude, et al. *Exercise, Fitness and Health*. Champagne, Illinois: Human Kinetics Books, 1990.

American Journal of Sports Medicine
Clinics in Sports Medicine
Medicine and Science in Sports and Exercise

PHYSIOTHERAPY

McKenzie, R.A. *The Lumbar Spine: Mechanical Diagnosis and Therapy*. Waikanae, New Zealand: Spinal Publications, 1981.

Australian Journal of Physiotherapy
Journal of Orthopaedic and Sports Physical Therapy
Physical Therapy
Physiotherapy Canada

CHIROPRACTIC/MANIPULATION

Altman, Nathaniel. *The Chiropractic Alternative*. Los Angeles: J.P. Tarcher, 1981.

Cyriax, James. Manipulation: *Past and Present*. London: Heinemann, 1975.

Haldeman, Scott, ed. *Modern Developments in the Principles and Practice of Chiropractic*. New York: Appleton-Century-Crofts, 1980.

Kelner, Merrijoy, Oswald Hall, and Ian Coulter. *Chiropractors: Do They Help?* Toronto: Fitzhenry & Whiteside, 1980.

Leach, Robert A. *The Chiropractic Theories: A Synopsis of Scientific Research*. Mississippi: Mid-South Scientific Publishers, 1980.

The Chiropractic Report (newsletter published by Fumio Publications, Toronto)

Journal of Manipulative and Physiological Therapeutics

Journal of the American Osteopathic Association

Journal of the Canadian Chiropractic Association

Topics in Clinical Chiropractic

HOLISTIC TREATMENTS

Berkeley Holistic Health Center. *The Holistic Health Handbook*. Berkeley, Calif.: And/Or Press, 1978.

Feldenkrais, Moshe. *The Potent Self*. New York: Harper & Row, 1985.

Jones, Frank Pierce. *Body Awareness in Action: A Study of the Alexander Technique*. New York: Schocken, 1976.

Zebroff, Kareen. *Back Fitness the Yoga Way*. Vancouver, B.C.: Fforbez Publications, 1982.

SURGERY

Genant, Harry K., ed. *Spine Update 1984: Perspectives in Radiology, Orthopaedic Surgery, and Neurosurgery*. San Francisco: Radiology Research and Education Foundation, 1984.

American Journal of Neuroradiology
American Journal of Surgery
Journal of Bone and Joint Surgery
Neurosurgery
Radiology

HEALTH POLICY

Rachlis, Kushner. *Second Opinion*. Toronto: Collins, 1989.

———. *Strong Medicine*, Toronto: HarperCollins, 1994.

Taylor, Malcolm G. *Health Insurance and Canadian Public Policy*. Montreal: Queen's University Press, 1978.

Thomas, Lewis. *The Youngest Science: Notes of a Medicine-Watcher*. New York: Bantam, 1984.

Wilcox, L. DeWitt. *Where Is My Doctor?* Toronto: Fitzhenry & Whiteside, 1977.

SPECIAL TOPICS

Fine, Judylaine. *Afraid to Ask: A Book About Cancer*. Toronto: Kids Can Press, 1984.

Notelovitz, Morris, and Marsha Ware. *Stand Tall: Every Woman's Guide to Preventing Osteoporosis*. Toronto: Bantam, 1985.

Pope, Malcolm H., John W. Frymoyer, and Gunnar Anderson. *Occupational Low Back Pain*. New York: Praeger, 1984.

Smith, Adam. *Powers of Mind*. New York: Summit Books, 1982.

Ergonomics
Occupational Medicine

Index